C000104336

Dictionary Of Medical
Abbreviations In Multiple
Languages

With More Than 200.000 Entries

In

French
English
German
Italian
Russian
Japanese
Chinese

Volume 2
Catherine-Chantal Marango

Dictionary Of The Medical Abbreviations In Multiple
Languages

With More Than 200.000 Entries In

French

English

German

Italian

Russian

Japanese

Chinese

Catherine-Chantal Marango

*

Table Of Contents

Introduction

Catherine Chantal Marango's Multilingual Book Of Medical Abbreviations Presents A Compilation Of Over 200.000 Entries In French, English, German, Spanish, Italian, Portuguese Russian, Chinese, Japanese, And Arabic Translations Of Terminology Used In The Various Fields Of Medicine, Medical Science And Technology.

This Comprehensive Multilingual Dictionary Is The Ideal Reference For All The Global Health Professionals And Medicine Students

A

M

French

MAF
Mouvements Actifs Foetaux
MAP
Menace D'accouchement Prématuré
MCE
Massage Cardiaque Externe
MDH
Maladie De Hodgkin
MDS
Myélodysplasie
MFIU
Mort Foetale In Utero
MGT
Maladie Gestationnelle Trophoblastique
MID
Membre Inférieur D, Mammaire Interne D
MIG
Membre Inférieur G, Mammaire Interne G
MM
Myélome Multiple
MMH
Maladie Des Membranes Hyalines (US=RDS)
MNI
Mononucléose Infectieuse
MSD
Membre Supérieur D
MSG
Membre Supérieur G
MSN
Mort Subite Du Nourrisson
MST

Maladie Sexuellement Transmissible
MTS
Maladie À Transmission Sexuelle

English

M4 Leukemia Monoblastic Differentiation
M4 Myelocyte At The Fourth Stage Of Maturation
M5 Monoblastic Leukemia
M5 Metamyelocyte
M6 Erythroleukemia With Dyserythropoiesis
And Megaloblastosis
M6 Band Form In The Sixth Stage Of Myelocyte
Maturation
M7 Megakaryoblastic Leukemia
M4 Leukemia Monoblastic Differentiation
M4 Myelocyte At The Fourth Stage Of Matura
M5 Monoblastic Leukemia
M5 Metamyelocyte
M6 Erythroleukemia With Dyserythropoiesis
And Megaloblastosis
M6 Band Form In The Sixth Stage Of Myelocyte
Maturation
M7 Megakaryoblastic Leukemia
M7 Polymorphonuclear Neutrophil
M/10 Tenth Molar Solution
M/100 Hundredth Molar Solution

M Electron Rest Mass; Electromagnetic Moment; Magnetic Moment; Magnetic Quantum Number; Male; Mass; Median; Melting [Temperature]; Metastable; Meter; Milli-; Minim; Minimum; Minute; Molality; Molar [Deciduous Tooth]; Mutated

M Lowercase Greek Letter Mu; Chemical Potential; Electrophoretic Mobility; Heavy Chain Of Immunoglobulin M; Linear Attenuation Coefficient; Magnetic Moment; Mean; Micro; Micrometer; Micron; Mutation Rate; Permeability

M−1 Per Meter

M2 Square Meter

M3 Cubic Meter

M8 Spin Quantum Number

MA Macrophage Aggregate; Malignant Arrhythmia; Management And Administration; Mandelic Acid; Martin-Albright [Syndrome]; Masseter; Master Of Arts; Maternal Age; Matrix; Maximum Amplitude; Mean Arterial; Mechanical Activity; Medial Amygdaloid; Medical Assistance; Medical Audit; Medical Authorization; Mega-Ampere; Megaloblastic Anemia; Megestrol Acetate; Membrane Antigen; Menstrual Age; Mental Age; Mentum Anterior; Metatarsus Adductus; Meterangle; Methacrylic Acid; Microadenoma; Microagglutination; Microalbuminuria; Microaneurysm; Microscopic Agglutination; Miller-Abbott [Tube]; Milliampere; Mitochondrial Antibody; Mitogen Activation; Mitotic Apparatus; Mixed Agglutination; Mobile Agent; Moderately Advanced; Monoamine;

Monoarthritis; Monoclonal Antibody; Motor Area; Movement Artifacts; Moving Average; Multiple Action; Muscle Activity; Mutagenic Activity; Myelinated Axon; Myoclonic Absences

MA-104 Embryonic Rhesus Monkey Kidney Cells

MA-111 Embryonic Rabbit Kidney Cells

MA-163 Human Embryonic Thymus Cells

MA-184 Newborn Human Foreskin Cells

M/A Male, Altered [Animal]; Mood And/Or Disease

MBDG Mesiobuccal Developmental Groove

MBE Medium Below Elbow [Cast]

MBEC Mouse Brain Endothelial Cell

MBF Medullary Blood Flow; Mesenteric Blood Flow; Muscle Blood Flow; Myocardial Blood Flow

MBFC Medial Brachial Fascial Compartment

MBFLB Monaural Bifrequency Loudness Balance

Mbfv Mite-Borne Filamentous Virus

MBG Marburg [Disease]; Mean Blood Glucose; Morphine-Benzedrine Group

MBH Medial Basal Hypothalamus

MBH2 Reduced Methylene Blue

MBHI Millon Behavioral Health Inventory

MBHO Managed Behavioral Health Care Organization

MBHR Mesh-Based Hernia Repair

MBI Maslach Burnout Inventory; Maximum Blink Index

MBK Methyl Butyl Ketone

MBL Mannose-Binding Lectin; Marine Biological Laboratory; Menstrual Blood Loss; Minimum Bactericidal Level

MBLA Methylbenzyl Linoleic Acid; Mousespecific

Bone-Marrow–Derived Lymphocyte
Antigen
Mblv Mite-Borne Latent Virus
MBM Meat And Bone Meal; Mineral Basal
Medium
MBNOA Member Of The British Naturopathic
And Osteopathic Association
MBO Management By Objectives;
Mesiobuccooclusal
MBO2 Oxymyoglobin
MBOV Mboke Virus
MBP Major Basic Protein; Maltose-Binding
Protein; Management By Policy; Mannosebinding
Protein; Mean Blood Pressure;
Melitensis, Bovine, Porcine [Antigen];
Mesiobuccopulpal;
Myelin Basic Protein
MBPM Modified Backward Prony Method
MBPS Multigated Blood Pool Scanning
Mbps Megabits Per Second; Myeloblastic
Syndrome
Mbq Megabecquerel
MBR Methylene Blue, Reduced
MBRT Methylene Blue Reduction Time
MBS Martin-Bell Syndrome; Media Broadband
Service; Modified Barium Swallow
MBSA Methylated Bovine Serum Albumin
MBSI Multichannel Blind System Identification
MBT Maternal Blood Type; Mercaptobenzothiazole;
Meridian-Based Therapy; Mixed Bacterial
Toxin; Myeloblastin
MCAB Monoclonal Antibody
MCAD Medium Chain Acyl-Coa Dehydrogenase
MCAF Monocyte Chemotactic And Activating
Factor

MCA/MR Multiple Congenital Anomaly/ Mental Retardation [Syndrome]
MCAO Middle Cerebral Artery Occlusion
MCAR Mixed Cell Agglutination Reaction
MCARE Managed Care
MCAS Middle Cerebral Artery Syndrome
MCAT Medical Chemical Advisory Team; Medical College Admission Test; Middle Cerebral Artery Thrombosis; Multimedia Cardiac Angiogram Tool; Myocardial Contrast Appearance Time
MCAV Macaua Virus
MCB Master Cell Bank; Membranous Cytoplasmic Body; Monochlorobimane
Mcb Mcburney [Point]
Domain; Minimal Brain Damage; Minimal Brain Dysfunction; Morquio-Brailsford Disease
MBDG Mesiobuccal Developmental Groove
MBE Medium Below Elbow [Cast]
MBEC Mouse Brain Endothelial Cell
MBF Medullary Blood Flow; Mesenteric Blood Flow; Muscle Blood Flow; Myocardial Blood Flow
MBFC Medial Brachial Fascial Compartment
MBFLB Monaural Bifrequency Loudness Balance
Mbfv Mite-Borne Filamentous Virus
MBG Marburg [Disease]; Mean Blood Glucose; Morphine-Benzedrine Group
MBH Medial Basal Hypothalamus
MBH2 Reduced Methylene Blue
MBHI Millon Behavioral Health Inventory
MBHO Managed Behavioral Health Care Organization
MBHR Mesh-Based Hernia Repair
MBI Maslach Burnout Inventory; Maximum

Blink Index
MBK Methyl Butyl Ketone
MBL Mannose-Binding Lectin; Marine Biological
Laboratory; Menstrual Blood Loss;
Minimum Bactericidal Level
MBLA Methylbenzyl Linoleic Acid; Mousespecific
Bone-Marrow–Derived Lymphocyte
Antigen
Mblv Mite-Borne Latent Virus
MBM Meat And Bone Meal; Mineral Basal
Medium
MBNOA Member Of The British Naturopathic
And Osteopathic Association
MBO Management By Objectives;
Mesiobuccoocclusal
MBO2 Oxymyoglobin
MBOV Mboke Virus
MBP Major Basic Protein; Maltose-Binding
Protein; Management By Policy; Mannosebinding
Protein; Mean Blood Pressure;
Melitensis, Bovine, Porcine [Antigen];
Mesiobuccopulpal;
Myelin Basic Protein
MBPM Modified Backward Prony Method
MBPS Multigated Blood Pool Scanning
Mbps Megabits Per Second; Myeloblastic
Syndrome
Mbq Megabecquerel
MBR Methylene Blue, Reduced
MBRT Methylene Blue Reduction Time
MBS Martin-Bell Syndrome; Media Broadband
Service; Modified Barium Swallow
MBSA Methylated Bovine Serum Albumin
MBSI Multichannel Blind System Identification
MBT Maternal Blood Type; Mercaptobenzothiazole;

Meridian-Based Therapy; Mixed Bacterial Toxin; Myeloblastin

Mgr Milligram

MGS Metric Gravitational System; Modified Gram-Schmidt Orthogonalization

MGSA Malignant Growth Stimulatory Activity

MGT Medical Guideline Technology; Multiple Glomus Tumors

MGUS Monoclonal Gammopathies Of Undetermined Significance

MGV Mean Gray Value

MGW Magnesium Sulfate, Glycerin, And Water

Mgy Milligray

Mgy Microgray

MH Malignant Histiocytosis; Malignant Hyperpyrexia; Malignant Hypertension; Malignant Hyperthermia; Mammotropic Hormone; Mannoheptulose; Marital History; Medial Hypothalamus; Medical History; Melanophorestimulating Hormone; Menstrual History; Mental Health; Mental Hygiene; Moist Heat; Monosymptomatic Hypochondriasis; Murine Hepatitis; Mutant Hybrid; Mycobacterium Haemophilum; Myohyoid

Mh Millihenry

Mh Microhenry

MHA Major Histocompatibility Antigen; May-Hegglin Anomaly; Mental Health America; Mental Health Association; Methemalbumin; Microangiopathic Hemolytic Anemia; Microhemagglutination; Middle Hepatic Artery; Mixed Hemadsorption; Mueller-Hinton Agar

MHAM Multiple Hamartoma
MHAQ Modified Health Assessment Questionnaire
M-HART Montreal Heart Attack Readjustment
Trial
MHA-TP Microhemagglutination–Treponema
Pallidum
MHAUS Malignant Hyperthermia Association
Of The United States
MHB Maximum Hospital Benefit; Mueller-
Hinton Base
Mhb Methemoglobin; Myohemoglobin
MHBSS Modified Hank Balanced Salt Solution
MHC Major Histocompatibility Complex;
Mental Health Care; Mental Health Center;
Mental Health Clinic; Myosin Heavy Chain
MHCS Mental Hygiene Consultation Service
MHCU Mental Health Care Unit
MHD Maintenance Hemodialysis; Mean Hemolytic
Dose; Mental Health Department;
Minimization Of Hypersurface Distance; Minimum
Hemolytic Dilution; Minimum Hemolytic
Dose
MHDI Minnesota Health Data Institute
MHPA Mild Hyperphenylalaninemia
MHPG 3-Methoxy-4-Hydroxyphenyl-Glycol
MHR Major Histocompatibility Region; Malignant
Hyperthermia Resistance; Maternal
Heart Rate; Maximal Heart Rate; Methemoglobin
Reductase
MHRA Medicines And Health Care Products
Regulatory Agency
MHRI Mental Health Research Institute
MHS Major Histocompatibility System; Malignant
Hyperthermia In Swine; Malignant
Hyperthermia Syndrome; Malignant Hypothermia

Susceptibility; Milan Hypertensive [Rat]; Minnesota Heart Survey; Modified Hybrid Sign; Multiple Health Screening; Multihospital System

MHSA Microaggregated Human Serum Albumin

MHSS Military Health Services System

MHT Mixed Hemagglutination Test

MHTS Multiphasic Health Testing Services

MHV Magnetic Heart Vector; Middle Hepatic Vein; Mouse Hepatitis Virus; Murine Hepatitis Virus

MHW Mental Health Worker

Mhx Medical History

Mhyg Master Of Hygiene

Mhz Megahertz

Mgr Milligram

MGS Metric Gravitational System; Modified Gram-Schmidt Orthogonalization

MGSA Malignant Growth Stimulatory Activity

MGT Medical Guideline Technology; Multiple Glomus Tumors

MGUS Monoclonal Gammopathies Of Undetermined Significance

MGV Mean Gray Value

MGW Magnesium Sulfate, Glycerin, And Water

Mgy Milligray

Mgy Microgray

MH Malignant Histiocytosis; Malignant Hyperpyrexia; Malignant Hypertension; Malignant Hyperthermia; Mammotropic Hormone; Mannoheptulose; Marital History; Medial Hypothalamus; Medical History; Melanophorestimulating Hormone; Menstrual History;

Mental Health; Mental Hygiene; Moist Heat; Monosymptomatic Hypochondriasis; Murine Hepatitis; Mutant Hybrid; Mycobacterium Haemophilum; Myohyoid

Mh Millihenry

Mh Microhenry

MHA Major Histocompatibility Antigen; May-Hegglin Anomaly; Mental Health America; Mental Health Association; Methemalbumin; Microangiopathic Hemolytic Anemia; Microhemagglutination; Middle Hepatic Artery; Mixed Hemadsorption; Mueller-Hinton Agar

MHAM Multiple Hamartoma

MHAQ Modified Health Assessment Questionnaire

M-HART Montreal Heart Attack Readjustment Trial

MHA-TP Microhemagglutination–Treponema Pallidum

MHAUS Malignant Hyperthermia Association Of The United States

MHB Maximum Hospital Benefit; Mueller-Hinton Base

Mhb Methemoglobin; Myohemoglobin

MHBSS Modified Hank Balanced Salt Solution

MHC Major Histocompatibility Complex; Mental Health Care; Mental Health Center; Mental Health Clinic; Myosin Heavy Chain

MHCS Mental Hygiene Consultation Service

MHCU Mental Health Care Unit

MHD Maintenance Hemodialysis; Mean Hemolytic Dose; Mental Health Department; Minimization Of Hypersurface Distance; Minimum Hemolytic Dilution; Minimum Hemolytic Dose

MHDI Minnesota Health Data Institute

MIP Macrophage Inflammatory Protein;
Major Intrinsic Protein; Maximum Inspiratory
Pressure; Maximum-Intensity Pixel; Maximum
Intensity Projection; Mean Incubation
Period; Mean Intravascular Pressure; Medical
Informatics Programme; Middle Interphalangeal;
Minimal Inspiratory Pressure; Minimally
Invasive Parathyroidectomy; Minimally
Invasive Procedure

Mip Minimum-Intensity Projection

Mip Macrophage Infectivity Potentiator,
Macrophage Infectivity Promoter

MIPA Macrophage Inflammatory Protein
Alpha

MIPB Macrophage Inflammatory Protein Beta

Mipcor Coronary Maximum-Intensity Projection

MIPO Minimally Invasive Plate Osteosynthesis

MIPP Maximum-Intensity Pixel Projection

MIPPO Minimally Invasive Percutaneous
Plate Osteosynthesis

MIPS Martinsried Institute Of Protein Sequences;
Mean Index Procedure Sum; Millions
Of Instructions Per Second; Munich
Information Center For Protein Sequences;
Myocardial Isotope Perfusion Scan

MIR Main Immunogenic Region; Multiple
Isomorphous Replacement

MIRACL Myocardial Ischemia Reduction
With Aggressive Cholesterol Lowering

MIRC Microtubuloreticular Complex

MIRD Medical Internal Radiation Dose

MIRL Medical Imaging Research Laboratory;
Membrane Inhibitor Of Reactive Lysis

MIRMO Medical Information Resources

Management Office

Mirna Micro–Ribonucleic Acid

MIRON Medical Information Resources On
The Net

MIG Measles Immune Globulin; Medicare
Insured Groups; Message Implementation
Guideline; Mitochondria Interest Group; Mo

MIL Mean Intercept Length Analysis

MILESTONE Multicenter Iloprost European
Study On Endangeitis

MILIS Multicenter Investigation Of The Limitations
Of Infarct Size

MILP Mitogen-Induced Lymphocyte Proliferation

MILS Medication Information Leaflet For Seniors

MILT Medical Laboratory Technician

MILT-AD Medical Laboratory Technician Associate
Degree

MILT-C Medical Laboratory Technician Certificate

MIM Mendelian Inheritance In Man; Message
Information Model; Multilateral Initiative
In Malaria

MIMC Multivane Intensity Modulation Compensator

MIMI Minimalist Immediate Mechanical Intervention

MIMIC Multivane Intensity Modulation
Compensation

MIMOSA Medical Image Management In
An Open System Architecture

MIMR Minimal Inhibitor Mole Ratio

MIMS Medical Information Management
System; Medical Inventory Management System;
Migraine And Myocardial Ischemia
Study

Mimyca Maternally Inherited Disorder
With Adult-Onset Myopathy And Cardiomyopathy

MIN Medial Interlaminar Nucleus; Medical

Information Network; Multiple Intestinal Neoplasia
MIRRACLE Myocardial Infarction Risk
Recognition And Conversion Of Life-
Threatening Events Into Survival [Trial]
MIRS Mean Index Resuscitation Sum
MIRSA Multicenter International Randomized
Study Of Angina Pectoris
MIRU Myocardial Infarction Research Unit
MIRU-VNTR Mycobacterial Interspersed Repetitive-
Unit Variable-Number Tandem Repeat
MIRV Mirim Virus
MIS Management Information System; Manager
Of Information System; Medical Information
Service; Medical Information System;
Meiosis-Inducing Substance; Minimally Invasive
Surgery; Motor Index Score; Müllerian
Inhibiting Substance
Misad Milan Study On Atherosclerosis And
Diabetes
MISC Multi–Interface Sensor Controlled
Misc Miscarriage; Miscellaneous
MISCHF Management To Improve Survival
In Congestive Heart Failure
MISG Modified Immune Serum Globulin
MISHAP Microcephalus, Imperforate Anussyndactyly,
Hamartoblastoma, Abnormal Lung
Lobulation, Polydactyly [Syndrome]
MISI Multiple Input–Single Input
MISJ Medical Instrument Society Of
Japan
MISNES Multicenter Italian Study On Neonatal
Electrocardiography And Sudden Infant
Death Syndrome
MISS Medical Image-Sharing System; Medical
Interview Satisfaction Scale; Minimally

Invasive Spinal Surgery; Modified Injury Severity
Scale

MIST Management Of Influenza In The
Southern Hemisphere Trials; Medical Information
Service By Telephone; Mibefradil
Ischemia Suppression Trial; Minimally Invasive
Surgery And Intervention Technology;
Multicenter Isradipine Salt Trial

MISU Maternal Interview Of Substance
Abuse

MIT Magnetic Induction Tomography; Male
Impotence Test; Marrow Iron Turnover;
Massachusetts
Institute Of Technology; Mean
Input Time; Melodic Intonation Therapy; Metabolism
Inhibition Test; Miracidial Immobilization
Test; Mitomycin; Monoiodotyrosine

Mit Mitral

MITF Microphthalmia-Associated Transcription
Factor

MITI Myocardial Infarction Triage And Intervention
[Project]

Mk Monkey

Mkat Millikatal

Mkat Microkatal

Mkat/L Millikatals Per Liter

MKB Medical Knowledge Database; Megakaryoblast

MKC Monkey Kidney Cell

MKF MEDLINE Knowledge Finder

M-Kg Meter-Kilogram

MKHS Menkes Kinky Hair Syndrome

Mkk Monkey Kidney

Mkl Megakaryoblastic Leukemia

MKMD Molecular Knowledge Of Metabolic
Diseases

MKP Monobasic Potassium Phosphate

MKS, Mks Meter-Kilogram-Second

MKSAP Medical Knowledge Self-Assessment
Program

MKT Mean Kinetic Temperature

MKTC Monkey Kidney Tissue Culture

MKV Killed Measles Vaccine

ML Licentiate In Medicine; Licentiate In
Midwifery; Malignant Lymphoma; Mandibular
Line; Marked Latency; Markup Language;
Maximum Likelihood; Medial Lemniscus; Median
Load; Mediolateral; Mesiolingual; Middle
Lobe; Midline; Molecular Layer; Motor Latency;
Mucolipidosis; Mucosal Leishmaniasis;

MIROW Modeling Of Immunization Registry
Operations Workgroup

MIRP Myocardial Infarction Rehabilitation
Program

MIRRACLE Myocardial Infarction Risk
Recognition And Conversion Of Life-
Threatening Events Into Survival [Trial]

MIRS Mean Index Resuscitation Sum

MIRSA Multicenter International Randomized
Study Of Angina Pectoris

MIRU Myocardial Infarction Research Unit

MIRU-VNTR Mycobacterial Interspersed Repetitive-
Unit Variable-Number Tandem Repeat

MIRV Mirim Virus

MIS Management Information System; Manager
Of Information System; Medical Information
Service; Medical Information System;
Meiosis-Inducing Substance; Minimally Invasive
Surgery; Motor Index Score; Müllerian
Inhibiting Substance

Misad Milan Study On Atherosclerosis And

Diabetes
MISC Multi–Interface Sensor Controlled
Misc Miscarriage; Miscellaneous
MISCHF Management To Improve Survival
In Congestive Heart Failure
MISG Modified Immune Serum Globulin
MISHAP Microcephalus, Imperforate Anussyndactyly,
Hamartoblastoma, Abnormal Lung
Lobulation, Polydactyly [Syndrome]
MISI Multiple Input–Single Input
MISJ Medical Instrument Society Of
Japan
MISNES Multicenter Italian Study On Neonatal
Electrocardiography And Sudden Infant
Death Syndrome
MISS Medical Image-Sharing System; Medical
Interview Satisfaction Scale; Minimally
Invasive Spinal Surgery; Modified Injury Severity
Scale
MIST Management Of Influenza In The
Southern Hemisphere Trials; Medical Information
Service By Telephone; Mibefradil
Ischemia Suppression Trial; Minimally Invasive
Surgery And Intervention Technology;
Multicenter Isradipine Salt Trial
MISU Maternal Interview Of Substance
Abuse
MIT Magnetic Induction Tomography; Male
Impotence Test; Marrow Iron Turnover;
Massachusetts
Institute Of Technology; Mean
Input Time; Melodic Intonation Therapy; Metabolism
Inhibition Test; Miracidial Immobilization
Test; Mitomycin; Monoiodotyrosine
Mit Mitral

MITF Microphthalmia-Associated Transcription Factor

MITI Myocardial Infarction Triage And Intervention [Project]

MLEM, ML-EM Maximum Likelihood Expectation Maximization

MLF Medial Longitudinal Fasciculus; Morphine-Like Factor

MLFF Multilayer Feed Forward

MLG Mesiolingual Groove; Mitochondrial Lipid Glycogen

MLGN Minimal Lesion Glomerulonephritis

ML-H Malignant Lymphoma, Histiocytic

MLI Mesiolinguoincisal; Mixed Lymphocyte Interaction

ML I, II, III, IV Mucolipidosis I, II, III, IV

MLL Mixed Lineage Leukemia; Multi-Level Logistic

Ml/L Milliliters Per Liter

MLLT1 Mixed Lineage Leukemia Translocated To 1

MLLT2 Mixed Lineage Leukemia Translocated To 2

MLM Map Of Local Minima; Medical Liability Monitor; Medical Logic Module

MLN Manifest Latent Nystagmus; Membranous Lupus Nephropathy; Mesenteric Lymph Node; Motilin

MLNS Minimal Lesion Nephrotic Syndrome; Mucocutaneous Lymph Node Syndrome

MLO Mediolateral Oblique; Mesiolinguoocclusal; Mycoplasma-Like Organism

MLP Left Mentoposterior; Match List Position; Maximum Lifespan Potential; Medical Language Processing; Mesiolinguopulpal;

Microsomal Lipoprotein; Midlevel Practitioner; Multilayer Perception; Multilocus
Probe
ML-PDL Malignant Lymphoma, Poorly Differentiated
Lymphocytic
MLR Mean Length Response; Middle Latency Response; Mineralocorticoid Receptor; Mixed Lymphocyte Reaction; Multilinear Regression; Multivariate Linear Regression
MLRD Microgastria–Limb Reduction Defects [Association]
MLS Maximum Length Sequence; Maximum Likelihood Estimator; Mean Lifespan; Median Lifespan; Median Longitudinal Section; Microphthalmia–Linear Skin Defects [Syndrome]; Middle Lobe Syndrome; Mouse Leukemia Virus; Multilevel Scheme; Multiple Line Scan; Myelomonocytic Leukemia, Subacute
MLS-ART Multilevel Scheme Algebraic Reconstruction
MLSB Mid–Left Sternal Border; Migrating Long Spike Burst
MLSI Multiple Line Scan Imaging
MLT Left Mentotransverse [Lat. Mento-Laeva Transversa]; Mean Latency Time; Median Lethal Time; Medical Laboratory Technician
MLT-AD Medical Laboratory Technician Associate Degree
Multiple Lentiginosis; Muscular Layer; Myeloid Leukemia
Myeloid
Leukemia
M/L Monocyte/Lymphocyte Ratio
M-L Martin-Lewis [Medium]

Ml Millilambert; Milliliter
Ml Milliliter
Ml Microliter
MLA Left Mentoanterior; Medical Library
Association; Mesiolabial; Monocytic Leukemia,
Acute
Mla Millilambert
MLAA Medical Library Assistance Act
MLAB Multilingual Aphasia Battery
MLAC Minimum Local Anesthetic Concentration
MLAEB Midlatency Auditory Evoked Potential
MLAEP Midlatency Auditory Evoked Potential
Mlai Mesiolabioincisal
MLAP Mean Left Atrial Pressure
Mlap Mesiolabiopulpal
MLB Microlaryngobronchoscopy; Monaural
Loudness Balance
Mlb Macrolymphoblast
MLBP Mechanical Low Back Pain
MLBPNN Multilayer Back Propagation Neural
Network
MLBW Moderately Low Birthweight
MLC Midline Catheter; Minimum Lethal
Concentration;
Mixed Leukocyte Culture; Mixed
Ligand Chelate; Mixed Lymphocyte Concentration;
Mixed Lymphocyte Culture; Morphinelike
Compound; Multilamellar Cytosome;
Multileaf Collimator; Myelomonocytic Leukemia,
Chronic; Myosin Light Chain
MLCCHF Multicenter Lisinopril Captopril
Congestive Heart Failure [Study]
MLCK Myosin Light Chain Kinase
MLCN Multilocular Cystic Nephroma
MLCO Member Of The London College Of

Osteopathy
MLCP Myosin Light-Chain Phosphatase
MLCQ Modified Learning Climate Questionnaire
MLCT Metal-To-Ligand Charge Transfer
MLD Manual Lymph Drainage; Masking Level
Difference; Mean Luminal Diameter; Median
Lethal Dose; Metachromatic Leukodystrophy;
Minimal Lesion Disease; Minimal Luminal Diameter;
Minimum Lethal Dose
MLD50 Median Lethal Dose
Ml/Dl Milliliters Per Deciliter
MLE Maximum Likelihood Estimation; Maximum
Likelihood Estimator; Midline Episiotomy
MLEE Multilocus Enzyme Electrophoresis
MLEI Most Likely Exposed Individual
MLEL Malignant Lymphoepithelial Lesion
Apothecaries
Mmsc Master Of Medical Science
MMSE Mini Mental State Examination
Mm/Sec Millimeters Per Second
MMSP Malignant Melanoma Of Soft Parts
Mm St Muscle Strength
MMT Alpha-Methyl-M-Tyrosine; Manual Muscle
Test; Microcephaly, Mesobrachydactyly,
Tracheoesophageal Fistula [Syndrome];
Mitochondrial
Membrane Potential; Mouse Mammary
Tumor
MMTA Methylmetatyramine
MMTB Multimedia Textbook
MMTP Methadone Maintenance Treatment
Program
MMTT Multicenter Myocarditis Treatment
Trial
MMTV Mouse Mammary Tumor Virus

MMU Medical Maintenance Unit; Mercaptomethyl Uracil

Mmu Millimass Unit

Mmulv Moloney Murine Leukemia Virus

MMV Mandatory Minute Ventilation; Mandatory Minute Volume; Medicines For Malaria Venture

MMVD Mixed Mitral Valve Disease

MMVF Man-Made Vitreous Fiber

MMVT Monomorphic Ventricular Tachycardia

MMWR Morbidity And Mortality Weekly Report

MMWV Modulated Morlet Wavelet Transform Vector Sum

MN A Blood Group In The MNS Blood Group System; Malignant Nephrosclerosis; Master Of Nursing; Maternal Newborn; Median Nerve; Meganewton; Melena Neonatorum; Melanocytic Nevus; Membranous Nephropathy; Membranous Neuropathy; Mesenteric Node; Metanephrine; Micronucleated; Micronucleus; Midnight; Mononuclear; Motor Neuron; Mucosal Neurolysis; Multinodular; Myoneural

M&N Morning And Night

Mn Manganese; Monocyte

Mn Millinewton; Millinormal

Mn Modal Number

Mn Nuclear Magneton

MNA Maximum Noise Area

MNAP Mixed Nerve Action Potential; Multineuron Acquisition Processor

MNB Mannosidase Beta; Multinucleated Blastomere; Murine Neuroblastoma

5-MNBA 5-Mercapto-2-Nitrobenzoic Acid

MNBCCS Multiple Nevoid Basal Cell Carcinoma

Syndrome
MNC Mononuclear Cell
MNCD Mild Neurocognitive Disorder
Mm/L Millimoles Per Liter
MMLV Moloney Murine Leukemia Virus;
Montana Myotis Leukoencephalitis Virus
MMM 3-M Syndrome; Marginal Metallophilic
Macrophage; Microsome-Mediated
Mutagenesis; Myelofibrosis With Myeloid
Metaplasia; Myelosclerosis With Myeloid
Metaplasia
Mmm Micromillimeter
Mmµ Meson
MMMF Manmade Mineral Fibers
MMMM Megalocornea, Macrocephaly, Motor
And Mental Retardation [Syndrome]
MMMSE Modified Mini-Mental State Exam
MMMT Malignant Mixed Müllerian Tumor
MMN Mismatch Negativity; Morbus Maculosus
Neonatorum; Multiple Mucosal Neuroma
MMNC Marrow Mononuclear Cell
MMNCB Multifocal Motor Neuropathy With
Conduction Block
MMNN Multimodular Neural Network
MMO Medical Management Office; Methane
Monooxygenase
MMOA Maxillary Mandibular Odontectomy
Alveolectomy
MMOB Molecular Modeling Database
M-Mode Motion Mode
Mmol Myelomonoblastic Leukemia
Mmol Millimole
Mmol Micromole, Micromolar
Mmol/L Millimoles Per Liter
MMP Matrix Metalloproteinase; Maximum

Maintained Pressure; Muscle Mechanical Power

4-MMPD 4-Methoxy-M-Phenylenediamine

MMPI Matrix Metalloproteinase Inhibitor; Minnesota Multiphasic Personality Inventory

MMPNC Medical Maternal Program For Nuclear Casualties

Mmpp Millimeters Partial Pressure

MMPR Methylmercaptopurine Riboside

MMPS Medicare Mortality Predictor System

MMR Major Molecular Response; Mass Miniature Radiography; Masseter Muscle Rigidity; Maternal Mortality Rate; Measles-Mumps-Rubella [Vaccine]; Megalocornea–Mental Retardation [Syndrome]; Mild Mental Retardation; Mobile Mass X-Ray; Mono-Methylorutin; Multimodal Reasoning; Myocardial Metabolic Rate

MMRB Mouth-To-Mouth Rescue Breathing

MMRS Mosoriot Medical Record System

MMRV Measles, Mumps, Rubella, Varicella [Vaccine]

MMS Mass Mammographic Screening; Master Of Medical Science; Methyl Methane Sulfonate; Mini Mental State [Examination

Media

Mom Multiples Of The Median

MOMA 3,4-Methylenedioxidemethylamphetamine; Methylhydroxymandelic Acid

MOMEDA Mobile Medical Data

MOMHR Metal-On-Metal Hip Resurfacing

Momlv, Mo-MLV Moloney Murine Leukemia Virus

MOMO Macrosomia, Obesity, Macrocephaly,

Ocular Abnormalities [Syndrome]
MO-MOM Mineral Oil And Milk Of Magnesia
MOMP Major Outer Membrane Protein
MOMS Multiple Organ Malrotation Syndrome
Mo-MSV Moloney Murine Sarcoma Virus
MOMX Macroorchidism–Marker X Chromosome
[Syndrome]
MON Monensin; Mongolian [Gerbil]
MONET Multiwavelength Optical Network
MONICA Monitoring Trends And Determinants
In Cardiovascular Diseases
Mono Monocyte; Mononucleosis
MONT Montelukast
MOOKP Modified Osteo-Odonto-Keratoprosthesis
MOOSE Meta-Analysis Of Observational
Studies In Epidemiology
MOOW Medical Officer Of The Watch
MOP Major Organ Profile; Medical Outpatient;
Memory Organization Packet
8-MOP 8-Methoxypsoralen
MOPD Microcephalic Osteodysplastic Primordial
Dwarfism
MOPEG 3-Methoxy-4-Hydroxyphenylglycol
MOPFC Medial And Orbital Prefrontal Cortex
MOPP Mechlorethamine, Oncovin, Procarbazine,
Prednisone; Mission-Oriented Protective
Posture [Clothing]
MOPS 3-Morpholino-Propanesulfonic Acid
MOPV Monovalent Oral Poliovirus Vaccine;
Mopeia Virus
Mopv Monovalent Oral Poliovirus Vaccine
Mor Matched Odds Ratio
Mor, Mor Morphine
MORAC Mixed Oligonucleotides Primed
Amplification Of Complementary DNA

MORC Medical Officers Reserve Corps
MORD Magnetic Optical Rotatory Dispersion
MORFAN Mental Retardation, Pre- And
Post-Natal Overgrowth, Remarkable Face,
Acanthosis Nigricans [Syndrome]
Morphol Morphology
MODV Modoc Virus
MODY Maturity-Onset Diabetes Of The
Young
MOF Marine Oxidation/Fermentation; Meta
Object Facility; Methotrexate, Oncovin, And
Fluorouracil; Multiple Organ Failure
Mof Moment Of Force
MOFE Multiple Organ Failure In The Elderly
MOFS Multiple Organ Failure Syndrome
MOG Myelin-Oligodendrocyte Glycoprotein
MO&G Master Of Obstetrics And Gynaecology
MOH Medical Officer Of Health; Ministry
Of Health
MOHSAIC Missouri Health Strategic Architectures
And Information Cooperative
MOI Master Object Index; Maximum Oxygen
Intake; Mechanism Of Injury; Multiplicity Of
Infection
Moi Multiplicity Of Infection
MOIVC Membranous Obstruction Of The Inferior
Vena Cava
MOJUV Moju Virus
MOKV Mokola Virus
MOL Method Of Limits; Molecular
Mol Mole; Molecular, Molecule
Molc Molar Concentration
Molfr Mole Fraction
Mol/Kg Moles Per Kilogram
MNCV Median Nerve Conduction Velocity;

Motor Nerve Conduction Velocity
MND Minimum Necrosing Dose; Minor Neurologic
Dysfunction; Modified Neck Dissection;
Motor Neuron Disease
MNER Multichannel Neural Ensemble Recording
Mng Morning
MNG/CRD/DA Multinodular Goiter, Cystic
Renal Disease, Digital Anomalies [Syndrome]
MNGIE Myo-, Neuro-, Gastrointestinal
Encephalopathy
MNH Maternal And Neonatal Health
MNJ Myoneural Junction
MNK Menkes Syndrome
MNL Marked Neutrophilic Leukocytosis;
Maximum Number Of Lamellae; Mononuclear
Leukocyte
MN/M2 Meganewtons Per Square Meter
Mn/M Millinewton Per Meter
MNMS Myonephropathic Metabolic Syndrome
MNNG N-Methyl N'-Nitro-N-Nitrosoguanidine
MNP Micellar Nanoparticle; Mononuclear
Phagocyte
MNPJSS Misener Nurse Practitioner Job
Satisfaction Scale
MNPV Multiple Nucleopolyhedrovirus
MNR Marrow Neutrophil Reserve; Multiple
Nucleoside Resistance
MNRH May Not Require Hospitalization
MNS Medial Nuclear Stratum; Melnick-
Needles Syndrome; Milan Normotensive
[Rat]; Moesin
Mn-SOD Manganese-Superoxide Dismutase
Mnss Blood Group System Consisting Of
Groups M, N, And MN
MNTBV Manitoba Virus

MNTD Maximum Nontoxic Dose
MNTV Minatitlan Virus
MNU N-Methyl-N-Nitrosourea
MO Macroorchidism; Manually Operated; Master Of Obstetrics; Master Of Osteopathy; Medical Officer; Mesio-Occlusal; Metastases, Zero; Mineral Oil; Minute Output; Modeling Object; Molecular Orbital; Monofunctional; Monooxygenase; Month; Morbid Obesity
MO2 Myocardial Oxygen
Mo Moloney [Strain]; Molybdenum; Monoclonal
Mo Mitral Opening
MΩ Megohm
Mo Mode; Month; Morgan
Mω Milliohm
Mo Permeability Of Vacuum
Mω Microhm
MOA Monoamine Oxidase
Moa Mechanism Of Action

German

M. - Musculus
Maj - Major
MAK - Maximale Arbeitsplatzkonzentration
MCV - Micro Corpuscular Volume
MDP - Magen-Darm-Passage (Röntgenverfahren Z.
Darstellung Magen-Darm-Trakt)
Med - Medial
MG - Molekulargewicht
MI - Cave! 2 Mögliche Bedeutungen: 1.
Myokardinfarkt, 2. Mitralinsuffizienz
Mibi - Mikrobiologie
MKE - Mitralklappenersatz
MLV - Mittellinienverlagerung (Bei Bewertung Eines
Ccts)
MR(T) - Magnetresonanztomographie
MSU - Mittelstrahlurin

Italian

Russian

M
Murmur
Шум
M
(1) Midnight
Полночь
(1) Monoclonal
Моноклональный
MAO
Monoamine Oxidase
Моноаминоксидаза (MAO)

MAP
Mean Arterial Pressure
Среднее Артериальное Давление
MAT
Multi-Focal Atrial Tachycardia
Мультифокальная Предсердная Тахикардия
Max
Maximum
Максимум, Максимальный
MBC
Minimum Bactericidal Concentration
Минимальная Бактерицидная Концентрация (МБК)
MCA
Middle Cerebral Artery
Средняя Мозговая Артерия
MCL
Midclavicular Line
Среднеключичная Линия
MCTD
Mixed Connective Tissue Disease
Смешанное Заболевание Соединительной Ткани
MCV
Mean Cell Volume
Средний Объем Клетки
MERSA, MRSA
Methicillin-Resistant Staphylococcus Aureus
Золотистый Стафилококк, [Штамм] Устойчивый К
Метициллину
Mets
Metastases
Метастазы
MH
Malignant Hyperthermia
Опухолевая Гипертермия
MI

Myocardial Infarction
Инфаркт Миокарда
MIBG
Meta-Iodobenzyl Guanidine
Мета-Йодобензилгуанидин
MIC
Minimum Inhibitory Concentration
Минимальная Ингибирующая Концентрация
Mixt
Mixture
Смесь
ML
Malignant Lymphoma
Злокачественная Лимфома
MPGN
Membrane Proliferative Glomerulonephritis
Мембранозный Пролиферативный
Гломерулонефрит
MPTP
Analog Of Meperidine (Used By Drug Addicts)
Аналог Меперидина, Используемый Наркоманами
MR
Mitral Regurgitation
Митральная Регургитация, Недостаточность
Митрального Клапана
MRI
Magnetic Resonance Imaging
Магнитно-Резонансная Томография (МРТ)
MRSA, MERSA
Methicillin-Resistant Staphylococcus Aureus
Золотистый Стафилококк, [Штамм] Устойчивый К
Метициллину
MS
(1) Multiple Sclerosis
Рассеяный Склероз

(2) Mitral Stenosis

Митральный Стеноз

(3) Mental Status

Психический Статус

MUGA Scan

Multigated Radionuclide Scan (Of Heart)

Многопроекционное Радиоизотопное
Исследование Сердца

MVP

Mitral Valve Prolapse

Пролапс Митрального Клапана

Chinese

M Medical 医 学的; 医疗的; 内科的

M Medicine ① 医学② 内科学③ 药品;
药物

M Melanocytic 黑素细胞

M Membrane 膜 ; 隔膜

M Metabolite 代射产物

M Meter (S) 米

M Methionine 蛋 氨酸; 甲硫氨酸

M Methotrexate 氨 甲喋呤

M Metoclopramide 灭吐灵; 胃复安

M Midvertebral Line 脊 椎中线

M Mitochondria 线 粒体

M Moniliformis 念珠棘虫属

M Monoclonal 单 克隆的

M Monocyte 单核细胞

M Morphine 吗 啡

M Morphoea 硬斑病

M Mother ①母(亲) ②人工孵卵器

M Mucor 毛 霉菌属; 白霉属

M Mucous 黏 液的

M Mucus 黏 液

M Multipara 经产妇

M Murmur 杂 音

M Muscle 肌肉

M Mutitas 〔拉〕浊音; 哑(症)

M Mycobacterium 分支杆菌属

M Mycoplasma 支 原体属; 支原菌属

M1 Myeloblast 原始粒细胞; 成髓细胞

M Myelocyte 髓 细胞; 中幼粒细胞

M Myelomatosis 骨 髓瘤病

M Myopia 近视

MA Mental Age 心 理(智力) 年龄【注释】〔与实
际年龄无关, 表示其智力
水平。智力测试是以大量正常例的统
计资料为依据〕

Mafojs Malformations 畸形

Mafu Malfunction 功能障碍; 功能不良

M-Ag Macrophage Associated Antigen
巨噬细胞相关抗原

MAG Maguari Virus 马 瓜里病毒

MAG Myelin-Associated G

Malic Malignancy 恶性

Mapl Mammoplasty 乳房成形术

MAS Malabsorption Syndrome 吸 收不
良综合征

MD Magnesium Deficiency 镁缺乏

Mebom Metabolism 新陈代谢

Meil Mentally Ill 精 神不健全

Meiln Mental Illness 精神病

Meno Melanoma 黑 色素瘤

Mepa Menopause 绝经期

MF Mutation Frequency 突变频率

MF Mutton Fat (Keratic Precipitates)
羊脂状 〔角膜后沉淀物〕

MF Mycosis Fungoides 蕈样真菌病【注释】 〔为皮
肤淋巴系的恶性肿瘤。首
先出现强烈的骚痒症状, 然后依次出现
扁平隆起、苔藓化及肿瘤, 最终衰弱〕

MF Myelinated Fiber 有髓鞘神经纤维

MF Myelofibrosis 骨髓纤维化

MF Myocardial Fibrosis 心肌纤维化

MF Myocardial Flow 心肌血流量

MH Medial Hypothalamus 内侧下丘脑

MH Melanophore Hormone 黑 素细胞
激素

MH Menst Rual History 月 经史

MH Mental Health 精神卫生; 心理保健

MI Menstrual Induction 月经诱导

MI Mental Illness 精神疾病

Micar Miscarriage 流产

Mmmc Mammographic 乳 房 X 线造影
的

Mmmy Mammography 乳 房 X 射线造
影术

Morp Morphine 吗啡

MR Magneresistant 磁阻

MR Magnetic Resonance 磁 共振

MR Measles And Rubella (Vaccine) 麻
疹与风疹疫苗

MR Medial Rectus 内直肌 〔解〕

MPG 404 MR

MR Medical Records 病 历

MR Medical Rehabilitation 医 学康复;
医疗康复【注释】〔在指导重新生活和重返社会
等

的训练过程中, 特指与治疗医学直接相
关的各种医疗康复〕

MR Medical Representatives 医 学情报
负责人【注释】〔为了从医学角度说明医药品、
药物副作用等情报而访问医院的制造
商专业人员〕

MR Menst Rual Regulation 月 经机制调
节

MR Mental Retardation 智力迟钝【注释】〔曾经被
称为精神薄弱。由于种
种原因导致智力发育迟缓〕

MR Muscle Relaxant 肌 肉松弛药

MRI Magnetic Resonance Imaging 磁
共振成像【注释】〔它是利用人体各细胞所具有
的
磁性, 即在强磁场中, 体内的氢原子(质
子) 中出现共振, 此外, 当关闭磁场装置
时, 恢复到质子的磁场状态。在这个期
间发生的变化可通过计算机进行影像
化。通过该方法使器官间或正常与异
常的鉴别上具有更加清楚的特征。目

前已在诊断中广泛应用。同时利用该
方法探索揭开机体的组织能量代谢和

MT Mammary Tumor 乳腺肿瘤

MT Medical Technologist 医疗技师

MT Medical T Reatment 药物治疗

Mure Muscle Relaxant 肌肉松弛药

Musc Multiple Sclerosis 多发性硬化症

Muscl Muddy Sclera 泥 沙样巩膜

Musd Muscled 肌肉发达的

Musk Musculoskeletal 肌 (与) 骨骼的

Musp Muscle Spasm 肌肉痉挛

Musps Muscle Spasms 肌肉痉挛

Muvi Multivitamin 多种维他命的

Muwea Muscle Weakness 肌肉无力

MV Measles Virus 麻疹病毒

MVI Multivitamin Infusion 多 种维生
素输液

Free 无 阻碍最大随意通气量

MW Mean Weight 平 均体重

MW Mediastinal Width 纵 隔宽度

MW Molecular Weight 分子量

MW Multiple Wounds 多 处伤

My Myopia 近视(眼)

Mygr Myasthenia Gravis 重 症肌无力

Myin Myocardial Infarction 心 肌梗塞

Japanese

M　　悪性 M a l i g n a n t 　　マリグナ
ント

□ モル濃度 Molar Concentration □ □

MA 運動性失語症 Motor Aphasia □

□ 僧帽弁閉鎖症 Mitral Atresia □

□ 精神年齢 Mental Age □

MAAS 過度羊水吸引症候群 Massive Mmnion Aspiration Syndrome □

MAC 最小肺胞内濃度 Minimum Alveolar Concentration □

□ 最小麻酔濃度 Mnimum Anesthetic Concentration □

□ 最大許容濃度 Maximum Allowable Cincentration □

□ 僧帽弁輪石灰化 Mitral Annulus Calcification □ □

MAD 最大許容線量 Maximum Allowable Dose □

MAHC 悪性腫瘍随伴性高カルシウム血症 Malignancy Associated Hypercalcemia □

MAP 僧帽弁輪形成術 Mitral Annuloplasty □

□ ヒト赤血球濃厚液 Mannitol-Adenine-Phospate Solution □

MAS　　　胎便吸引症候群　　Ｍｅｃｏｍｉｕｍ□Ａｓｐｉｒａｔｉｏｎ□Ｓｙｍｄｒｏｍｅ□
□　大量吸引症候群　　Ｍａｓｓｉｖｅ□Ａｓｐｉｒａｔｉｏｎ□Ｓｙｎｄｒｏｍｅ　マッシブ□アスピレイション□シンドローム

MAT　　　多源性心房性頻脈　Ｍｕｌｔｉｆｏｃａｌ□Ａｔｒｉａｌ□Ｔａｃｈｙｃａｒｄｉａ　　マルチフォーカル□アトリアル□タキアルディア

MB、Mb　ミオグロビン　　　Ｍｙｏｇｌｏｂｉｎ　ミオグロビン

MBC　　　最大換気量　Ｍａｘｉｍｕｍ□Ｂｒｅａｔｈｉｎｇ□Ｃａｐａｃｉｔｙ　　マキシマム□ブリージング□キャパシティ

□　最大膀胱容量　　　Ｍａｘｉｍｕｍ□Ｂｌａｄｄｅｒ□Ｃａｐａｃｉｔｙ　□

MBD　　　微細脳損傷　Ｍｉｎｏｒ□Ｂｒａｉｎ□Ｄａｍａｇｅ　マイナー□ブレイン□ダメージ

□　微細脳障害　Ｍｉｎｉｍａｌ□Ｂｒａｉｎ□Ｄｙｓｆｕｎｃｔｉｏｎ　□

MBP、Mbp　　平均血圧　　Ｍｅａｎ□Ｂｌｏｏｄ□Ｐｒｅｓｓｕｒｅ　　　ミーン□ブラッド□プレッシャー

MCA　　　中大脳動脈　Ｍｉｄｄｌｅ□Ｃｅｒｅｂｒａｌ□Ａｒｔｅｒｙ　　　　□

Mcb　　　マックバーニ圧痛点　　Ｍｃｂｕｒｎｅｙ'Ｓ□（Ｐｏｉｎｔ）　　マックバーイズ□ポイント

ＭＣＣ　　平均赤血球ヘモグロビン濃度　Ｍｅａｎ□Ｃｏｒｏｕｓｃｕｌａｒ□Ｈｅｍｏｇｌｏｂｉｎ□Ｃｏｎｃｅｎｔｒａｔｉｏｎ□　□

ＭＣ□Ｆｌａｐ　　筋皮弁　Ｍｕｓｃｕｌｏｃｕｔａｎｅｏｕｓ□Ｆｌａｐ　□

ＭＣＨＣ　　平均赤血球ヘモグロビン濃度　Ｍｅａｎ□Ｃｏｒｏｕｓｃｕｌａｒ□Ｈｅｍｏｇｌｏｂｉｎ□Ｃｏｎｃｅｎｔｒａｔｉｏｎ□　□

ＭＣＬＳ　　急性皮膚粘膜リンパ節症候群・川崎病　Ｍｕｃｏｃｕｔａｎｅｏｕｓ□Ｌｙｍｐｈ□Ｎｏｄｅ□Ｓｙｎｄｒｏｍｅ　　□

ＭＣＴ　　平均循環時間　Ｍｅａｎ□Ｃｉｒｃｕｌａｔｉｏｎ□Ｔｉｍｅ　ミーン□サーキュレイション□タイム

ＭＤ　医師・医学博士　Ｍｅｄｉｃａｌ□Ｄｏｃｔｏｒ　メディカルドクター
□　躁うつ病　Ｍａｎｉｃ□Ｄｅｐｒｅｓｓｉｖｅ　　□

ＭＤ５０　　５０％有効量　Ｍｅａｎ□Ｅｆｆｅｃｔｉｖｅ□Ｄｏｓｅ　　ミーン□エフェクティブ□ドーズ

ＭＤＣ　　最大拡散能力　Ｍａｘｉｍａｌ□Ｄｉｆｆｕｓｉｎｇ□Ｃａｐａｃｉｔｙ　　マキシマル□ディフュージング□キャパシティ

ＭＤＩ　　躁うつ病　Ｍａｎｉｃ－Ｄｅｐｒｅｓｓｉｖｅ□Ｉｌｌｎｅｓｓ　□
□　定量噴霧吸入器　Ｍｅｔｅｒｅｄ－Ｄｏｓｅ□Ｉｎｈａｌｅｒ　　□

ＭＤＲ　　一日最低必要量　Ｍｉｎｉｍｕｍ□Ｄａｉｌｙ□Ｒｅｑｕｉｒｅｍｅｎｔ　□

□　　多剤耐性　　Ｍｕｌｔｉｐｌｅ□Ｄｒｕｇ□
Ｒｅｓｉｓｔａｎｃｅ　　□

ＭＤＲＴＢ　多剤耐性結核　　　Ｍｕｌｔｉｐｌ
ｅ□Ｄｒｕｇ□Ｒｅｓｉｓｔａｎｃｅ□Ｔｕｂｅ
ｒｃｕｌｏｓｉｓ　□

ＭＥＤ　　　最小有効量　Ｍｉｎｉｍｕｍ□Ｅｆ
ｆｅｃｔｉｖｅ□Ｄｏｓｅ　　ミニマム□エフ
ェクティブ□ドーズ

ＭＥＦ　　　最大呼気流量　　Ｍａｘｉｍａｌ□
Ｅｘｐｉｒａｔｏｒｙ□Ｆｌｏｗ　　マキシマ
ル□エクスピラトリー□フロー

ＭＥＦＲ　　　最大呼気速度　　Ｍａｘｉｍａｌ□
Ｅｘｐｉｒａｔｏｒｙ□Ｆｌｏｗ□Ｒａｔｅ　マ
キシマル□エクスピラトリー□フロー□レイト

ＭＥＦＶ　　　最大努力性呼気流量　　　Ｍａｉｍ
ａｌ□Ｅｘｐｉｒａｔｏｒｕ□Ｆｌｏｗ□Ｖｏｌ
ｕｍｅ　　　マキシマル□エクスピラトりー□フ
ローボリューム

ＭＥＧ　　　脳磁図　　　Magnetoencepalogram
□

ＭＥＰ　最大呼気圧　Maximal□Expiratory□Pressure
マキシマル□エクスピラトりー□プレッシ
ャー

ＭＥＳ　最大眼球速度　　　Maximal□Eyes□Speed
マキシマル□アイズ□スピード

Ｍｅｔａ　　　癌の転位　　Ｍｅｔａｓｔａｓｉｓ
メタスタシス

ＭＥＴＴ　　　最大負荷試験　　　Ｍａｘｉｍｕｍ□
Ｅｘｅｒｃｉｓｅ□Ｔｏｌｅｒａｎｃｅ□Ｔｅｓ
ｔ　　□

MF　マイトマイシンＣとフルオロウラシルの併用化学療法　Ｍｉｔｏｍｙｃｉｎ□Ｆｌｕｏｒｏｕｒａｃｉｌ　　マイトマイシン□フルオロウラシル

MFD　最小致死量　Minimum Fetal Dose □

MFP　循環系平均充満圧　Mean Circulatory Filling Pressure　　　□

MFT　運動機能テスト　Motor Function Test □

MG　重症筋無力症　Myasthenia Gravis □

Mg　マグネシウム　Magnesium □

MGN 膜性糸球体腎炎　Membranous Glomerulonephritis □

MH　悪性高体温症、悪性高熱症　Malignant Hyperthermia □

MHV 中肝静脈　Middle Hepatic Vein □

MI　心筋梗塞　Myocardial Infarction□

□　精神疾患　Mental Illness □

□　僧帽弁閉鎖不全(症) Mitral Insufficiency □

MICU ドクターカー　Mobile Intensive Care Unit □

MID　多発梗塞性痴呆　Multi-Infarct-Dementia □

MIF　最大吸気流量　Maximum Inspiratory Flow □

MIP　最大吸気圧　Maximum Inspiratory Pressure □

ML　悪性リンパ腫　Malignant Lymphoma □

□　肺中葉　Middle Lobe Of Lung □

MLD　最小致死量、最低致死量　Minimum Lethal Dose □

□　中間致死量　Mean(Median)Lethal Dose □

MLG 脊髄腔造影(法)　　Myelography □

MLNS急性皮膚粘膜リンパ節症候群、川崎病
(Acute)Mucocutaneous Lymphnode Syndrome
□

MM　悪性黒色腫　Malignant Melanoma □

□　　多発性骨髄腫　　　Multiple Myeloma　　□

MMC　マイトマイシンC　Mitomycin C □

MM(E)F　　最大中間呼気流量　Maximal
Midexpiratory Flow　□

MMFR　　　最大中間呼気流速　Maximum
Midexpiratory Flow Rate　　□

MMR 麻疹、おたふくかぜ(流行性耳下腺炎)、風
疹の混合ワクチン　Measles-Mumps-
Rubella(Vaccine)　　□

MMST　　　簡易知能試験　　Mini-Mental
State Test　□

MMT　徒手筋力テスト　Manual Muscle Testing
□

MMV 強制分時換気量　　Mandatory Minute
Volume　　□

MOD 成人型糖尿病　　Maturity Onset Diabetes
Mellitus　　□

MODS多臓器不全症候群　Multiple Organ
Dysfunction Syndrome　　□

MODY　　　小児成人型糖尿病　Maturity Onset
Diabetes Mellitus Og Young People □

MOF 多臓器不全　Multiple Organ Failure　　□

MOI　感染多重度　Mutiplicity Of Infection　　□

Mol　モル　Mole　□

Mole　胞状奇胎　□　　　□

Mortal 死亡率　　Mortality　　□

MPA　主肺動脈　Main Pulmonary Artery　　□

Mpap 平均肺動脈圧　　　　Mean Pulmonary Arterial Pressure　　□

MPC 最大許容濃度　　　　Maximum Permissible Concentration □

MPI 心筋血流像(イメージング) Myocardial Perfusion Imaging　　□

M ・ Pn　　　マイコプラズマ肺炎

　　　　　Mycoplasma Pneumonia　　□

MPV 門脈本幹　　Main Portal Vein　　□

MR 医療情報担当者　　Medical Representative □

□　　精神(発達)遅滞　　Mental Retardation　□

□　　僧帽弁逆流(症)　　Mitral Regurgitation　□

□　　麻疹・風疹ワクチン　　　　　Measles-Rubella(Vacine)　　□

MRA 悪性関節リウマチ　Malignant Rheumatoid Arthritis　　□

□　　磁気共鳴血管造影(法)　　Magnetic Resonance Angiography　　□

MRDM　　栄養障害関連糖尿病

　　　Malnutrition Related Diabetes Mellitus　　□

MRF 中脳網様体　Mesencephalic Reticular Formation　　□

MRI 磁気共鳴撮像法　　Magnetic Resonance Imaging　　□

MRM おたふくかぜ(流行性耳下腺炎)、風疹、麻疹3種混合ワクチン　　　　Mumps.Rubella And Measles(Vaccine)　　□

Mrna 伝令リボ核酸、メッセンジャー RNA

　　　Messenger Ribonucleic Acid □

Mrnp 伝令リボ核蛋白、メッセンジャー RNP

　　　Messenger Ribonucleoprotein　　□

MRS(A)　　メチシリン耐性黄色ブドウ球菌
Methicillin-Resistant Staphylococcus (Aureus) □

MRV 分時呼吸量　Minute Respiratory Volume □

MS 精神状態　Mental Status □

□ 僧帽弁狭窄(症)　Mitral Stenosis □

□ 多発性硬化症　Multiple Sclerosis □

□ メニエール症候群　Meniere's Syndrome □

MSI 僧帽弁狭窄兼閉鎖不全症　Mitral Stenoinsufficiency □

MSR 僧帽弁狭窄兼閉鎖不全症　Mitral Stenoregurgitation □

MSSA メチシリン感受性黄色ブドウ球菌
Methicillin-Sensitive Staphylococcus Aureus □

MST 50％生存期間　Median Survival Time □

MSUD メープルシロップ尿症　Maple Syrup Urine Disease □

MSVR 最大胃液分泌量　Maximal Secretion Volume Rate □

MSW 医療ソーシャルワーカー　Medical Social Worker □

MT 母体搬送　Maternal Transport □

MTX メトトレキサート　Methotrexate □

MV 機械的人工換気　Mechanical Ventilation □

□ 僧帽弁　Mitral Valve □

□ 分時換気量　Minute Ventilation □

MVA 僧帽弁弁口面積　Mitral Valve Area □

MVD 微小血管神経減圧法　Microvascular Decompression □

MVO 心室中部閉塞症　Midventricular Obstruction　□
MVP 僧帽弁逸脱(症)　Mitral Valve Prolapse □
□　僧帽弁形成(術)　Mitral Valvuloplasty　□
MVR 僧帽弁置換(術)　Mitral Valve Replacemant　□
MVV 最大換気量　Maximal Voluntary Bventilation　□
My　近視　Myopia　　□
Myelo 脊髄造影　　Myelography

N

French

NFS Numération Formule Sanguine
NK Natural Killer
NLPC Néphrolithotomie Percutanée
NN Nouveau-Né

English

NAT N-Acetyltransferase; Natal; Nateglinide;
Neonatal Alloimmune Thrombocytopenia; Network
Address Translation; No Action Taken;
Nonaccidental Trauma; Nucleic Acid Testing

Nat Sodium Tartrate

Nat Native; Natural

NATCO North American Transplant Coordinator
Organization

Natr Sodium [Lat. Natrium]

NATSAL National Survey Of Sexual Attitudes
And Lifestyles

NAVAPAM National Association Of Veterans
Affairs Physician Ambulatory Care
Managers

NAVEL Naloxone, Atropine, Valium, Epinephrine,
Lidocaine

NAVL Nerve, Artery, Vein, Lymphatic

NAPNES National Association For Practical
Nursing Education And Services

NAPP Nerve Agent Pyridostigmine Pretreatment

NAPPH National Association Of Private
Psychiatric Hospitals

NAPPS Nerve Agent Pyridostigmine Pretreatment
Set

NAPQI N-Acetyl-P-Benzoquinone Imine

NAPS12 NLRP12-Associated Periodic Syndrome

NAPT National Association For The Prevention
Of Tuberculosis

NAQAP National Association Of Quality
Assurance Professionals

NAR Nasal Airway Resistance; National Association

For Retarded [Children, Citizens];
No Action Required; Nutrient Adequacy Ratio
NARA Narcotics Addict Rehabilitation Act;
National Association Of Recovered Alcoholics
NARAL National Abortion Rights Action
League
NARC Narcotic; National Association For
Retarded Children; Nucleus Arcuatus
NARCF National Association Of Residential
Care Facilities
Narco Narcotic, Narcotic Addict; Drug Enforcement
Agent
NARD National Association Of Retail Druggists
NARES Nonallergic Rhinitis-Eosinophilia
Syndrome
NARF National Association Of Rehabilitation
Facilities
NARHC National Association Of Rural
Health Clinics
NARIC National Rehabilitation Information
Center
NARL No Adverse Response Level
NARMA Nonlinear Autoregressive Moving
Average
NARMAX Nonlinear Autoregressive Moving
Average With Exogenous [Input]
NARMH National Association For Rural
Mental Health
NARP Neuropathy, Ataxia, Retinitis Pigmentosa
[Syndrome]
NARS National Acupuncture Research Society
NARSAD National Alliance For Research
On Schizophrenia And Depression
NARSD National Alliance For Research On
Schizophrenia And Depression

NARX Nonlinear Autoregressive Model With Exogenous Input

NAS Narcotics Assistance Section; Nasal; National Academy Of Sciences; National Association Of Sanitarians; Neonatal Abstinence Syndrome; Neonatal Airleak Syndrome;

NGF Nerve Growth Factor

NGFA Nerve Growth Factor Alpha

NGFB Nerve Growth Factor Beta

NGFG Nerve Growth Factor Gamma

NGFIA Nerve Growth Factor–Induced Clone A

NGFIC Nerve Growth Factor–Induced Clone C

NGFR Nerve Growth Factor Receptor

NGGR Nonglucogenic/Glucogenic Ratio

NGI Nuclear Globulin Inclusion

NGL Neutral Glycolipid

Ng/Ml Nanograms Per Milliliter

NGNA National Gerontological Nursing Association

NGO Nongovernmental Organization

NGOV Ngoupe Virus

NGPA Nursing Grade Point Average

NGR Narrow Gauze Roll; Nasogastric Replacement

NGS Next-Generation Software; Normal Goat Serum

NGSA Nerve Growth–Stimulating Activity

NGSF Nongenital Skin Fibroblast

NGT Nasogastric Tube; Nominal Group Technique; Normal Glucose Tolerance

NGU Nongonococcal Urethritis

NGVL National Gene Vector Laboratories

NH Natriuretic Hormone; Naval Hospital; Neonatal Hemochromatosis; Neonatal Hepatitis; Neurologically Handicapped; Nocturnal Hypoventilation; Node Of His; Nonhuman;

Nursing Home
N(H) Proton Density
NHA National Health Association; National
Hearing Association; National Hemophilia
Association; Nonspecific Hepatocellular Abnormality;
Nursing Home Administrator
NHAAP National Heart Attack Alert
NHEFS National Epidemiologic Follow-Up
Study
NHES National Health Examination Survey
NHF National Health Federation; National
Heart Foundation; National Hemophilia
Foundation; Nonimmune Hydrops Fetalis;
Normal Human Fibroblast
NHG Normal Human Globulin
NHGB Net Hepatic Glucose Balance
NHGJ Normal Human Gastric Juice
NHGRI National Human Genome Research
Institute
NHH Neurohypophyseal Hormone
NHHCS National Home And Hospice Care
Survey
NHI National Heart Institute; Nuclear Hepatobiliary
Imaging
NHIC National Health Information Council
[Canada]
NHIF National Head Injury Foundation
NHIS National Health Interview Survey
NHIS-YRB National Health Interview
Survey–Your Risk Behavior
NHK Normal Human Kidney
NHL Nodular Histiocytic Lymphoma; Non-
Hodgkin Lymphoma
German
N. - Nervus

NAP - Nervenaustrittspunkt
NI - Niereninsuffizienz
NIDDM - Non-Insulin-Dependend-Diabetes-Mellitus
NL - Nierenlager
NLKS - Nierenlagerklopfschmerz
NNH - Nasennebenhöhlen
Nukl. - Nuklearmedizinisch

Italian

NE Nutrizione Enterale
NIV Invasive Ventilation (Ventilazione Non Invasiva)
NP Nutrizione Parenterale
NRS (Acronimo Inglese)Numeric Rating Scale (Scala
Di Valutazione Numerica)

Russian

NAPA
(1) N-Acetyl-Procainamide
N-Ацетилпрокаинамид
(1) N-Acetyl-Paraaminophenol
N-Ацетилпарааминофенол
NAS
No Added Sodium
Без Добавления Натрия, Не Содержит Натрия
NB
Newborn
Новорожденный
NCI
National Cancer Institute
Национальный Институт Рака (США)
Neg
Negative
Отрицательный
Neuro
Neurology
Неврология
NG
Nasogastric
Назогастральный
NGU
Nongonococcal Urethritis
Негонококковый (Негонорейный) Уретрит
NHL
Non-Hodgkin's Lymphoma
Неходжкинская Лимфома

NHLBI
National Heart Blood Lung Institute
Национальный Институт Сердца, Крови И Легких
(США)
NIDDM
Non Insulin Dependent Diabetes Mellitus
Инсулиннезависимый Сахарный Диабет
NIH
National Institutes Of Health
Национальный Институт Здоровья (США)
NLM
National Medicine Library
Национальная Медицинская Библиотека (США)
NM
Neuromuscular
Нейромышечный
No
Number
Номер
Noc
Night
Ночь
NS
Normal Saline
Физиологический Раствор
NSAID
Nonsteroidal Antiinflammatory Drug
Нестероидное Противовоспалительное Средство
(НПВС)
NSILA
Nonsuppressable Insulin-Like Activity
Неподавляемая Исулин-Подобная Активность
NSR
Normal Sinus Rhythm
Нормальный Синусовый Ритм [ЭКГ]

NTG
Nitroglycerin
Нитроглицерин

Chinese

N

N Nano 纤 ; 纳

N Negative 照 相底片; 底片; 消极的;
负; 负的; 阴

N Neisseria 奈瑟氏菌属

N Nephrectomy 肾切除术

N Nephron 肾单位

N Neuroticism 神经过敏症

N Neutrophil 嗜中性粒细胞; 中性白细
胞; 中性粒细胞

N Nocardia 诺 卡氏菌属; 奴卡氏(放线)
菌属

N Nonmalignant 良 性的; 非恶性的 〔指
肿瘤〕

NA Nalidixic Acid 萘啶(酮) 酸

NA Nasal Allergy 鼻 变态反应

NA Nervous Apnea 神经性呼吸暂停

NA Neuraminidase 神 经氨酸酶; 神经氨
(糖) 酸苷酶; 唾液酸苷酶

NA Neurological Age 神 经系统的年龄
(寿命)

NA Neut Ralizing Antibody 中 和抗体

NA Neutrophil Antibody 嗜 中性白细胞
抗体

NA Nicotinic Acid 吡啶甲酸

NA Nitrous Acid 亚 硝酸

NA Nomina Anatomica 解 剖学名词

NA Nonalcoholic 不 含酒精的; 非酒精

性的

NA Noradrenalin 去甲肾上腺素

NA Nucleic Acid 核酸

NAA Neutral Amino Acid 中性氨基酸

NAA Nicotinic Acid Amide 烟酰胺

NAAC National Association Of Agricultural
Cont Ractors 国家农业承包人协会

NAACP Neoplasia, Allergy , Addison□s
(Disease) , Collagen (Vascular Disease)
, Parasites 瘤形成, 变态反应, 阿
狄森氏病, 胶原(血管病) 及寄生虫

Naano Narcotics Anonymous 无名麻醉
剂

Naans Narcotic Analgesics 麻醉性镇痛
药

Nabes Nail Beds 甲床

NABMNC Nonadherent Bone Marrow
Nucleated Cell 非黏附性骨髓有核细胞

NABR National Association For Biomedical
Research 国家生物医学研究学会

NABS (Nabs) Normal Active Bowel
Sounds 正常活动性肠鸣音

NAC Accessory Nucleus 副 (神经) 核

NAC N Acetyl Cysteine N 乙酰半胱氨
酸

NAC Nonadherent Cell 非黏附性细胞

Naca Navel Cannula 脐导管

Nacav Nasal Cavity 鼻腔

NACFT National Association Of Cattle
Foot Trimmers 全国牛脚装饰者学会

Nacl Sodium Chloride 氯化钠

Naco Nasal Congestion 鼻塞; 鼻充血

Nacos Narcotics 麻醉毒品

NAD Nadolol 萘羟心安

NAD New Antigenic Determinant 新抗原决定簇

NAD Nicotinamide Adenine Dinucleotide 烟酰胺腺嘌呤二核苷酸; 辅酶 I

NAD Nicotinic Acid Dehydrogenase 烟酸脱氢酶

NAD No Abnormality Demonst Rable 无异常可见

NAD No Active Disease 无活动性病变

NAD No Acute Distress 无急性痛苦; 无急性病痛; 无急性窘迫

NAD No Apparent Distress 无明显窘迫; 无明显病痛; 未查出疾病

NAD Nothing Abnormal Detected 检查无异常; 未见异常

NADC Nandrolone Decanoate 癸酸诺龙; 长效多乐宝灵

NADC National Animal Disease Center (US Department Of Agriculture) 国家动物疾病中心〔美国农业部〕

Nade Nasal Deformity 鼻畸形

NADH Nicotinamide Adenine Dinucleotide 烟酰胺腺嘌呤二核苷酸; 辅酶 I

NADH Reduced Form Of Nicotinamideadenine Dinucleotide 还原型烟酰胺二核苷酸

NADH Reduced Nicotinamide Adenine Dinucleotide 还原型烟酰胺腺嘌呤酸二

核苷酸

Nadi Nasal Discharge 鼻液; 鼻漏; 鼻汁

NADIS National Animal Disease Information
Service 国 家动物疾病信息中心

NADP(H) Nicotinamide Adenine Dinucleo-
Tide Phosphate 烟酰胺腺嘌呤二核
苷酸磷酸; 辅酶 II

NADP (H) Reduced Form Of Nicotinamide-
Adenine Dinucleotide Phosphate
还 原型烟酰胺腺嘌呤二核苷酸磷酸
(还原型辅酶 II)

NADPH Reduced Nicotinamide Adenine
Dinucleotide Phosphate 还 原型辅酶 II

NAE Neoplastic Angioendotheliomatosis
瘤性血管内皮瘤病

NAE Nonamblyopic Eye 非弱视眼

NAEMSP National Association Of EMS
Physicians 国家电子显微镜医师协会

NAERIC Nor Th American Equine
Ranching Information Council 北美洲
马牧场信息委员会

NAF Nafcillin 乙 氧萘青霉素; 萘夫西
林; 新霉素 III

Nafo Nasolabial Fold 鼻 唇皱襞

NAG N- Acetyl-B-D-Glucosamidase N-
乙酰-B-D 氨基葡萄糖酶; 肾小管上皮细胞
溶血卵磷脂酶【注释】〔在肾小管出现障碍时, 通
过尿
液排出的 NAG 量增加, 它是一种反应
近曲小管机能状况的酶〕

NAG N- Acetylglucosamine N- 乙酰氨基

葡萄糖

NAG Narrow Angle Glaucoma 狭 角性青光眼

NAG Nonagglutinable (Vibrios) 非 凝集的(孤菌)

Naga Nasogastric 鼻胃的

NAGD Naloxone , Activated Charcoal, Glucagon , Doxapram 纳 洛酮、活性炭、高血糖素和吗乙苯吡酮(治疗有关药物过量引起的昏迷)

NAH Nicotinic Acid Hydrazide 烟酰肼

NAHIS National Animal Health Information System (Aust Ralia) 国 家动物保健信息中心

NAHMS National Animal Health Monitoring Service (USA) 国 家动物保健监测系统

NAHMS National Animal Health Monitoring Systems 国家动物保健监测系统

NAI Neuraminidase Inhibition 神 经氨酸酶抑制作用

NAI No Acute Inflammation 无 急性炎症

NAI Nut Ritional Assessment Index 营养评价指数

NAIA National Animal Interest Alliance 全国动物兴趣联盟

NAD 413 NAI

NAIAD Nerve Agent Immobilized Enzyme Alarm And Detector 神 经性(毒) 剂固定酶警报器

NAIVPP National Association Of Independent Veterinary Practices And Practitioners (USA) 全国独立兽医实习和 开业者学会

NAL Non- Adherent Leukocyte 非黏附性 白血球

NAL Nonadherent Lymphocytes 非 黏附 淋巴细胞

Nala Nasolacrimal 鼻泪的

Nalab Nasolabial 鼻唇的

Nale Narcolepsy 发 作性睡病

NALL Null (Cell Line Of) Acute Lymphocytic Leukemia 急 性淋巴细胞白血病的 无标记细胞系

NALP Neutrophilic Alkaline Phosphatase 嗜中性白细胞碱性磷酸酶

NAMA National Agri-Marketing Association (USA) 国家农业销售协会

NAME National Association Of Medical Examiners 全 国法医协会

NAMI Non-Atherosclerotic Acute Myocardial Infarction 非 动脉粥样硬化性 急性心肌梗塞

Namu Nasal Mucosa 鼻 黏膜

NANA N- Acetylneuraminic Acid N- 乙 酰神经氨酸

NANBH Non-A, Non-B Hepatitis 非 甲 非乙型肝炎

NANB-PTH Non A And Non B-Post Transfusion Hepatitis 输 血后非甲非乙 型肝炎

NANC Non- Adrenergic Non-Cholinergic (Nerves) 非肾上腺素能非胆碱能神经【注释】〔有许多物质参与支气管哮喘症的发生, 但是, 近年来发现, 除交感神经和副交感神经以外, 还有以呼吸道中的神经肽为神经传递物质的神经。其中之一就是不属于交感神经, 也不属于副交感神经的所谓第三自律神经系假说。有人认为, 它可能与以往的肾上腺素能神经和胆碱能神经间相互作用或具有共同的递质〕

Naovo Nausea Or Vomiting 恶心与呕吐

NAP Nerve Action Potential 神经动作电位

NAP Neut Rophilic Alkaline Phosphatase 嗜中性白细胞碱性磷酸酶

NAPA N- Acetyl Procaine Amide N-乙酰普鲁卡因酰胺

NAPA N-Acetyl-P- Aminophenol 扑热息痛; N- 乙酰对氨基苯酚(退热镇痛药)

NAPA Network Against Psychiatric Assault 精神病防治网

NAPCC National Animal Poison Control Center (USA) 国家动物中毒控制中心

NAR Nasal Airway Resistance 鼻通气阻力; 鼻气导阻力

NARES Nonallergic Rhinitis With Nasal Eosinophilia 鼻嗜酸性细胞增多性非变应性鼻炎

NARP Nonaqueous Reverse Phase Chromatography

非水反相色谱法

NARS National Acupuncture Research Society 全国针灸研究会

NART Nasal Airway Resistance Tester 鼻腔气道阻力测量器

Nasa Sodium Salicylate 水杨酸钠

NASDA National Association Of State Departments Of Agriculture 全国州农业部学会

Nase Nasal Septum 鼻中隔 Se Ptum N Asale〔拉〕

NASE National Association For The Study Of Epilepsy 全国癫痫研究协会

NASEAN National Association For State Enrolled Assistant Nurses 全国州注册 NAI 414 NAS 助理护士协会

NASHA Non-Animal Stabilized Hyaluronic Acid 非动物稳定性透明质酸

NASN National Air Sampling Network 全国大气取样网

NASN National Air Surveillance Net - Work 全国大气监视网; 国家空中监视网

Nasp Nasal Spray 鼻腔喷雾

NASPHV National Association Of State Public Health Veterinarians 全国公共卫生兽医协会

NASS National Agriculture Statistics Service (USA) 国家农业统计局

NAT Natal 分娩的; 生产的

NAT National Tuberculosis Association

全国结核病协会; 全国防痨协会

NAT Neut Ralizing Antibody Titer 中 和
抗体效价; 中和抗体滴度

NAT Nonaccidental T Rauma 非 意外创
伤

NAT Noradrenalin Theophylline 去 甲肾
上腺素茶碱

NATP Neonatal Alloimmune Thrombocytopenia
新生儿同种免疫性血小板减少
症

NAV Nucleus Anteroventralis 〔拉〕前
腹核

NAVBC National Agricultural And Veterinary
Biotechnology Centre (Ireland)
国家农业与兽医生物技术中心

NAVCA North American Veterinary
College Administ Rators 北 美兽医学院
行政管理员

NAVLE Nor Th American Veterinary
Licensing Examination 北 美兽医执照
考试

Navo Nausea And Vomiting 恶心与呕吐

NAWAD National Assembly For Wales
Agriculture Depar Tment 威 尔士农业
部国民议会

Nax Nasopharynx 鼻 咽 Pars Nasalis
Ph Aryngis 〔拉〕

Naxl Nasopharyngeal 鼻咽的

NB Negri Bodies 内基氏小体〔为确诊狂
犬病的依据〕

NB Nervus Buccalis 颊 神经

NB Newly Formed Bone 新骨; 新生骨

NB Nitrobenzene 硝基苯

NB Nitrogen Balance 氮 平衡

NB Noise Burst 噪声猝发; 噪声冲击

NB Normoblast 正成红细胞; 幼红细胞

NB Novobiocin 新 生霉素

NB Nuclear Bag (Certain Intrafusal Muscle
Fiber Nuclei Of A Neuromuscular Spindle)
核 袋 〔在一个神经肌肉肌梭内的某
些肌纤维的核〕

NB Nutrient Broth 营 养肉汤

NBA National Beef Association 全国牛
肉学会

NBAS Neonatal Behavioral Assessment
Score 新 生婴儿行为评价法【注释】 〔由有关新生
婴儿行为的 18 个项

目和诱发反应的 17 个项目构成。给新
生婴儿各种刺激, 并对其反应进行评
价〕

NBBG Nebraska Behavioral Biology
Group 内布拉斯加行为生物委员会

NBC Nasobiliary Catheterization 鼻 胆
管插管术

NBC National Broiler Council 全 国烤
肉师委员会

NBC Natural Bir Th Cont Rol 自然节育

NBC Newborn Center 新生儿中心

NBC Nonbacterial Conjunctivitis 非 细
菌性结膜炎

NBCC Nevoid Basal Cell Carcinoma 痣
样基底细胞癌

NBCCS Nevoid Basal Cell Carcinoma Syndrome
痣样基底细胞癌综合征

NAS 415 NBC

NBCD Nuclear , Biological And Chemical
Warfare Defense 核 、 生物、化学战防护;
三防

NBD Neurogenic Bladder Dysfunction
神经原性膀胱功能障碍

NBD No Brain Damage 非 脑损伤; 无脑
损伤

NBEC National Board Examination
Commit Tee For Veterinary Medicine
全国兽医考试委员会

NBEI Synd (R) Non-Butanol Extractable
Iodine Syndrome 非 正丁醇可提取的碘
综合征

NBF Not Breast Fed 非 母乳喂养

NBI Non-Battle Injury 非战伤

NBI Neut Rophil Bactericidal Index 中性
白细胞杀菌指数

NBI Nit Rogen Balance Index 氮 平衡指
数

NBIF National Biotechnology Informa -
Tion Center (USA) 国家生物技术信息
中心

NBL Neuroblastoma 成神经细胞瘤

NBL Newborn Larva 新生蚴

NBM Normal Bone Marrow 正 常骨髓

NBM Nothing By Mouth 禁 食

NBME National Board Of Medical
Examiners (美国) 医师国家考试委员

会 【注释】〔以往, 美国、加拿大和波多黎各的医学院毕业生的资格考试分为 Par T Ⅰ、Ⅱ、Ⅲ, 1992 年进行了修改, 和 F SMB 一起, 由被称为 USML E 的组织统一进行〕

NBME Normal Bone Marrow Ext Ract 正常骨髓提取物

NBN Narrow Band Noise 窄带噪音

NBN Newborn Nursery 新生儿病房

NB (Nb) Newborn ① 新生儿; 新生的 ②新生仔畜; 初生仔畜

NBP National Blood Policy 国家血液政策; 国家献血政策

NBP Needle Biopsy Of Prostate 前列腺针吸活检

NBP Nitrobenzylpyridine 硝基苄基吡啶

NBP Nonbacterial Pharyngitis 非细菌性咽炎

N .B .S . National Bureau Of Standards 国家标准局

NBS Neri-Barre Syndrome 尼内-巴雷综合征

NBS Neurobehavioral Scale 神经行为量表

NBS Neut Ral Buffered Saline 中性缓冲盐水

NBS No Bacteria Seen 无细菌可见

NBS Normal Blood Serum 正常血清

NBS Normal Brain Stem 正常脑干

NBSM Nut Rient Broth Sporulation Medium
孢子形成营养肉汤培养基

NBS (Nbs) Normal Bowel Sounds 正常
肠鸣者

NBT Nitrobenzene Thiocyanate 硝 基苯
硫氰酸酯; 硫氰酸硝基苯酯

NBT Nit Roblue Tetrazolium 四 唑氮蓝;
氮蓝四唑; 硝基蓝四唑; 四唑硝基蓝

NBT Nitro-Blue Tetrazolium (Test) 四
唑氮蓝(试验) 【注释】 〔当白细胞吞噬微生物后,
其代
谢被活化, 增加与杀菌有关的活性氧的
生成。然后, 通过氧化还原反应, NBT
被还原后呈现蓝色为指标, 测定活性氧
产量, 由此间接地测定杀菌能力〕

NBT Normal Breast Tissue 正 常乳房组
织

NBTE Nonbacterial Thrombotic Endocardits
非细菌性血栓性心内膜炎【注释】 〔癌患者脑缺
血发作的 27 % 病例
为形成栓塞所致〕

NBTNF Newborn Term Normal Female
新生(儿) 足月顺产女婴

NBC 416 NBT

NBTNM Newborn Term Normal Male
新生(儿) 足月顺产男婴

NBW Normal Bir Th Weight 正 常出生重
量; 出生体重正常

NC Nasal Cannula 输氧鼻管

NCA Natural Chromosome Aberration
自然染色体畸形

NCA Neurocirculatory Asthenia 神 经性
循环衰弱症; 心神经官能症【注释】〔伴有体格瘦
小、易疲劳、速脉、
心悸、眩晕等症状〕

NCA Neutrophil Chemotactic Activity
中性细胞趋化活性

NCA Nodulocystic Acne 结 囊性痤疮

NCA Nonspecific Cross-Reacting Antigen
非特异性交叉反应抗原

NCAST Nucleus Commissurae Anterioris
Et Striae Terminalis 〔拉〕终纹及前连合
核

NCAT Normal Cephalic Atraumatic 正
常头侧无损伤的

NC/ AT Normocephalic / Atraumatic
(Head Not Injured) 正 常头的/ 无创伤
的

Ncbs No Carotid Bruits 无颈动脉杂音

NC-BVDV Noncytopathogenic Bovine
Viral Diarrhea Virus 非细胞病变性牛病
毒性腹泻病毒

NCC Network Cont Rol Center 网 络控
制中心; 网控中心

Ncce No Clubbing , Cyanosis Or Edema
无杵状指、无紫绀、无水肿

NCCP Non-Cardiac Chest Pain 非 心脏
性胸痛【注释】〔具有狭心症样症状(胸痛) , 但
看不到心脏异常〕

NCD National Commission On Diabetes
全国糖尿病委员会

NCD Normal Childhood Diseases 正 常

儿童期疾病

NCD Normal Childhood Disorders 正常
儿童期机能失调

NCD Unbroken Cells 非破碎细胞

NCDCV Neonatal Calf Diarrhea Coronavirus
新生小牛腹泻冠状病毒

NCDV Nebraska Calf Diarrhea Virus 内
布拉斯加牛腹泻病毒

NCE Negative Contrast Echocardiography
负差超声心动图; 负性对比超声心动图

NCE Noncardiogenic Edema 非 心源性
肺水肿

NCE Nonconvulsive Epilepsy 非 惊厥性
癫痫

NCE Normal Chick Embryo 正常小鸡胚
胎

N Cell Natural Cell 天 然细胞

N Cell Null Cell 无标记细胞; 裸细胞

NCEP National Cholesterol Education
Program 全美胆固醇教育计划

NCF National Cancer Foundation 全国
癌症基金会〔美〕

NCF Neut Rophil Chemotactic Factor 中
性粒细胞趋化因子

NCF No Cold Fluids 非 寒冷液; 不冷
(冻) 液

NCF Normal Colposcopic Findings 阴 道
镜所见正常

NCGL Nucleus Corporis Geniculai Lateralis
外侧膝状体核

NCH Noncirrhotic Hepatocellular Carcinoma

非硬化性肝细胞癌

NCH Normal Childhood Diseases 正 常
儿童期疾病

NCI Naphthalene, Creosote , Iodoform
Powder (Licetreatment) 萘、杂酚油、碘
仿粉剂〔灭虱用〕

N .C .I . National Cancer Institute 国
立癌症研究所〔美〕

NCI Netherlands Cancer Institute 荷
兰癌症研究所

NCI Nuclear Contour Index 核 形指数
NBT 417 NCI

NCI Nucleus Colliculi Inferioris 下丘核

NCIP Nonclassifiable Interstitial Pneumonia
无法分类的间质性肺炎【注释】〔经活体开胸剖
检的结果, 从病

理学上无 UI P, 也没有 DIP、LIP、DAD
的原因不明的间质性肺炎〕

NCL Neuronal Ceroid Lipofuscinosis 神
经元蜡样脂褐质沉积症

NCLM Nodular Cutaneous Lupus Mucinosis
皮肤结节性狼疮黏蛋白症【注释】〔在 LE 患者的
真皮内, 由于黏
蛋白的沉积而出现的丘疹, 形成结节〕

Ncm Normal Circumcised Male 正 常包
皮环切男性

NCM Nucleus Centralis Medialis 〔拉〕
中央内侧核

NCMC Natural Cell-Mediated Cytotoxicity
天 然细胞介导的细胞毒性

NCMC Natural Killer Cell-Mediated Cytotoxicity

天 然杀伤细胞介导的细胞毒性

NCNCA Normochromic Normocytic Anemia
正 色性正常红细胞性贫血

Ncob Near Cavity Obliteration 近腔闭塞

NCP Nitro-Chlorophenol 硝基氯苯酚

NCP Non-Cellulosic Polysaccharide 非
纤维素多糖类

NCP Nonclonogenic Proliferating (Cells)
非克隆性增生(细胞)

NCP Noncollagen Protein 非 胶原蛋白

NCP Nucleus Commissurae Posterioris
〔拉〕后连合核

NCPE Noncardiogenic Pulmonary Edema
非心源性肺水肿

NCPF Noncirrhotic Portal Fibrosis 非 硬
变性肝门纤维化

NCPR New Cardiopulmonary Resuscita -
Tion 新的心肺复苏术

NCR Nuclear-Cytoplasmic Ratio 核质比

NCRR National Center For Research
Resources (USA) 国家研究资源中心

NCS National Cancer Survey 全 国癌症
调查

NCS Neocarcinostatin 新 制癌菌素

NCS Newborn Calf Serum 新生牛血清

NCS Noncircumferential Stenosis 非 周
围性狭窄

NCS Noncoronary Sinus 无冠窦

NCS Non-Cured Sarcoidosis 非 治愈性类
肉瘤病; 不能治愈的类肉瘤病

Ncsts Nerve Conduction Studies 神 经传

导研究

NCSU North Carolina State University
北卡罗莱纳州大学

NCT Neural Crest Tumor 神经脊肿瘤

NCT Non-Contact Tonometer 不接触式
眼压计

NCT Nucleus Corporis Trapezoidei 〔拉〕
斜方体核

NCT Number Connection Test 数字连接
试验

NCV Nerve Conduction Velocities 神经
传导速率

NCVD Noncardiovascular Death 非心血
管病死亡

NCVMA Nor Th Carolina Veterinary
Medical Association 北卡罗来纳州兽
医医学会

NCV(Ncv) Nerve Conduction Velocity
神经传导速率【注释】〔应用于末梢神经障碍的
诊断。
对于感觉神经和运动神经分别用肌电
极测定〕

NCVQ National Council For Vocational
Qualifications 国家职业资格委员会〔美
国〕

Ncvs Nerve Conduction Velocities 神经
传导速率

NCWVI Noncondylomatous Cervical
Wart Virus Infection 非湿疣性颈疣病
毒感染

ND Doctor Of Nursing 护理学博士

NCI 418 ND

ND Nasal Deformation 鼻畸形

ND Nasal Drain 鼻腔引流管

ND Nasolacrimal Duct 鼻泪管

ND Natural Death 自然死亡; 非病理死亡

ND Neonatal Death 新生儿死亡

ND Neoplastic Disease 肿瘤性疾病

ND Nerve Deafness 神经性聋

ND Nervous Debility 神经性无力

ND Neurological Disability 神经失能

ND Neurotic Depression 官能性抑郁症; 神经症性忧郁病

ND Newcastle Disease 新城病 〔鸡的病毒性肺炎及脑脊髓炎〕

ND Nifedipine 硝苯吡啶; 心痛定

ND Nondiabetic 非糖尿病的

ND Non-Distended 无扩张的

ND Normal Delivery 正常分娩

ND Normal Diet 正常膳食

ND Normal Dose 正常量; 标准剂量

ND Not Diagnosed 未诊断的

ND Not Distended 非扩张的

N .D . Numerus Digitorum 指数辨别【注释】〔用视力表不能测定的条件下,
以手指为辨别物, 用辨别距离的远近表示视力好坏〕

ND Nursing Diagnosis 护理诊断

NDA National Dental Association 全国牙科协会

NDA New Drug Application 新药应用

NDA No Demonstrable Antibodies 无抗体显示; 未显示抗体

NDA No Detectable Activity 未能检出活性

NDB Normal Vaginal-Delivery Babies 正常分娩婴儿

NDC National Dairy Council 全国乳品业联合会〔美国〕

NDC Nondifferentiated Cell 未分化细胞

NDC Nuclear Dehydrogenating Clost Ridia 脱氢梭状芽胞杆菌核

NDE Near-Death Experience 濒死体验; 临近死亡经历【注释】〔病情已不能治愈恢复而等待死亡的患者, 称为临死患者。虽然患者处于病危状态, 但偶尔出现意识恢复, 有时需要在这种状态下进行体检〕

NDE Nondeviating Eye 非偏斜眼

NDE Nondiabetic Extremity 非糖尿病肢端

NDF Neut Ral Detergent Fiber 中性去污剂纤维

NDI Nasal Deformity Index 鼻畸形指数

NDI Nephrogenic Diabetes Insipidus 肾原性尿崩症

NDI Nerve Deficit Index 神经缺损指数

NDI Nondestructive Inspection 非破坏性检验; 无损伤性检查

NDIR Nondispersive Infrared Analyzer 非色散红外分析仪

NDL Nuclear Defense Laboratory 核防护实验室

NDM Neoplasm Embryonic Antigen 癌胚抗原

NDM No Evidence Of Abnormality 无畸形征象; 无异常症象

NDM Nucleus Dorsomedialis 〔拉〕背内侧核

NDR Neonatal Death Rate 新生(仔)畜死亡率

NDV Newcastle Disease Virus 新城疫病毒

NE Nerve Ending 神经末梢〔解〕Te Rmin Atio Ne Ur Alis 〔拉〕

NE Norepinephrine 去甲肾上腺素

NEA Neoplasm(Carcino) Embryonic Antigen 胎儿性癌抗原【注释】〔广泛地存在于内脏各种腺癌和
胎儿的正常消化道组织中, 是对结肠癌细胞具有特异性的抗原〕

NEAA Non-Essential Amino Acid 非必
ND 419 NEA
需氨基酸

NEB Neuroendocrine Body 神经内分泌体

NEB Neuroepithelial Body 神经上皮小体

Nebl Nerve Block 神经传导阻滞; 神经阻滞术

Nebr Nervous Breakdown 精神崩溃

Nebz Nebulization 喷雾法

NECA 5′-N- Ethylcarboxyami-Doadenosine 5′-N- 乙基羧基酰胺基腺苷【注释】〔腺苷 5′取代同系物, 腺苷 A2 受体选择性拮抗剂〕

NECL Non Epitheliot Ropic Cutaneous Lymphosarcomas 非 亲上皮细胞性皮肤淋巴肉瘤

Necon Nephrology Consultation 肾 脏病学会诊

Necr Necrosis 坏 死

Necrc Necrotic 坏死的

NED No Evidence Of Disease 无 疾病迹象〔病案记录用语〕

NEEE Norethisterone Enathate 庚 酸炔诺酮

NEEP Negative End- Expiratory Airway Pressure 呼气终末气道负压

NEEP Negative End-Expiratory Pressure 呼 气终末负压【注释】〔为了避免循环受到抑制, 用机械进行人工呼吸时, 降低呼吸道的平均内压, 进行间歇性平压换气, 为此使终末呼气道处于负压。 由于可能导致无气肺, 所以很少利用〕

NEF Nephritic Factor 肾炎因子

NEF Neurite Extension Factor 神经轴突伸长因子

NEFA Non Esterified Fat Ty Acid 非脂化脂肪酸【注释】〔机体内的脂肪酸几乎都是以脂化或与氨基酸结合后的酰化形式存在,

但是, 存在于食物中的脂肪酸是以水解的非脂化脂肪酸或单酸甘油脂的形式被小肠吸收〕

Nefas Necrotizing Fasciitis 坏 死性筋膜炎

Nefi Neurofibromatosis 神经纤维瘤病

Nege Nephrogenic 肾原性的; 肾发生的

Negr Nerve Graft 神经移植物

Neho Nerve Hook 神经钩

Neis Neisseria 奈瑟菌属

NEJM New England Journal Of Medicine 新 英格兰医学杂志

Neles Neuroleptics 神 经安定剂

Neli Nephrolithiasis 肾 结石

Nelit Nephrolithotomy 肾 石切除术

Nelo Needle Localization 针 刺定位

NEM No Evidence Of Malignancy 无 恶变征象; 无恶变证据

NEM Normal Ethyl Morpholine 标 准乙基吗啉

Nema Neuromalignant 神 经恶性的

NEMD Nonspecific Esophageal Motor Disorder 非 特异性食管运动失调

NEMD Nonspecific Esophageal Motor Dysfunction 非特异性食管运动机能障碍

Nemu Neuromuscular 神经肌肉的

Nen Nervousness 神 经质; 神经过敏

Neopc Neoplastic 新 生物的; 赘生的; (肿) 瘤的; 瘤形成的

Neopm Neoplasm 肿瘤

Neopms Neoplasms 新生物(肿瘤)

NEP Negative Expiratory Pressure 呼气
负压

NEP Nephrology 肾病学

NEP Nepuyo Virus 尼 普约病毒

Nepa Nephropathy 肾病

Nepal Nerve Palsy 神 经瘫

NEPD No Evidence Of Pulmonary Disease
无肺病证据

Nepe Neutropenia 中性粒细胞减少症

NEB 420 Nep

Nepec Neutropenic 中 性粒细胞减少的

Nephc Nephrectomy 肾切除术

Nephcs Nephrectomies 肾切除术

Nephpa Nephropathy 肾病

Nephs Neutrophils 中性粒细胞

Nepht Nephrologists 肾 病学家

Nephy Nephrology 肾 脏病学

Nepl Neoplasia 瘤形成; 新生物形成

NER Nit Rogen Efficiency Ratio 氮 功效
比值

NER Normal Estrogen Responders 正 常
雌激素应答者

NERC Natural Environmental Research
Council 自 然环境研究委员会

NERD No Evidence Of Recurrent Disease
无疾病复发征象

Nero Nerve Root 神 经根 〔解〕 Radix Ne Rvi
〔拉〕

NES Neurosurgery 神经外科学

NES Newborn Emergency Service 新生儿急救科

Nesa Neosalpingostomy 新输卵管切开术

Nesas Neosalpingostomies 新输卵管切开术

Nesc Nephrosclerosis 肾硬化; 肾硬变 (病)

Nesin Nearsightedness 近视

Nesv Nephrology Service 肾脏病科

Nesy Near-Syncope 几乎晕厥

Nesyn Nephritic Syndrome 肾病综合征

NET Nerve Excitability Test 神经兴奋性试验

NET Nerve Excitability Threshold 神经兴奋阈

NET Neuroendocrine Tumor 神经内分泌瘤

NET No Evidence Of Tumor 无肿癌证据

NETA Nasal Endot Racheal Anesthesia 鼻气管内麻醉

NETBIOS Network Basic I/ O System 网络基本输入输出系统

Neti Necrotic Tissue 坏死组织

Neto Nephrotoxin 溶肾素

Netoc Nephrotoxic 肾中毒的

Netos Nephrotoxins 肾毒素

Netoy Nephrotoxicity 中毒性肾损害

Netr Neurotrophic 神经营养的

Netu Nephrectomy Tube 肾盂引流管

Netus Nephrectomy Tubes 肾造口导管

Neule Neuroleptic 神经安定的

Neules Neuroleptics 神经安定剂

Neva Neovascular 新血管的

NEVA Nor Th Of England Veterinary Association 英格兰以北兽医学会

Nevaj Neovascularization 新血管形成; 血管再生

Nevay Neurovascularly 神经血管的

NF1 Nuclear Factor 1 细胞核因子 1 【注释】〔一个转录因子家族, 与回文对

称部位 TGG X/ A NNNNNGCCAA 或回文对称部位 TGGCA 相结合。最初认为是腺病毒复制所需的因子, 也是某些病毒基因表达的转录因子, 调节多种细胞基因的表达, 如脂肪细胞特异性增强子活性、乳腺细胞特异性基因的表达、肝特异性转录等〕

NF Native Ferritin 天然铁蛋白

NF Neurofibromatosis 神经纤维瘤病; 多发性神经纤维瘤

NF Neurofilament 神经微丝的

NF Neurological Function 神经功能

NF Neut Ral Fraction 中性部分; 中性分段; 中性馏分

NF Nitrofurazone 呋喃西林

NF Noise Factor 噪声系数

NF Nuclear Factor 核因子

NFAP Nerve Fiber Action Potential 神

经纤维动作电位 NFB

NF-Kb Nuclear Factorκb 核 因子 Kb

Nep 421 NFB

NFH No Family History Of 无 …… 家族
病史

NFL Nerve Fiber Layer 神 经纤维层(眼
科学)

NFL Non-Fatty Liver 非脂肪肝

NFM Nonfamilial Myocardiopathy 非
家族性心肌病

NFM Nor Thern Fowl Mite 林 禽刺螨

NFO National Farmers Organization
(USA) 全 国农场主联合会

NFP Furyl-Propionate Nortestosterone
呋喃丙酸去甲睾酮

NFP Nandrolone Furylpropionate 呋 喃
丙酸诺龙

NFP Neurofilament Protein 神 经丝蛋
白

NFPH Nonfamilial Parathyroid Hyperplasia
非家族性甲状旁腺增生

NFT Neurofibrillary Tangle 神经纤维缠
结; 神经原纤维紊乱

NFT Nit Razine Fern Test 硝 嗪蕨试验

NFTD Normal Full Term Delivery 正 常
足月分娩

NFTSD Normal, Full Term, Spontaneous
Delivery 正 常足月自然分娩

NFU National Farmers Union 全 国农
场主联合会

NG Did Not Receive Therapy Or Drug For

对…… 未接受治疗或药物

NG Nasogastric Tube 鼻胃管

NG Nephrography 肾 X 线照相术; 肾造
影术

NGA Neogalactoalbumin 新 半乳糖白蛋
白

NGA Neuroglandular Antigen 神 经腺抗
原

NGA Normal Glucose Albumin 正 常糖
白蛋白

NGA Normogonadotropic Amenorrhoea
促性腺激素正常性闭经

NGF Nerve Growth Factor 神 经生长因
子【注释】〔在培养的神经节和发育中的交
感神经节中, 具有明显促神经纤维生长
和再生作用的因子。此外, 它又是一种
引起细胞数增多的增殖因子〕

NGFA National Grain And Feed Association
(USA) 全国谷类和饲料学会

NGGR Nonglucogenic/ Glucogenic Ratio
非生成葡萄糖与生成葡萄糖比率

NGIF Neuroblastoma Growth Inhibitory
Factor 成神经细胞瘤生长抑制因子; 神
经母细胞瘤生长抑制因

NG(Ng) Nasogast Ric 鼻 胃的

NGP Normal Glycoprotein 正常糖蛋白

NGSA Nerve Growth Stimulating Activity
促进神经生长活性

NGT Normal Glucose Tolerance 正常(标
准) 葡萄糖耐量

NGT(Ngt) Nasogast Ric Tube 鼻 胃管

NGU Nongonococcal Urethritis 非 淋菌
性尿道炎

NH No History Of 无……病史

NH Nursing Home 家 庭护理; 疗养院;
私人医院

NHC Neonatal Hypocalcemia 新 生儿低
血钙

NHC Nonhistone Chromosomal (Protein)
非 组蛋白染色体(蛋白)

NHG Normal Human Globulin 正 常人
球蛋白

NHL Non-Hodgkin□s Lymphoma 非 何
杰金氏淋巴瘤【注释】〔和何杰金氏病相比, 用化
学疗
法也难以奏效〕

NHM Natural History Museum 自 然
历史博物馆

NHP Nonhemoglobin Protein 非血红蛋
白蛋白质

Nhp Nursing Home Placement 安 置在疗
养院

NFH 422 Nhp

NHR Neonatal Heart Rate 新生儿心率

NHS Neonatal Hepatitis Syndrome 新生
儿肝炎综合征

NHS Normal Human Serum 标 准人血清

NI Noise Induced 噪声诱发的

NIA, Nia . Niacin 烟 酸; 尼克酸; 抗糙
皮病维生素; 维生素 P P

NIA Nephelometric Inhibition Assay 浊

度抑制测定

NIA Nutrient Intake Analysis 营养素摄
入量分析

NIAB National Institute Of Agricultural
Botany 全国农业植物学会

NIBP Non-Invasive Blood Pressure 非
侵害性血压

NIBSC National Institute For Biological
Standards And Cont Rol (UK) 生物标
准与控制研究会〔英国〕

NIC Neonatal Intensive Care 新生儿特
护病房

NICE National Institute For Clinical Excellence
全国临床优秀研究所

Nico Nicotine 尼古丁〔抗疥螨药〕

NICU Neonatal Intensive Care Unit 新
生儿集中治疗室【注释】〔新生儿期, 由于受子宫
外的许
多致病因子的影响而常发病或死亡率
增高, 因此有必要对所谓高度危险婴儿
进行特殊护理。对于这些婴儿进行集
中管理的治疗室, 就称为新生儿集中治
疗室。见于大医院〕

NICVBP National Institute For Control
Of Veterinary Bioproducts And Pharma -
Ceuticals 全国兽医生物制品与医药品研
究会

NIDA Nut Ritional Iron Deficiency Anemia
营养性缺铁性贫血

NIDDM Non Insulin Dependent Diabetes

Mellitus 非 胰岛素依赖性糖尿病【注释】〔在糖尿病中所占的比率最高,
占糖尿病患者总数的 90 %。可分为非
肥胖型和肥胖型两个亚型。在发病时,
机体对胰岛素分泌反应低下和组织对
胰岛素的感受性下降〕

Nidi Nipple Discharge 乳 头溢液

NIF Negative Inspiratory Force 阴 性吸
气力【注释】〔将压力计连接到气管内进行测
定的肺弹力学检测〕

NIF Nifedipine 利 心平〔冠状血管扩张
药〕

Nifun Nissen Fundoplication 尼 森胃底
折叠术

NIG National Institute Of Genetics Genetic
Resources Laboratory (Japan)
全国遗传学与遗传资源检验学会〔日本〕

Nigl Nit Roglycerin 硝 酸甘油〔血管扩张
药〕

NIH National Institutes Of Health
(USA) 全国卫生研究院〔美国〕

NIHL Noise Induced Hearing Loss 噪 声
性聋

Niin Nipple Inversion 乳头内翻

NIMH National Institute Of Mental
Health 全 国精神卫生研究所

NI , N II, Etc Cranial No I , No II , Etc
第一对脑神经, 第二对脑神经等

Nipa Nitroglycerin Patch 硝 酸甘油贴片

Nipas Nit Roglycerin Paste 硝 酸甘油膏剂

NIPPV Non-Invasive Positive Pressure

Ventilation 非损伤性正压呼吸【注释】〔为不需在气管内插入导管就可
进行正压换气的呼吸管理法。它具有
对气管无刺激, 不需镇静药等优点, 但
是同时由于气管和食管不能分离, 存在
不易吸痰等难以管理的缺点。不过对
患者损伤小〕

Nire Nipple Retraction 乳头内陷

Niri Ninth Rib 第九肋

Nis Neck Is Supple 颈部柔软

Nisws Night Sweats 盗 汗

Nitm Nicked In The Midline 中线缺口

NHR 423 Nit

Nitr Nit Rate 硝酸盐; 硝酸酯

Nitrs Nitrates 硝酸盐

NIVA North Of Ireland Veterinary Association 北爱尔兰兽医学会

NIVF Natural Cycle In Vitro Fer Tilization 自然循环体外授精

NK Natural Killer 天然杀伤性细胞【注释】〔作为免疫疗法, 主要通过药物
投与来促进癌患者的细胞性免疫, 无抗
原特异性地杀伤肿瘤细胞〕

NKA No Known Allergies 不 明变态反
应; 无已知过敏史

NK-CELL Natural Killer Cell 天 然杀伤
细胞; NK 细胞

NKDA No Known Drug Allergies 无 已
知药物过敏史

Nkex Neck Examination 颈部检查

Nkh No Known History 无已知病史

Nkl Necklace 项圈; 动物颈部花纹

Nkma Neck Mass 颈部肿块

Nkpa Neck Pain 颈痛

Nkst Neck Stiffness 颈强直

NKT Natural Killer T (Cell) NKT 细胞【注释】
〔以前, 对于淋巴细胞系只知道
所谓的 B 细胞、T 细胞和 NK 细胞等。
最近发现了存在于胎儿组织中的完全
不同类型的淋巴细胞。认为此淋巴细
胞对免疫系统进行自我调节〕

Nkves Neck Veins 颈静脉

NL Normolipemic 正常脂血(症)

NLA Neuroleptanalgesia 安 定镇痛【注释】 〔通过
强效镇痛药和镇静药, 使
患者保持清醒意识, 医师边和患者沟通
边进行手术〕

NLA Neuroleptanesthesia 安 定镇痛麻
醉【注释】 〔在用安定镇痛法(NLA) 的同时
并用氧和一氧化二氮(笑气) , 使患者处
于丧失意识的状态〕

NLA Normal Lactase Activity 正 常乳糖
酶活性

Nlb Needle-Localization Biopsy 针 刺定
位活组织检查

NLD Necrobiosis Lipoidica Diabeticorum
〔拉〕糖尿病脂性渐进性坏死

NLDL Normal Low Density Lipoprotein
正常低密度脂蛋白

NLE Neonatal Lupus Erythematosus 新

生儿红斑狼疮

Nlf Nasolabial Fold 鼻 唇皱襞

NLI Natural Language Interface 自 然语言接口

NLL Nodular Lepromatous Leprosy 结节性瘤型麻风

NLMC Nocturnal Leg Muscle Cramp 夜间腿肌痉挛

Nlmno No Lymphadenopathy 无 淋巴结病

NLP No Light Perception 无光感

NLPA National Livestock Producers Association (USA) 全 国家畜生产者协会 〔美〕

NLT Normal Lymphocyte Transfer Test 正常淋巴细胞转化试验

NM Neomycin 新 霉素

NM Neuromuscular 神经肌肉的

NM Nit Rogen Mustard 氮芥

NM Nodular Melanoma 结 节性黑色素瘤

NM Nonmalignant 非 恶性的

NM Not Measurable 不 能测定的(不能检查的)

NM Nuclear Medicine 核医学【注释】 〔为利用各种同位素进行诊断和
治疗的医学〕

NMA National Meat Association 全国肉类联盟

NMA Neurogenic Muscular Atrophy 神

经源性肌萎缩

神经肌肉

接点

NMR Neonatal Mortality Rate 新 生儿
死亡率

NMR Nuclear Magnetic Resonance 核
磁共振(测定法) 【注释】 〔是一种与电子自转共
振同时的
磁场共振。氢、氮、磷和碳等具有核磁
力的原子和具有核自转的原子核置于
外部的磁场时, 从其相互作用的电磁波
变化中, 观测到核磁共振吸收和其光
谱。于是在医学上, 通过利用获得的其
吸收带的强度、位置、幅度等情报, 应用
于疾病的诊断〕

NMRI Nuclear Magnetic Resonance
Imaging 核磁共振成像; 核磁共振显影

NMS Neonatal Maladjustment Syndrome
新生畜调节不良综合征

NMS Neuroleptic Malignant Syndrome
神经安定剂诱发的恶性综合征

NMSD Neuro Muscular Spindle 神 经肌
梭

NMT Neuro Muscular Transmission 神
经肌肉传递

NMT Neuro Myo Tonia 神经性肌强直

NMU Neuromuscular Unit 神 经肌肉单
位【注释】 〔肌肉收缩的功能单位, 为一个
运动神经元和其所支配的肌纤维群〕

NMV Nasal Mask Ventilation 鼻 罩人工

呼吸法【注释】〔是一种不同于气管内插管法的人工呼吸补助管理法〕

NMVMA New Mexico Veterinary Medical Association 新 墨西哥州兽医医学学会

NMWA New Mexico Wildlife Association 新 墨西哥州野生动植物协会

NN Necrobiotic Nodules 渐 进性坏死结节

NN Neural Network 神 经网络

NNE Neonatal Necrotizing Enterocolitis 新生儿坏死性小肠结肠炎

NNM Nanaomycin 七 尾霉素

NNM Neonatal Mortality 初 生(仔) 畜死亡(率)

NNP Neonatal Nurse Practitioner 新 生儿护士开业者

NO Nasal Obstruction 鼻 塞; 鼻闭

NO Nitric Oxide 一 氧化氮; 氧化亚氮; 笑气【注释】〔它一直被认为是环境污染物, 容易与血红蛋白结合, 近年来由于对其血管扩张作用的各种药理作用备受关注, 有些学者探讨将该物质在病理性收缩状态的肺血管扩张和一般微循环系的血流改善中应用〕

Noad No Adenopathy 无 淋巴腺增大

NOAH AVMA Network Of Animal NMD 425 NOA Health 美国兽医协会动物保健网

NOAH National Office Of Animal Health 国家动物保健办公室

Noals No Allergies 无 过敏

Noar No Ar Thritis 无 关节炎

Noas No Asterixis 无扑翼样震颤

NOBAS No-Numbered BASIC For Advanced
St Ructures 无 编号高级结构的
BASIC

Nobl Nosebleed 鼻 出血; 衄血

Nobls Nosebleeds 鼻 出血(鼻衄)

NOCAD Non-Obst Ructive Coronary Artery
Disease 非阻塞性冠状动脉病

Nocoms No Complications 无 并发症

Noct . Nocturia 夜尿症

Nodgc Nondiagnostic 非 诊断性的

Nodi Nondistended 无扩张的

Nodis Nondisplaced 无位移的

Nodl Nodular 小结的; 结的; 小结状的

Nodr Nondrinker 非 饮酒者

Nodus Nodules 瘤状体

Noed No Edema 无水肿

Noer No Erythema 无 红斑

Noev No Evidence 无 迹象

NOF Neck Of Femur 股骨颈

Nofe(S) No Fever(S) 无发热

Nofo Nonfocal 非病灶的

NOHL Non-Organic Hearing Loss 非 器
质性耳聋

Nohsm No Hepatosplenomegaly 无 肝脾
肿大

Noin Noninvasive 非扩散的; 非侵害的

Nomen No Meningismus 无 假性脑脊膜

炎

NOMI Nonocclusive Mesenteric Infarction
非阻塞性肠系膜梗塞

NON-REM Nonrapid Eye Movement
非快眼动相; 无迅速眼球运动(睡眼)

Nonsegs . Nonsegmented (Neut Rophils) 未
分叶的(中性粒细胞)

NONSTOP Permit For T Ransit Of Contaminated
Area 允 许通过污染地区

NOPC Neutral Organophosphorus Compounds
中 性有机磷化合物

Nopn Nosocomial Pneumonia 院 内获得
性肺炎

Nopr Nonproductive 非 生产的; 非生产
性; 非生产性的; 非生产性支出

Nora No Rash 无 皮疹

Nore Nonreactive 非电抗性的

Noseq No Sequelae 无后遗症

Nosm Nonsmoker 不 抽烟的人

Nost No Stone 无 结石

Noste Nonsteroidal 非类固醇性

Nostes Nonsteroidals 非类固醇性药物

Notc Notch 切 口

Noten No Tenderness 无 压痛

Nothr No Thrush 无鹅口疮

Nothy No Thyromegaly 无甲状腺肿大

Notu Nocturia 夜尿

Novi No Vitreous 无 玻璃体的

NP Nafenopin 降脂素

NP Nasopharyngeal 鼻 咽的

Np Nasopharynx 鼻咽

NP Neuropsychiatric / Neuropsychiatrique 神经精神病学的

NP Neutropenia 中性粒细胞减少症

NP Nifedipine 硝苯吡啶; 心痛定

NP Nit Rophenide 双 (间硝基苯) 二硫; 硝基苯基金属

NP Nit Roprusside 硝普盐

NP Nodal Point 结点【注释】 〔一般地说, 从垂直经过透镜中
心面的主轴上某一点发出的点, 或者从
此点进入的光, 通过透镜系统后, 存在
有和主轴其他定点完全相同方向而去
的两个定点, 称为结点〕

NP Nosocomial Pneumonia 医院性肺炎 〔在医院感染的肺炎〕

NP Not Perceptible 未 察觉到的

NOA 426 NP

NP Nucleoprotein 核蛋白【注释】 〔为核酸和蛋白质的复合体, 其
蛋白质部分已知的有盐基性蛋白(组蛋
白、精蛋白) 和酸性蛋白〕

NP Nucleoside Phosphorylase 核 苷磷酸化酶

NPA Near Point Of Accommodation 调节近点

NPAF Nasopharyngeal Angiofibroma 鼻咽血管纤维瘤

NPC Nasopharyngeal Carcinoma 鼻 咽癌

NPC Near Point Of Convergence 集合近

点; 会聚的近点

NPC Nodal Premature Contraction 结节性期前收缩

NPD Narcissistic Personality Disorder 自恋性人格障碍

NPD Niemann-Pick(□s) Disease 尼曼皮克病〔神经鞘磷脂沉积病〕

NPD No Pathologic Diagnosis 无病理诊断

NPDL Nodular , Poorly Differentiated Lymphocytes 结节性低分化淋巴细胞

NPDLL Nodulaar , Poorly Differentiated Lymphocytic (Lymphoma) 结节性低分化淋巴细胞性(淋巴瘤)

NPDR Non-Proliferataive Diabetic Retinopathy 非增生性糖尿病性视网膜病变

NPE Neurogenic Pulmonary Edema 神经原性肺水肿【注释】〔在肺水肿中, 由于血管神经性原因引发的疾病, 非常罕见〕

NPH Neut Ral Protamine Hagedorn (Insulin) 中性鱼精蛋白锌(胰岛素) ; 中效低精蛋白(胰岛素)〔用于糖尿病治疗〕

NPH Normal Pressure Hydrocephalus 常压性脑积水【注释】〔它与脑脊液回流障碍有关, 常见于老年初期。出现行走障碍、痴呆、尿失禁、脑室系扩张, 由于是正常脑脊液压, 所以, 可通过短路术加以缓解〕

NPHI Neut Ral Protamine Hagedorn Insulin 中性鱼精蛋白哈格多恩氏胰岛素

Nphi NPH Insulin 中性鱼精蛋白锌胰岛
素

Nphy Normal-Pressure Hydrocephalus
正常压力性脑水肿

NPIA National Pet Insurance Association
国家宠物保险协会

NPK Non Protein Kilocalorie 非蛋白大
卡

NPL Noise Pollution Level 噪声污染级

NPLC National Pedigreed Livestock
Council (USA) 全国纯种家畜委员会
〔美国〕

NPMA Neural Progressive Muscle At Rophy
神经性进行性肌萎缩

Npmi Normal Point Of Maximal Impulse
正常最大搏动点

NPN Non-Protein Nit Rogen 非蛋白氮【注释】〔除
血清蛋白以外, 存在于血液
中的尿素、尿酸、肌酸、肌酸苷、氨等氮
化合物的总称。在胃功能不全时含量
增高〕

NPPC National Pork Producers Council
(USA) 国家猪肉生产者委员会

NPPNG Nonpenicillinase-Producing Neisseria
Gonorrheae 不产生育霉素酶的淋
病奈瑟氏菌

NPR Net Protein Ratio 蛋白质净比值

NPR Noise Power Ratio 噪声功率比

N-Pros Nervous Prost Ration 神经衰弱;
神经性虚脱

NPT Nocturnal Penile Tumescence 夜间

阴茎勃起

NPU National Pharmaceutical Union
全国药学联合会; 全国制药联合会

NPU Net Protein Utilization 蛋白质净
利用; 净蛋白质利用

NPW National Pet Week 国家宠物周

NP 427 NPW

NPY Neuropeptide Y 神经肽 Y 【注释】 〔为一种
存在于肠壁神经丛内的
肽神经元, 与黏膜内反射和蠕动反射有
关〕

NQA Nursing Quality Assurance 护理质
量保险

NR Neut Ral Red 中性红

NR Nonreactive 非电抗性的

NRA National Registration Authority
For Agricultural & Veterinary Chemicals
(Australia) 全国农业和兽医化学
注册当局 〔澳大利亚〕

NRAAC National Reptile And Amphibian
Advisory Council (USA) 全国爬
行类和两栖类动物

Nrax Normal Axis 垂直轴

Nrb Non Rebreathe 非重复呼吸

NRBC Normal Red Blood Cell 正常红细
胞

Nrbc Nucleated Red Blood Cells 有核红
细胞

NRC National Research Council (USA)
国家研究中心 〔美国〕

NRC Normal Retinal Correspondence 视

网膜正常对应

Nrch Normochromic 色 正常的; 血色素
含量正常的

NRCR Nonrenal Clearance Rate 非 肾清
除率

Nrcy Normocytic 正常红细胞的

NREM Non Rapid Eye Movement Sleep
非快速眼动睡眠【注释】〔又称徐波睡眠, 眼球无
快速活
动的深度睡眠状态, 脑波呈平缓波形〕

NREM Nonrapid Eye Movements 非 快
速眼球运动; 非快速眼动期

NRF Neutrophil Releasing Factor 中 性
白细胞释放因子

NRFC Nonrosette-Forming Cell 玫 瑰花
环形成细胞

NRFM Non Rebreathing Face Mask 非
再呼吸面罩

NRG Normal Rabbit Globulin 正 常兔球
蛋白

NRGC Nucleus Reticularis Gigantocellularis
〔拉〕网状巨核细胞

NRI Nuclear Resonance Imaging 核共振
成像

NRI Nut Ritional Risk Index 营 养学上的
手术危险指数

NRIC National Rehabilitation Information
Center 全 国康复情报中心

NRM Non Rebreathing Mask 非 再呼吸
面罩

NRM Nucleus Raphe Magnus 大缝际核

NROM(Nrom) Normal Range Of Motion
正常运动范围

NRPB National Radiological Protection
Board 国家放射性保护委员会

NRR Net Reproductive Rate 净生殖率;
净再生产率

NRR Noise Reduction Rating 噪音减弱
等级; 低噪声级

NRS Nonimmunized Rabbit Serum 非免
疫兔血清

NRS Normal Rabbit Serum 正常兔血清

NRT Neutron Radiation Therapy 中子辐
射治疗; 中子放射治疗

Nrtv Normotensive ① 血压正常的② 血
压正常者

Nrves Normal Vessels 正常血管

Nrvol Normovolemic 血量正常的

NS Nephritic Syndrome 肾病综合征

NS Nervous System 神经系统

NS Neurosurgery 神经外科学

NS Nonsmoker 不抽烟的人

NS Normal Saline 生理盐水

NS Nuclear Sclerosis 核硬化

Nsa No Spider Angiomata 无蜘蛛血管瘤

NSAID Non-Steroidal Anti-Inflammatory
Drug 非类固醇性抗炎药物; 非甾体抗

NPY 428 NSA
炎药

Nsaids Nonsteroidal Anti- Inflammatory
Drugs 非类固醇性抗炎药物

NSAVA Norwegian Small Animal

Veterinary Association 挪威小动物兽医学会

NSC-64826 Azetepa 氮替派; 阿替派〔抗肿瘤药〕

NSC-119875 Cisplatin 顺氯氨铂; 氯氨铂〔抗肿瘤药〕

NSC-145688 Cyclocytidine 环胞苷〔抗肿瘤药〕

NSC-82151 Daunomycin (Daunorubicin) 柔红霉素; 红比霉素〔抗肿瘤药〕

NSC-7365 6-Diazo-5-Oxo-L-Norleucine 重氮氧代正亮氨酸

NSC-80439 Etoglucid 环氧甘醚; 乙环氧啶〔抗肿瘤药〕

NSC-3364 Filipin 菲里平〔抗真菌抗生素〕

NSC-148958 Ftorafur 呋氟尿嘧啶〔抗肿瘤药〕

NSC-1895 Guanazole 胍唑; 二氨二唑〔抗肿瘤药〕

NSC-13875 Haxamethylmelamine 六甲蜜氨〔抗肿瘤药〕

NSC-11905 Lapachol 拉伯醇; 拉伯醌〔抗疟药, 抗肿瘤药〕

NSC Nonspecific Suppressor Cell 非特异性抑制细胞

NSC-135758 Piperazinedione 哌嗪双酮〔抗肿瘤药〕

Nscc Non-Small-Cell Carcinoma 非小细胞癌

Nsche Nonspecific Cholinesterase 非 特
异性的胆碱脂酶

NSD Nominal Standard Dose 统 一标准
线量【注释】〔为获得同一放射线照射效果的
统一线量单位〕

NSD Normal Spontaneous Delivery 正 常
自然分娩

NSD Normal Standard Dose 标 准剂量
(射线)

NSE Neuron Specific Enolase 神 经元特
异性烯醇化酶【注释】〔一种肠肿瘤标记〕

NSF National Science Foundation
(USA) 国家科学基金会

NSFNET National Science Foundation
Network 国 家科学基金网

NSFNET National Security Foundation
Network 国 家安全基金会网络

NSFTD Normal Spontaneous Full Term
Delivery 正常自然足月分娩

NSH Nasal Septal Hematoma 鼻 中隔血
肿

NSH National Society For Histotechnology
(USA) 国 家组织学技术学会

NSHA National Swedish Herpetological
Association 瑞典国家爬虫类学会

NSHD Nodular Sclerosing Hodgkin□s Disease
结 节硬化性何杰金氏病

Nshs No Splinter Hemorrhages 无 裂片
形出血

NSILA Non-Suppressible Insulin Like Activity
非抑制性胰岛素样活性; 不可抑

制的类胰岛素活性

NSLF Normal Sheep Lung Fibroblast 正常绵羊肺成纤维细胞

NS(N/ S) Normal Saline (I .E . 0 .9% Nacl) 生理盐水

NSPCA National Council Of Societies For The Prevention Of Cruelty To Animals (Republic Of South Africa) 全国预防残忍对待动物委员会〔南非〕

NSR Normal Sinus Rhythm 正常窦性节律

NSS Normal Saline Solution 生理盐水溶液

NSS Nut Ritional Support Service 营养支

NSA 429 NSS

持设施

NST Non-Stress Test 无应激试验; 非应激试验【注释】〔在分娩开始前, 诊断高度危险妊娠的滞留性胎儿假死的方法。为一种胎儿心搏系统〕

Nsto Normal Sphincter Tone 正常括约肌张力

NSU Nonspecific Urethritis 非特异性尿道炎【注释】〔除淋菌等特殊感染外, 通过某种病原体感染引起的感染性尿道炎, 一般用此诊断名。近来将其与非淋菌性尿道炎一同看待〕

NSV Nonspecific Vaginitis 非特异性阴道炎

NSVD Normal, Spontaneous Vaginal Delivery 正常阴道自然分娩

NSVT Nonsustained Ventricular Tachycardia
非持续性室性心动过速

N & T Nose And Throat 鼻 和喉

NT Naso- Tracheal 鼻 气管的

NT Neut Ralization Test 中 和试验

NT Non- Tender 无压痛

NTA Natural Thymocytotoxic Autoantibody
天 然性胸腺细胞毒性自身抗体【注释】〔为一种
小鼠的自身抗体。在以
胸腺细胞为靶细胞的补体依赖性细胞
损伤性试验中被检出。由于其与 T 细
胞机能下降有关而备受关注〕

NTA Nephrotoxic Antibody 肾 毒抗体

NTC Neuroepithelioma Teratoides Ciliare
畸胎样神经上皮瘤

NTD Neural Tube Defect 神经管缺陷

NTF National Turkey Federation
(USA) 全 国火鸡联合会〔美国〕

NTG Nitroglycerin 硝 酸甘油〔血管扩张
药〕

NTG Nontoxic Goiter 非毒性甲状腺肿

NTL Netilmicin 小 诺米星

NTN Nephrotoxic Nephritis 肾 毒性肾
炎

NTP,N . T . P& (R) Normal Temperature
And Pressure 正 常体温和血压; 常
温常压

NTP,N . T . P& (R) Normal Temperature
And Pulse 正 常体温和脉搏

NTR Negative Therapeutic Reaction 阴
性治疗反应

NTR Neonatally Thymectomized Rats
新生期胸腺切除的大鼠

NTX Nephrotoxicity 肾毒性

NU-445 Gant Risin (Sulfisoxazole) 磺胺
异□唑

Nubl Neurogenic Bladder 神经原性膀胱
障碍

Nuc Nucleus 神经核〔解〕Nucle Us〔拉〕

Nuca Neurocardiogenic 神经心脏起源的

Nucon Neurological Consultation 神经科
会诊

Nucos Neurological Complaints 神经性
主述

NUD Non-Ulcer Dyspepsia 非溃疡性消
化不良

Nuex Neurological Examination 神经科
检查

Nufo Neural Foramen 神经孔

NUG Necrotizing Ulcerative Gingivitis
坏死性溃疡性牙龈炎

Nug Numbing 引起麻木的

Nuge Neurogenic 发生神经的; 神经原
(性) 的

Nugr Nulligravida 未孕妇

Nuin Nut Ritional Insufficiency 营养不足

Nul Neurological 神经学上的

Nule Neuroleptic 神经安定的

Nules Neuroleptics 神经安定剂

Nulic Neurological 神经病学的; 神经学
的; 神经系统的

Nulot Neurologist 神经病学家; 神经学家

NST 430 Nul

Nulps Nulliparous 未经产的

Nulpy Nulliparity 未经产

Nuly Neurologically 神经病学的

Nulys Neurolysis 神经松解术; 神经组织崩解; 神经疲惫

Numed Nuclear Medicine 核医学

Nune Numbness 麻木

Nuop Neuroophthalmology 神经眼科学

Nupa Neuropathy 神经障碍

Nuph Neut Rophil 嗜中性粒细胞

Nupr Neurapraxia 神经失用症〔外伤后功能性麻痹〕

Nupra Nurse Practitioner 护士开业者

Nups Neuropsychiatry 神经精神病学

Nupsc Neuropsychiat Ric 神经精神病学的

Nupst Neuropsychiatrist 神经精神病学家

Nusn(S) Neurosurgeon（S）神经外科医师

Nust Neurological Status 神经状态

Nusv Neurology Service 神经科

Nusy Neurosurgery 神经外科(学)

Nutcon Nut Rition Consultation 营养学会诊

Nuti Numbness And Tingling 麻木并刺痛

Nutr Nutrition 肠 道喂养

Nuva Neurovascular 神经血管的

Nuy Neurology 神经学; 神经病学

NV Naked Vision 裸 眼视力

N/ V Nausea And Vomiting 恶心和呕吐

N&V Nausea & Vomiting 恶心与呕吐

N/ V Nausea/ Vomiting 恶心/ 呕吐

NV Near Vision 近距视觉; 近视力

Nv Neurovascular 神经血管的

NVA Near Visual Acuity 近距视敏度
血管束

N/ V/ D Nausea / Vomiting / Diarrhea 恶
心、呕吐与腹泻

Japanese

N 好中球 Neutrophilic Leukocyte

所属リンパ節転移の程度 Regional Lymph Nodes

窒素 Nitrogen

NA 壊死性血管炎 Necrotizing Angiitis

ノルアドレナリン Noradrenaline

NAA 異常なし No Apparent Abnormalities

NAD 検査異常なし Nothing Abnormal Detected

特記すべき疾患なし No Appreciable Disease

NAD ノルアドレナリン Noradrenaline

NANB、NANAH 非 A 非 B 型肝炎 Non-A Non-B 肝炎 Hepatitis

NANDA 北米看護診断協会 North American Nursing Diagnosis Association

NAP 好中球アルカリフォスファターゼ Neutrophil Alkaline Phosphatase

神経活動電位 Nerve Action Potential

NB 神経芽腫 Neuroblastoma

新生児 Newbone

N-B 鼻・胆道チューブ Naso-Biliary（Tube）

NBAS 新生児行動評価 Newbone Behavioral Assessment Scale

NBM 経口摂取不可 Nothing By Mouth

NBN 新生児室 Newborn Nursery

NBTE 非細菌性血栓性心内膜炎　Non-Bacterial□
Thrombotic□Endocarditis　　□
NC　　訴えなし　　　No□Complaints　　　□
　□　　特記なし　　　Non-Contributory　　　□
　□　　不変　No□Change　□
NCC　無冠状動脈弁尖　　　Non□Coronary□Cusp
　　　□
NCCHD　　　非チアノーゼ性先天性心疾患
　　　　Non-Cyanotic□Congenital□Heart□Disease
　　　　□
NCE　非痙攣性てんかん　Nonconvulsive□
Epilepsy　　　□
N-CPAP　　　経鼻持続的陽圧呼吸　　　　Nasal□
Continuous□Positive□Ai R Way□Pressure　□
NCU　神経疾患集中治療室　　　　Neurologic□
（Intensive）□Care□Unit　　　□
　□　　新生児集中治療室　Neonatal□（Intensive）□
Care□Unit　　□
ND　　看護診断　　Nursing□Diagnosis　　□
　□　　神経性うつ病　　　Neurotic□Depression□
　□　　神経難聴　　Nerve□Deafness　　　□
NDI　腎性尿崩症　Nephrogenic□Diabetes□
Inspidus　□
NE　　ノルエピネフリン　Norepinephrine　　□
NF　　神経線維腫症　　　Neurofibromatosis　　□
NEC　壊死性腸炎　Necrotizing Enterocolitis　　□
NEEP 呼気終末陰圧　　　Negative□End-
Expiratory□Pressure　□
Neg　陰性の　　　Negative　　　□
Neutro 好中球　　Neutrophilic□Leukocyte　　□
NF　　中性脂肪　Neutral□Fat　□
NG　　腎造影法　Nephrography□

NGB　神経因性膀胱　　　Neurogenic□Bladder□

NHC　非ケトン高浸透圧性昏睡　Non-Ketotic□
Hyperosmolar□Coma　　　□

NHL　非ホジキンリンパ腫　　Non-Hodgkin's□
Lymphoma　　□

NHP　非ヘモグロビン蛋白　　Non-Hemoglobin□
Proteins　　　□

NICU　神経疾患集中管理室　　Neurologic□
Intensive□Care□Unit　　　□

□　　新生児集中治療室　Neonatal□Intensive□
Care□Unit　　□

NIDDM　　　インスリン非依存型糖尿病
　　　Non-Insulin-Dependent Diabetes Mellitus　□

NK　　NK(ナチュラルキラー)細胞　　　Natural
Killer(Cell)　□

NL　　正常範囲　　Normal Limits　　　□

NLA　ニューロレプト麻酔、神経遮断麻酔、神経
弛緩麻酔　Neuroleptanesthesia(Analgesia)　　□

NLD　糖尿病性脂肪類壊死症　　□　　　□

NLE　新生児エリテマトーデス　Neonaral Lupus
Erythematosus　　　□

NLP　失明、視力零　　No Light Perception□

NM　核医学　　Nuclear Medicine　　□

NMR　核磁気共鳴　Nuslear Magnetic Resonance□

NN　神経鞘腫　Neurinoma　　□

NO　笑気　Nitrous Oxide□

NP　鼻ポリープ　Nasal Polyp　□

NPC　鼻咽頭癌　Nasopharygeal Carcinoma　　□

NPH　NPHインスリン、中間型インスリン
　　　Neutral-Protamine-Hagedorn(Insulin)　　□

□　　正常圧水頭症　　Normal Pressure
Hydrocephalus　　　□

☐ 椎間板ヘルニア Nucleus Pulposus Herniation ☐

NR 正常範囲 Normal Range ☐

NS(S) 生理食塩水 Normal Saline(Solution) ☐

NSAID 非ステロイド系抗炎症剤 Non-Steroidal Anti-Inflammatory Drug ☐

NSD 経膣自然分娩 Normal Spontaneous Delivery ☐

NSR 正常洞調律 Normal Sinus Rhythm ☐

NST ノンストレステスト Non Stress Test ☐

☐ 栄養サポートチーム Nutrition Support Team ☐

NTG ニトログリセリン Nitroglycerin ☐

NTP 常温１気圧 Normal Temperature And Pressure ☐

N&V 悪心、嘔吐 Neusea And Vomiting ☐

Ny 眼振 Nystagmus

O

French

OAP

Oedème Aigu Pulmonaire

OMI

Oedème Des Membres Inférieurs

OMS
Organisation Mondiale De La Santé

English

OAD Obstructive Airway Disease; Organic Anionic Dye

OADC Oleate-Albumin-Dextrose-Catalase

OAE Otoacoustic Emission

OAF Off-Axis Factor; Off-Axis Ratio; Open-Air Factor; Osteoclast Activating Factor

OAFNS Oculo-Auriculofrontonasal Syndrome

OAG Open-Angle Glaucoma

OAH Ovarian Androgenic Hyperfunction

OAIS Outcomes And Information Set

OAISO Overaction Of The Ipsilateral Superior Oblique

OAK Kjer Optic Atrophy

OALF Organic Acid Labile Fluid

OALL Ossification Of Anterior Longitudinal Ligament

OAM Office Of Alternative Medicine; Outer Acrosomal Membrane

OAP Office Of Adolescent Pregnancy; Oldage Pension/Pensioner; Ophthalmic Artery Pressure; Osteoarthropathy; Oxygen At Atmospheric Pressure; Precocious Osteoarthrosis

OAPP Office Of Adolescent Pregnancy Programs

OAR Organ At Risk; Ottawa Ankle Rule

OARS Older Americans Research And Service; Older Americans Resources And Services; Optimal Atherectomy Restenosis Study

OAS Old-Age Security; Ongoing Abuse Screening; Oral Allergy Syndrome; Osmotically Active Substance

OASD Ocular Albinism, Sensorineural Deafness [Syndrome]

OASDHI Old Age, Survivors, Disability And Health Insurance

OASDI Old Age Survivors And Disability Insurance

OASI Old Age And Survivors Insurance

OASIS Older Adults Service And Information System; Organization To Assess Strategies For Ischemic Syndromes; Outcome And Assessment Information Set; Overweight And Seeking Infertility Support

OASP Organic Acid Soluble Phosphorus

Oastv Ovine Astrovirus

OAT O-Acetyltransferase; Ochanomizu Aspirin Trial; Oligoasthenoteratozoospermia; Open Artery Trial; Organic Anion Transporter; Ornithine Aminotransferase

OATL Ornithine Aminotransferase-Like

OATP1B1 Organic Anion-Transporting Polypeptide 1B1

OATR Organism Attribute

OAV Oculoauriculovertebral

OAVS Oculoauriculovertebral Syndrome

OAVD Oculoauriculovertebral Dysplasia

OAW Oral Airways

OB Obese [Mouse]; Obese, Obesity; Objective Benefit; Obliterative Bronchiolitis; Obstetrics,

O&A Observation And Assessment

OA1 Ocular Albinism Type 1

O2a Oxygen Availability

OAA Old Age Assistance; Older Americans Act; Opticians Association Of America; Oxaloacetic Acid

OAAD Ovarian Ascorbic Acid Depletion

OAAS Observer's Assessment Alertness/ Sedation Scale

OAAV Ovine Adeno-Associated Virus
Oadv Ovine Adenovirus
Oadv-A, B, C Ovine Adenoviruses A, B, C
OAB Old-Age Benefits; Overactive Bladder
OABP Organic Anion Binding Protein
OA/BVM Oral Airway/Bag-Valve-Mask
OAC Omeprazole, Amoxicillin, Clarithromycin
OACT Occupational Activity
O&A Observation And Assessment
OA1 Ocular Albinism Type 1
O2a Oxygen Availability
OAA Old Age Assistance; Older Americans
Act; Opticians Association Of America; Oxaloacetic
Acid
OAAD Ovarian Ascorbic Acid Depletion
OAAS Observer's Assessment Alertness/
Sedation Scale
OAAV Ovine Adeno-Associated Virus
Oadv Ovine Adenovirus
Oadv-A, B, C Ovine Adenoviruses A, B, C
OAB Old-Age Benefits; Overactive Bladder
OABP Organic Anion Binding Protein
OA/BVM Oral Airway/Bag-Valve-Mask
OAC Omeprazole, Amoxicillin, Clarithromycin
OACT Occupational Activity
O&B Opium And Belladonna
Ob Obese [Mouse]
OBA Office-Based Anesthesia; Office Of
Biotechnology
Activities
OBAD Optimal Biologically Active Dose
OBB Oriented Bounding Boxes; Own Bed
Bath
OBD Organic Brain Disease
OBCAM Opioid-Binding Cell Adhesion Molecule

OBE Office Of Biological Education

OBET Odor-Baited Entry Trap

OBF Organ Blood Flow

OBG, Obg Obstetrics And Gynecology, Obstetrician-Gynecologist

OBGS Obstetric And Gynecologic Surgery

OB-GYN, Ob-Gyn Obstetrics And Gynecology, Obstetrician-Gynecologist

Obj Objective

Obl Oblique

OBMT Omeprazole, Bismuth, Metronidazole, Tetracycline

OBOV Obodhiang Virus

OBP Odorant-Binding Protein; Ova, Blood, Parasites

OBR Obesity Gene Receptor

OBRA Omnibus Reconciliation Act

OBS Obesity; Obstetric Service; Office-Based Surgery; Organic Brain Syndrome

Obs Observation, Observed; Obstetrics, Obstetrician

Obs Obsolete

Obst Obstetrics, Obstetrician

Obst, Obstr Obstruction, Obstructed

OBT Optimized Background Therapy

OB-US Obstetric Ultrasound

OC Obstetric Conjugate; Occlusocervical; [O]Esophageal Candidiasis; Office Call; On Call; Only Child; Optical Colonoscopy; Optic Chiasma; Oral Contraceptive; Orbicularis Oculi; Order Communication; Organ Culture; Organochlorine; Original Claim; Orofacial Cleft; Outer Canthal [Distance]; Ovarian Cancer; Oxygen Consumed

O&C Onset And Course

O/C Ornithine/Citrulline Ratio

OCA Octylcyanoacrylate; Oculocutaneous Albinism;
Olivopontocerebellar Atrophy; Opticalclearing
Agent; Oral Contraceptive Agent
Oca Ovarian Carcinoma
OCA1A Oculocutaneous Albinism Type 1a
OCA1B Oculocutaneous Albinism Type 1b
OCA2 Oculocutaneous Albinism Type 2
OCA3 Oculocutaneous Albinism Type 3
OCA4 Oculocutaneous Albinism Type 4
OCAD Occlusive Carotid Artery Disease
O2cap Oxygen Capacity
OW Once Weekly; Open Wedge; Outcome
Washing; Outer Wall; Oval Window; Overweight
O/W, O/W Oil In Water
OWCL Old World Cutaneous Leishmaniasis
OWI Office Of Worksite Initiatives
OW/O Overweight And Obesity
O/W/O Oil In Water/Oil
OWR Osler-Weber-Rendu [Syndrome]; Ovarian
Wedge Resection
OWS Outerwear Syndrome
OX Optic Chiasma; Orthopedic Examination;
Oxacillin; Oxalate; Oxide; Oxytocin
Ox Oxygen
Ox Oxidized
OXA Oxaprotiline
OXCHECK Oxford And Collaborators
Health Check [Trial]
OXIPHOS Oxidative Phosphorylation
Oxldl, Ox-LDL Oxidized Low-Density Lipoprotein
OXMIS Oxford Myocardial Infarction Incidence
Study
Oxo Oxanosine
8oxoa 8-Oxoadenine
8oxog 8-Oxoguanine

OXP Oxypressin
OXPHOS Oxidative Phosphorylation
OXT Oxytocin
OXTR Oxytocin Receptor
OXY Oxytocin
OXY, Oxy Oxygen
OYE Old Yellow Enzyme
OYS Oslo Youth Study
Oz Ounce
Oz Ap, Oz Apoth Apothecary Ounce
OZD Optic Zone Diameter
Oz T, Oz Tr Troy Ounce
OU Observation Unit; Oppenheimer-Urbach
OU Observation Unit; Oppenheimer-Urbach
[Syndrome]
Ou Both Eyes Together [Lat. Oculi Unitas]
OUAV Ouango Virus
OUB Ouabain
OUBIV Oubi Virus
OUBR Ouabain Resistance
OULQ Outer Upper Left Quadrant
OUME Operative Unit Of Medical Herpetology
OUR Oxygen Uptake Rate
OURQ Outer Upper Right Quadrant
OURS Oxford University Research Study;
Oxygen Utilization Rate Study
OURV Ourem Virus
OUS Overuse Syndrome
OUTCLAS Outpatient Coronary Low-
Profile Angioplasty Study
OUTI Other Urinary Tract Infections
OV Oculovestibular; Office Visit; Oncovirus;
Osteoid Volume; Outflow Volume; Ovalbumin;
Ovary; Overventilation; Ovulation
Ov Ovary

Ov Ovum
OVA Ovalbumin
Ova Ovariectomy
OVAT Ongoing Violence Assessment Tool
OVC Ovarian Cancer
OVD Occlusal Vertical Dimension; Ophthalmic
Viscosurgical Device
Ovdf Ovarian Dysfunction
Ovhv Ovine Herpesvirus
OVLT Organum Vasculosum Of The Lamina
Terminalis
OVRV Oak-Vale Virus
OVSMC Ovine Vascular Smooth Muscle
Cell
OVX Ovariectomized

German

OA - Oberarm
O.B. - Ohne Befund
OGTT - Oraler Glukose-Toleranztest
OS - Oberschenkel
OSG - Oberes Sprunggelenk

Italian

O

ORL
Otorinolaringoiatria
OSS
) Operatore Socio-Sanitario
Per Os
Per Via Orale

Russian

OAF
Osteoclast Activating Factor
Фактор, Активирующий Остеокласты
OB
Obstetrics
Акушерство
OD
(1) Overdose
Передозировка
(2) Oculus Dextra (Latin)
Правый Глаз
OGTT
Oral Glucose Tolerance Test
Оральный Тест На Толерантность К Глюкозе
(ОТТГ)
17-OHCS
17-Hydroxycorticosteroid
17-Гидроксикортикостероид
OHSS
Ovarian Hyperstimulation Syndrome
Синдром Гиперстимуляции Яичников
Ophth
Ophthalmology
Офтальмология
OR
Operating Room
Операционная
Orth, Ortho
Orthopedics
Ортопедия
OS
Oculus Sinistra (Latin)

Левый Глаз
Osm
Osmolality
Осмоляльность
OT
Occupational Therapy
Вид Медицинской Помощи В США, Примерно
Соответствующий Физиотерапии Или
Реабилитационной Медицине. Сочетает
Физические Упражнения, Массаж, Кинезо- И
Психотерапию. Проводится Специальным
Персоналом (Не Врачами И Не Медсестрами).
OU
Each Eye
Каждый Глаз

Chinese

O Blood Group In ABO System O 型血
O Occipital 枕 骨的; 枕部的; 属于枕骨
的; 位于枕骨附近的
O Opium 鸦 片; 阿片
O Osteomyelitis 骨 髓炎
O Oxidant 氧化剂
O Oxytocinase 催产素酶; 缩宫素酶
O Respirations 呼 吸(麻醉记录)
OA Occipito- Anterior 前 端后头位【注释】 〔表示
胎位的产科用语〕
OA Optic At Rophy 视神经萎缩
OA Osteoarthritis , Degenerative Joint
Disease 骨关节炎; 退行性关节病
OAA Oxaloacetic Acid 草酰乙酸【注释】 〔三羧酸
循环中的一个中间产

物, 起着将糖代谢、氨基酸代谢、脂肪代谢与三羧酸循环联系在一起的作用。是天冬氨酸氨基转移酶的底物, 也是三羧酸循环的一个限速因子〕

Oac Osteoarthritic 骨 关节炎的

OAD Obstructive Airway Disease 呼 吸道阻塞疾病

OAD Occlusive Arterial Disease 闭 塞性动脉疾患

OAF Osteoclast Activating Factor 破 骨细胞激活因子

OAG Ocular Angiography 眼 血管造影术

OAG(Oag) Open Angle Glaucoma 开 角型青光眼

OAM The Office Of Alternative Medicine (NIH) 备选医学局 〔在 NIH(美国国立卫生研究所) 内 1992 年设立的一个局, 主要推进被现代医学忽视的民间疗法的开展〕

OA(Oa) Osteoar Thritis 变 形性关节炎【注释】〔又叫骨关节炎, 因关节的退行性变化而变形, 是一种主诉为运动障碍的慢性疼痛性关节炎〕

OAP Oncovin (Vincristine) , Ara-C (Cytarabine) , And Prednisone 长 春新碱、阿糖胞苷和强的松(化疗方案)

OAP Ophthalmic Ar Tery Pressure 眼 动脉压

OASPL Overall Sound Pressure Level 总 声压级

OAT Ornithine-Oxo-Acid Amino ACID T Ransferase 鸟氨酸-氧代酸-氨基酸转移酶

OAVT Ontario Association Of Veterinary Technicians 安大略兽医技师协会

OB Obstetrical 产科的

OB Occult Blood 潜血; 隐血

Obfo Obturator Fossa 闭孔肌凹

OB-GYN Obstetrics And Gynecology 妇产科学

Obhx Obstet Rical History 婚育史

Obja Obst Ructive Jaundice 阻塞性黄疸; 梗阻性黄疸

Obma Obtuse Marginal 钝边缘

OBN Octave Band Of Noise 噪声倍频带; 噪声青阶频带

Obne Obturator Nerve 闭孔神经〔解〕

Ne Rvus Obturatorius 〔拉〕

Obpa Obstipation 顽固性便秘

OBRA Oregon Biomedical Research Association 俄勒冈州生物医学研究协会

OBS Organic Brain Syndrome 器质性脑综合征

Obst . Obstipation 顽固性便秘

Obst Obst Ruct , Obst Ruction 梗阻; 阻塞

Obsy Organic Brain Syndrome 器质性脑综合征

OBT Occult Blood Test 隐血试验; 潜血试验

Obtur Obturator 阻塞器

Obturs Obturators 闭孔肌

Obva Observation 观测(值)

Oby Obesity 肥胖症

OC Optic Chiasm 视交叉

OC Oral Cavity 口腔

OC Oral Cholecystography 口服胆囊造
影术

OC Oral Contraceptive(S) 口服避孕药

OC Osteocalcin 骨钙素【注释】〔含有骨Γ羧基
谷氨酸的蛋白质

(BGP)〕

OC Ovarian Cancer 卵巢癌

OC Oxytocin 催产素

OC[A] Oral Cont Raceptive Agent 口服
避孕剂

O2 Cap . Oxygen Capacity 氧容量

OCAR Occlusion Of The Cent Ral Ar Tery Of
The Retina 视网膜中央动脉闭塞

Ocbl Occult Blood 潜血; 隐血

OCC Oat Cell Carcinoma 燕麦形细胞癌

Occi Occiput 枕 (鸟) (动)

Occil Occipital 枕骨的; 枕部的; 属于枕
骨的; 位于枕骨附近的

Occlug Occluding 咬合架

OCCPR Open-Chest CPR 开胸心肺复
苏

OCD Osteochondritis Dissecans 剥脱性
骨软骨炎

OCD Obsessive Compulsive Disorder 强

制性障碍【注释】〔指有强迫意念或强迫行为的症状〕

Ocd Obsessive-Compulsive Disorder 强迫观念与行为疾病

OCD Osteochondritis Dissecans 〔拉〕剥脱性骨软骨炎; 分离性骨软骨炎【注释】〔又称解离性骨软骨炎, 关节软骨下海绵骨的一部分坏死, 产生关节游离体(关节鼠) , 引起疼痛和功能障碍〕

Ocdr Occlusive Dressing 包扎疗法

OCG Oral Cholecystography 口服胆囊造影(术)

OCP Oral Cont Raceptive Pill 口服避孕药丸

Ocpar Occipitoparietal 枕顶的

OCPD Occult Constrictive Pericardial Disease 隐性狭窄性心包疾病

Ocpo Occipitoposterior 枕后位

OCR Oculocephalic Reflex 眼脑反射

OCR Oxygen Consumption Rate 耗氧率; 氧气消耗率

OCRS Oculo-Cerebro-Renal Syndrome 眼、脑、肾综合征(又称眼、脑、肾发育不良综合征, Lowe-Blckl 二氏综合征)

OCS Obstetric Crush Syndrome 产科挤压综合征; Young- Paxson 综合征

OCS Oculocraniosomatic (Dyst Rophy) 眼脑体〔营养障碍〕

OCS Oral Cont Raceptive Steroid 口服类

固醇避孕药

OCS Ovine Chorionic Somatomammot
Ropin 羊绒毛膜生长催乳激素

OCT Oxytocin Challenge Test 催产素负
荷试验【注释】〔一种在无子宫收缩时投与催产
素, 观察胎儿心跳的试验〕

OCT Oxytocin Contraction Test 催产素
收缩试验

OCTD Ornithine Carbamoylt Ransferase
Deficiency 鸟氨酸氨基甲酰转移酶缺乏
症

Octr Occipitot Ransverse 枕横的

OBS 434 Oct

OCVE La Organización Colegial Veterinaria
Espanola (Spanish Veterinary Association
) 西班牙兽医学会

OD Occupational Dermatitis 职业皮肤
炎

OD Occupational Disease 职业病

OD Oculus Dexter 右眼

O .D . Oculus Dexter 右眼

OD Optical Density 光密度; 吸光度

OD Or Thostatic Dysregulation (Disturbance
) (Disfunction) 站立性共济失调【注释】 〔为自律
神经失调症, 有头晕、不
能久立、易心悸心焦、午前不适等症状〕

OD Oxygen Demand 需氧量

ODA Oklahoma Department Of Agriculture
俄克拉何马州农业部

ODBMS Open Database Management
System 开放式数据库管理系统

ODC Oxygen Dissociation Curve 氧 解离
曲线【注释】〔表示氧分压与血红蛋白氧饱和
度相互关系的曲线, 呈 S 型〕

ODE Old-Dog Encephalitis 老年狗脑炎

ODG Opthalmodynamography 眼 底血
压检查法【注释】〔利用一种可与上臂血压同时
测
定的眼底血压计, 从两眼睑上面用气囊
同时压迫眼球, 通过分析产生的脉冲波
动来测出眼底血压的方法。比上臂血
压低 5～10mmhg , 比较左右两侧的眼
底血压, 可分析有无颈内动脉闭塞症〕

ODN Ophthalmodynamometry 视 网膜
血管血压测定法

OD(O .D .) Outside Diameter 外径

ODS Octadecyl Silane 十八(烷) 基硅烷

ODS Open Distal System 开 放的末梢系
统

ODSG Ophthalmic Doppler Sonogram
眼多普勒超声图

ODT Occipitodextra T Ransversa 第 2 头
位【注释】〔产科学中表示胎位的用语〕

ODT Occulusive Dressing Technique 密
封疗法【注释】〔在皮肤病病灶处涂抹甾体激素
等软膏, 然后用塑料薄膜覆盖, 使之完
全密封, 以促进药物浸透〕

Odt On Direct Testing 直 接检验时

Ody Odynophagia 吞 咽痛

OE Otitis Externa 外 耳炎

OEP Original Endotoxin Protein 菌体内

毒蛋白〔菌体内毒素蛋白〕

OER Osmotic Erythrocyte 红细胞渗透(压)

OER Oxygen Enhancement Ratio 氧增强比(率)【注释】〔将放疗时的氧增强效果, 用低氧状态下的必需放射剂量与生理氧状态下的必需放射剂量之比来表示, 比值为 2～3〕

OF Occipitofrontal 枕骨和前额的

OF Osteitis Fibrosa 纤维性骨炎

OFA Oncofetal Antigen 癌胚抗原

OFA Orthopedic Foundation For Animals 动物矫形基金会

OFD Occipitofrontal Diameter 枕额径

OFD Oral-Facial-Digital (Syndrome) 口面指(综合征)

O-FHA (OF-HA) Occipitofrontal Headache 枕额部头痛

OFI Ocular Fixation Index 注视抑制指数

OFLX Ofloxacin 氧氟沙星

OG Osmolality Gap 克分子渗透压浓度差【注释】〔脏器功能不全时的异常代谢所产生的蓄积, 肝功能不好时可导致此差值增大〕

Ogh Ob/ Gyn History 妇产科病史

OGTT Oral Glucose Tolerance Test 口服萄萄糖耐量试验【注释】〔口服一定量的葡萄糖, 测定血

OCV 435 OGT

糖高低和持续时间。将 50 克或 100 克
(WHO 建议 75 克) 葡萄糖溶于水中饮
下, 在 180 分钟里检测血糖和尿糖〕

OH Obstructive Hypopnea 阻 塞性呼吸
不足

OH Occupational Health 职业保健

OHA Oral Hypoglycemic Agent 口 服降
糖药

O-Hb Oxyhemoglobin 氧合血红蛋白

OHCS Hydroxycorticosteroids 羟 皮质
类固醇; 羟皮质甾醇

17-OHCS 17-Hydroxycosteroids 17- 羟
基皮质类固醇【注释】〔大部分来自肾上腺皮质
的糖皮

质激素。这些甾醇激素在体内转化成
各种代谢产物, 多数以结合型、而少数
则以游离型从尿中排出。它可作为检
查肾上腺皮质功能的重要指标〕

OHD Organic Heart Disease 器 质性心脏
病

17α-OHP 17α- Hydroxyprogesterone
17α- 羟基孕酮

OHP Oxygen Under High Pressure 高 压
氧疗法【注释】〔在高压氧舱(2～ 3 个气压) 内吸
入氧气, 以提高溶解氧浓度〕

OHPP Occluded Hepatic Portal Pressure
阻断性肝门静脉压

17 OH Preg 17 Hydroxy Pregnenolone
羟 基孕烯醇酮

17-OHS 17-Hydroxysteroid (17-Hydroxycor

Ticosteroid) 羟 皮质类固醇

OHSS Ovarian Hyperstimulation Syndrome
卵巢过度刺激综合征

OHT Ocular Hyper Tension 高眼压症

OI Oppor Tunistic Infection 机遇性感染;
机会性感染【注释】〔指原本致病力弱的低致病
性微
生物所导致的感染。其感染是由于宿
主体虚弱、免疫抑制和滥用抗生素导致
共生菌群失调等。近年有增加趋势〕

OI Opsonic Index 调理素指数

OI Osteogenesis Imperfecta 成 骨不全

OI Oxygenation Index 氧合指数

OI Oxytocin Induction 催 产素引产

OI Oxygenation Index 氧化指数
俄亥俄切斯特改良白猪

OID Ovine Interdigital Dermatitis 绵羊
趾间皮炎

O-Ig Ophthalmopathic Ig 眼 病性免疫
球蛋白

OIH Ovulation Inducing Hormone 排卵
诱导激素【注释】〔通过 FSH 和 LH 的刺激,成熟
卵泡从卵巢中排出。HMG 和 HCG 作
为强效促排卵激素而被使用〕

OKAN Optokinetic After-Nystagmus 视
动性后遗眼球震颤; 眼运动性继发性眼球
震颤

OKN Optokinetic Nystagmus 视 动性眼
球震颤【注释】〔指从运动的车窗向外观望,盯
住一个目标注视追踪时所发生的眼球

震颤〕

OKP Optokinetic Pattern 视 动性眼震
方式【注释】〔一种注视旋转圆筒内的黑线使
眼球震颤的检查, 为节省记录时间, 将
其缩写为 OKP〕

OKT Ornithine Ketoacid Transaminase
鸟氨酸酮酸转氨酶

OL Oleandomycin 夹竹桃霉素

OLD Obstructive Lung Disease 阻 塞性
肺病

Olhy Oligohydramnios 羊水过少

Olin Old Incision 旧 切口

Olme Oligomenorrhea 月 经稀发

OM Occipitomental 枕 骨和颏部的

OM Osteomalacia 骨 质软化; 软骨病

OH 436 OM

OM Osteomyelitis 骨髓炎

OM Otitis Media 中 耳炎

OMAC Otitis Media Acute Catarrhal 急
性卡他性中耳炎

OMAD Oncovin (Vincristine) ,
Methotrexate (And Citrovorum Factor) ,
Adriamycin (Doxorubicin) , And Dactinomycin
(Actinomycin D) 长 春新碱、
氨甲喋呤、阿霉素和放线菌素 D(化疗方
案)

Omads Omental Adhesions 大网膜粘连

OMCC Otitis Media, Catarrhal , Chronic
慢性卡他性中耳炎

OMD Ocular Muscle Dyst Rophy 眼 肌营
养不良; 眼肌萎缩

Omd Organic Mood Disorder 器质性情
感障碍

OMI Old Myocardial Infarction 陈旧性
心肌梗死

Oml Omental 网膜的

OMPA Otitis Media Purulenta Acute 急
性化脓性中耳炎

OMPC Otitis Media Purulenta Chronica
慢性化脓性中耳炎

OMSA Otitis Media, Suppurative , Acute
急性化脓性中耳炎

OMSC Otitis Media, Secretory (Or Suppurative)
Chronic 慢性分泌性中耳炎

OMSCO Organic Milk Suppliers Cooperative
组织牛奶供应者合作团体

Omte Omentectomy 网膜切除术

OMV Ordem Dos Médicos Veterinários
(Por Tugese Veterinary Association)
葡萄牙兽医学会

OMV Oronasal Mask Ventilation 口鼻
面罩人工呼吸法【注释】〔不用插管而是使用覆
盖口鼻的
面罩的非侵入性辅助性呼吸方法〕

ON Optic Nerve 视神经

ON Optic Neuritis 视神经炎

ON Osteonecrosis 骨坏死

Oncy Oncology 肿瘤学

Oncyt Oncologist 肿瘤学家

Onlys Onycholysis 爪脱离; 爪松离

Onmy Onychomycosis 爪癣

ONTG Oral Nit Roglycerin 口服硝酸甘油

Onymy Onychomycosis 爪癣

OOP Out Of Plaster 去 石膏

OP Optical Probe 光学探头

Op Oral Pharynx 口咽

Opfis Operative Findings 手术所见

OPH Obliterative Pulmonary Hyper Tension 闭塞性动脉高压

Oph Ophthalmology 眼 科学

Ophc Ophthalmic 眼的

OM 437 Oph

Ophgc Ophthalmologic 眼科学的

Ophma Ophthalmic Manner 用 眼习惯

Ophpr Ophthalmic Procedure 眼 科操作 过程

Ophsu Ophthalmic Surgery 眼 科手术学

Opht Ophthalmologist 眼科学家

Ophth Ophthalmology 眼 科学

Opin Opportunistic Infection 机 会性感 染

Opins Oppor Tunistic Infections 条 件感 染

Opiv Operative Intervention 手术干预

Opla Operative Laparoscopy 手术腹腔镜 检

OPLL Ossication Of Posterior Longitudinal Ligament 后 纵韧带骨化【注释】〔脊柱后纵韧带 的病理性肥厚、 骨化,伤及神经根时则表现出相应的神 经症状,颈椎部位的发病率高,病程为 慢性渐进性〕

Opmi Operating Microscope 手 术显微镜

Opms Oral Pain Medications 口 服镇痛
药

Opne Optic Nerve 视 神经〔动〕

Opre Open Reduction 切 开复位(术)

OPRT Orotate Phosphoribosyl Transferase
乳 清酸磷酸核糖(基) 转移酶; 乳
清酸转磷酸核糖(基) 酶

OPS Adipositas- (Hyper Thermia) Oligomenorrhea
Parotitis Syndrome AOP 综
合征, 即指肥胖; 月经过少; 腮腺炎综合
征(间脑调节障碍)

Opsc Ophthalmoscope 眼 底镜

Opscc Ophthalmoscopic 检 眼镜的

Opscy Ophthalmoscopy 检眼镜检查术

OPV Oral , (At Tenuated) Poliovirus Vaccine
口服脊髓灰质炎减毒疫苗

OPV Oral Poliovirus 口 腔脊髓灰质炎病
毒

Opwi Opiate Withdrawal 鸦 片戒断

Opwu Open Wound 开 放性创伤

OR Optimum Requirement 最 适需要量

OR Oxygen Requirement 需 氧量

Orab Oral Antibiotic 口服抗生素

OS Osteosarcoma 骨肉瘤

Osot Osteotomy 截 骨术

Osots Osteotomies 截骨术

Ospa Osteoarthropathy 骨关节病

Ospe Osteopenia 骨质稀少; 骨质减少

Osph Osteophyte 骨 赘

Osphs Osteophytes 骨赘

Ospo Osteoporosis 骨 质疏松(症)

Ost Ostomy 造 瘘术; 造口术

Osto Osteotome 骨凿

OT Occupational Therapist 职业治疗师【注释】
〔康复医学的一种专业技术职
称, 通过有目的的操作, 增强病人返回
社会的能力和信心。 进行这种操作指
导的人即称为 OT〕

OT Occupational Therapy 职业疗法

OT Olfactory Tobercle 嗅结(节) ; 嗅球

OT Operating Theatre 手术教室

OT Optic Tract 视 (神经) 束

OT Oxytocin 催产素

量(放射量)

Ovar Ovary 卵 巢〔解〕Ovar Ium 〔拉〕

Ovca Ovarian Cancer 卵巢癌

Ovcy(S) Ovarian Cyst (S) 卵巢囊肿

Ovlaj Ovulation 排卵

Ovlas Ovulates 排卵

Ovma Ovarian Mass 卵 巢肿块

Ovn Ovarian ① 卵巢的②子房的

Ovo Ovocyte 卵母细胞

Ovos Ovocytes 卵 母细胞

Oxnaj Oxygenation 充氧作用

Oxsa(S) Oxygen Saturation (S) 氧 饱和
度

Japanese

略語　日本語の意味　　スペル

O　　酸素　Oxygen

OA　　後頭動脈　　Occipital
　　　前方後頭位（胎位）
　　　Occipitoanterior(Position)

OAC　直視下大動脈弁交連切開（術）　　Open
Aortic Commissurotomy

OALL 前縦人体骨化症　　Ossification Of Anterior
Longitudinal Ligament

OA-PICA　　後頭動脈・後下小脳動脈吻合（術）
　　　Occipital Artery-Posterior Inferior Cerebellar
Artery(Anastomosis)

OB　　潜血　　Occult Blood

Ob　　斜位　　Oblique

OBD　器質性脳疾患　　Organic Brain Disease

OBS　器質性脳症候群　　Organic Brain Syndrome

OC　　経口避妊薬　Oral Contraceptive
　　　酸素消費量　Oxygen Consumption
　　　視神経交叉　Optic Chiasma

O&C　発症と経過　Onset And Course

OCD　強迫性障害　Obsessive-Compulsive Disorder

OCG　経口胆嚢造影（法）　　Oral
Cholecystography

OCT　オキシトシン負荷試験　　Oxytocin
Challenge Test

OCU　分娩監視装置　　Obstetric Care Unit

OCV　硝子体混濁　Opacitas Corporis Vitrei(ラ)

OD　起立性調節障害　Orthostatic Dysregulation

ODA　右前方後頭位（胎位）　Occipitodextra Anterior(Position)

ODC　酸素解離曲線　Oxygen Dissociation(Saturation)Curve

OEF　酸素摂取率　Oxygen Extraction Fraction

OER　酸素増感比　Oxygen Enhancement Ratio

OGI　骨形成不全症　Osteogenesis Imperfecta

OGTT 経ロブドウ糖負荷試験　Oral Glucose Tolerance Test

OH　起立性低血圧（症）　Orthostatic Hypotension

OHP　高圧酸素療法　Oxygen Of Hyperbaric Pressure，Oxygen Under High Pressure

OI　オキシトシン分娩誘導　Oxytocin Induction

　　骨形成不全（症）　Osteogenesis Imperfecta

　　日和見感染症　Opportunistic Infection

OICU 産科集中監視室　Obstetric Intensive Care Unit

Oint　軟膏　Ointment

OKN　視運動性眼振　Optokinetic Nystagmus

OLA　左頭前方位（胎位）　Occipitolevoanterior(Position)

OLF　黄色靭帯骨化（症）　Ossification Of Ligamentum Flavum

OLP　左後頭後方位（胎位）　Occipitolevoposterior(Position)

OLT　左後頭横位（胎位）　Occipitolevotransverse(Position)

OM　鈍縁枝　　Obtuse Marginal(Coronary Artery)

OMC　直視下僧帽弁交連切開（術）　　Open Mitral Commissurotomy

OMD　器質性精神疾患　　Organic Mental Disorder

OME　滲出性中耳炎　　Otitis Media With Effusion

OMI　陳旧性心筋梗塞　　Old Myocardial Infarction

OP　浸透圧　　Osmotic Pressure

Ope　手術　Operation

OPLL　後縦靱帯骨化（症）　　Ossification Of Posterior Longitudinal Ligament

OPV　経口ポリオワクチン　　Oral Polio Vaccine

OR　オッズ比　　Odds Ratio

ORIF　観血的整復と内固定　　Open Reduction And Internal Fixation

OS　後頭仙骨位（胎位）　　Occipitosacral (Position)

　　骨肉腫　　Osteosarcoma

　　僧帽弁開放音　　(Mitral Valve)Opening Snap

OSAS　閉塞性睡眠時無呼吸症候群　　Obstructive Sleep Apnea Syndrome

Osteo　骨髄炎　　Osteomyelitis

OT　見当識検査　Orientation Test

　　後頭横位（胎位）　Occiput Transverse

　　作業療法(士) Occupational Therapy

OTCA　術中経管的冠状動脈形成（拡張）術　　Operative Transluminal Coronary Angioplasty

Ova Ca　　卵巣癌　　Ovarian Carcinoma

OYL　黄色靭帯骨化症　　Ossification Of Yellow
Ligament

P

French

PAC Pontage Aorto-Coronaire

PBH Ponction-Biopsie Hépatique

PBR Ponction-Biopsie Rénale

PC Périmètre Crânien, Perte De Connaissance

PCR Polymerase Chain-Reaction, Protéine C-Réactive

PDF Produits De Dégradation De La Fibrine

PDGF Platelet-Derived Growth Factor

PL Ponction Lombaire

PM Poids Moléculaire, Pace-Maker

PMA Procréation Médicalement Assistée

PMD Psychose Maniaco-Dépressive

PNB Olynucléaires Basophiles

PNE Polynucléaires Éosinophiles

PP Polynucléaires Neutrophiles

PNO Pneumothorax

Popérimètre Ombilical

PP Lacenta Praevia

Prlprolactine PS

Ponction Sternale

PSA Prostatic Specific Antigen

PSF Ponction De De Sang Foetal

PUPH

PVA

Prothèse Valvulaire Aortique

PVC

Pression Veineuse Centrale

English

PWLV Posterior Wall Of Left Ventricle

PWM Pulse With Modulation

Pw-MW Prewhitening [Of Data] Multiple
Window

PWP Patient Word Processing; Prentice,
Williams, And Peterson [Model]; Pulmonary
Wedge Pressure

PWRQ Parental Worry Of Recurrent Abdominal
Pain Questionnaire

PWS Port Wine Stain; Physician Workstation;
Prader-Willi Syndrome

PWS/AS Prader-Willi Syndrome/Angelman
Syndrome

PWT Physician Waiting Time; Posterior Wall
Thickness; Pseudo–Winger Transform

Pwt Pennyweight

PWTT Pulsed Wave Transit Time

PWV Pulsed Wave Velocity

PX Pancreatectomized; Peroxidase; Physical
Examination

Px Past History; Peroxidase; Physical Examination;
Pneumothorax; Prognosis

Px Pancreas, Pancreatic

PXA Pleomorphic Xanthoastrocytoma

PXE Pseudoxanthoma Elasticum

PXM Projection X-Ray Microscopy;
Pseudoexfoliation
Material

PXMP Peroxysomal Membrane Protein

PXS Pseudoexfoliation Syndrome

PXT Piroxantrone

Pxy Propagation Delay

Py Phosphopyridoxal; Polyoma [Virus];
Pyridine; Pyridoxal
Py Pack-Years
PYA Psychoanalysis
Pyc Pyogenic Culture
PYCR Pyrroline-5-Carboxylate Reductase
PYD N-Terminal Pyrin Domain
PYE Peptone Yeast Extract
PYG Peptone, Yeast Extract, Glucose
PYGM Peptone, Yeast, Glucose, Maltose
PYLL Potential Years Of Life Lost
PYM Psychosomatic
Pynpase Pyridine Nucleoside Phosphorylase
PYP Pyrophosphate
Pyr Pyridine; Pyruvate
Pyrp Pyridoxal Phosphate
Pyv Polyomavirus, Polyomavirus
PZ Pancreozymin; Phthalazinone; Pregnancy
Zone; Proliferative Zone; Protamine Zinc
Pz 4-Phenylazobenzylycarbonyl; Parietal
Midline Electrode Placement [ECG]
Pz Pièze
PZA Pyrazinamide
PZ-CCK Pancreozymin Cholecystokinin
PZD Partial Zona Dissection
PZE Piezoelectric
PZI Protamine Zinc Insulin
PZP Pregnancy Zone Protein
PZQ Praziquantel
PZT Lead Zirconate Titanate
Venous Confluence; Pulmonary Venous Congestion
PVCM Paradoxic Vocal Cord Motion
PVCO2 Partial Pressure Of Carbon Dioxide In
Mixed Venous Blood
PVD Patient Very Disturbed; Peripheral Vascular

Disease; Portal Vein Dilation; Posterior
Vitreous Detachment; Postural Vertical Dimension;
Premature Ventricular Depolarization;
Pulmonary Valvular Dysplasia; Pulmonary
Vascular Disease
PVDF Polyvinyl Diisopropyl Fluoride;
Polyvinylidene
Difluoride
PVE Partial Volume Effect; Perivenous
Encephalomyelitis;
Periventricular Echogenicity;
Postvaccinial Encephalopathy; Premature
Ventricular Event; Premature Ventricular Extrasystole;
Prosthetic Valve Endocarditis
PV-ECF Plasma Volume/Extracellular Fluid
[Ratio]
PVEM Postvaccinial Encephalomyelitis
P-VEP Pattern Visual Evoked Potential
PVF Peripheral Visual Field; Portal Venous
Flow; Primary Ventricular Fibrillation
PVFS Postviral Fatigue Syndrome
PVG Periventricular Gray Matter; Pulmonary
Valve Gradient
PVH Paraventricular Hyperintensity; Pulmonary
Venous Hypertension
PVI Patient Video Interview; Peripheral Vascular
Insufficiency; Perivascular Infiltration;
Positron Volume Imaging; Protracted Venous
Infusion
PVK Penicillin V Potassium
PVL Perivalvular Leakage; Periventricular
Leukomalacia; Permanent Vision Loss
PVM Parallel Virtual Machine; Pneumonia
Virus Of Mice; Proteins, Vitamins, And Minerals;
Pulmonary Vascular Marking

Pvmed Preventive Medicine
PVMR PRODIGY Virtual Medical Record
PVN Paraventricular Nucleus; Predictive Value Negative
PVNPS Post–Viet Nam Psychiatric Syndrome
PVNS Pigmented Villonodular Synovitis
PVNZ Parapoxvirus Of Red Deer In New Zealand
PVO Pulmonary Venous Obstruction
PVO2 Partial Oxygen Pressure In Mixed Venous Blood
PVOD Pulmonary Vascular Obstructive Disease; Pulmonary Venoocclusive Disease
PVP Penicillin V Potassium; Peripheral Vein Plasma; Peripheral Venous Pressure; Polyvinylpyrrolidone;
Portal Venous Phase; Portal Venous Pressure; Predictive Value Of Positive Results; Pulmonary Vein Potential; Pulmonary Venous Pressure
PVP-I Polyvinylpyrrolidone-Iodine
PVR Peripheral Vascular Resistance; Perspective Volume Rendering; Poliovirus Receptor; Postvoiding Residual; Pulmonary Valve Replacement Or Repair; Pulmonary Vascular Resistance; Pulse Volume Recording
Pvr Perspective Volume Rendering
PVRI Pulmonary Vascular Resistance Index
PVS Partner Violence Screening; Percussion, Vibration, Suction; Percutaneous Vascular Surgery; Peritoneovenous Shunt; Permanent Vegetative State; Persistent Vegetative State; Persistent Viral Syndrome; Plummer-Vinson Syndrome; Poliovirus Susceptibility; Polyvinyl Sponge; Premature Ventricular Systole;

Programmed Ventricular Stimulation; Pulmonary
Valvular Stenosis

Pvs Pulmonary Venous Systolic

PVSA Percutaneous Vasal Sperm Aspiration

PVSG Polycythemia Vera Study Group

PVST Prevertebral Soft Tissue

PVU Pueblo Viejo Virus

PVT Paroxysmal Ventricular Tachycardia;
Periventricular Thalamic [Nucleus]; Portal
Vein Thrombosis; Pressure, Volume, And
Temperature;

Private Patient; Psychomotor Vigilance
Task

PVTT Portal Vein Tumor Thrombosis; Portal
Vein Tumor Thrombus

PVW Posterior Vaginal Wall

Pvz Pulverization

PW Peristaltic Wave; Plantar Wart; Posterior
Wall; Pressure Wave; Psychological Warfare;
Pulmonary Wedge; Pulsed Wave; Pulse
Width

Pw Progesterone Withdrawal; Pulsed Wave;
Whole-Cell Pertussis [Vaccine]

Pw Picowatt

PWA Person With AIDS; Pulse Wave Analysis

PWB Partial Weight Bearing

PWBC Peripheral White Blood Cell

PWBRT Prophylactic Whole-Brain Radiation
Therapy

PWBT Partial Weight-Bearing Therapy

PWC Peak Work Capacity; Physical Work
Capacity

PWCA Pure White Cell Aplasia

PWCR Prader-Willi Chromosome Region

PWCT Perfusion-Weighted Computed Tomography

PWD Posterior Wall In Diastole; Printed Wiring Board

Pwd Powder

PWDS Postweaning Diarrhea Syndrome

PWDU Pulsed Wave Doppler Ultrasound

PWE Posterior Wall Excursion

PWI Perfusion-Weighted Imaging; Posterior Wall Infarct

PTV Patient-Triggered Ventilation; Planning Target Volume; Porcine Teschovirus; Posterior Terminal Vein; Posterior Tibial Vein; Punta Toro Virus

PTV2 Planning Target Volume 2

Ptv Pneumotropic Virus

PTVT Planning Target Volume Tool

PTVV Ponteves Virus

PTX Palytoxin; Pentoxifylline; Picrotoxinin; Pneumothorax

Ptx Parathyroidectomy; Pelvic Traction

Ptx Pneumothorax

Ptx No Evidence Of Primary Tumor

PTXT Pointer To Text

PTZ Pentylenetetrazol

PU Palindromic Unit; Passed Urine; Patient Unit; Pepsin Unit; Peptic Ulcer; Perfusion Unit; Polyurethane; Pregnancy Urine; 6-Propyluracil; Prostatic Urethra

Pu Plutonium; Purine; Purple

PUA Patient Unit Assistant

Pub Public

PUBS Percutaneous Umbilical Blood Sampling; Perforations, Ulcers, And Gastrointestinal Bleeds; Purple Urine Bag Syndrome

PUC Pediatric Urine Collector; Premature Uterine Contractions

PUCV Puchong Virus
PUD Peptic Ulcer Disease; Pudendal
Pud Pulmonary Disease
PUF Polyurethane Foam; Pure Ultrafiltration
PUFA Polyunsaturated Fatty Acid
PUF-HAL Polyurethane Foam–Hybrid Artificial
Liver
PUH Pregnancy Urine Hormones
PUI Platelet Uptake Index; Posterior Urethral
Injury
PUJO Pelviureteric Junction Obstruction
PUL Percutaneous Ultrasonic Lithotripsy
PUL, Pul Pulmonary
PULHEMS Physique, Upper Extremity,
Lower Extremity, Hearing And Ears, Eyes And
Vision, Mental Capacity, Emotional Stability
Pulm Pulmonary
PULSES Physical Condition, Upper Limb
Function, Lower Limb Function, Sensory Component,
Excretory Function, And Mental
Status/Support Factors
Pulv. Powder [Lat. Pulvis]
PUM Peanut-Reactive Urinary Mucin
PUMF Public Use Microdata File
PUMP Putative Metalloproteinase
PUMS Patient Utility Measurement Set; Permanently
Unfit For Military Service
PUN Plasma Urea Nitrogen
PUO Pyrexia Of Unknown Origin
PUP Previously Untreated Patient; Previously
Untreated Product
Pupid Paternal Uniparental Isodisomy
PUPPP Pruritic Urticarial Papules And
Plaques Of Pregnancy
PUR Polyurethrane

Pur Purple
Pur Purulent
Purg Purgative
Purr Purine Repressor
PURSUIT Platelet Glycoprotein Iib/Iiia Underpinning
The Receptor For Suppression Of
Unstable Ischemia Trial; Platelet Glycoprotein
Iib-Iiia In Unstable Angina: Receptor
Suppression Using Integrilin Therapy
PURV Purus Virus
PUT Provocative Use Test; Putamen
PUU Puumala [Virus]
PUUV Puumala Virus
PUV Posterior Urethral Valve
PUVA Psoralen Ultraviolet-A Range
PV Pancreatic Vein; Papilla Of Vater; Papillomavirus;
Paramyxovirus; Parapoxvirus;
Paraventricular; Paravertebral; Partial Volume;
Parvovirus; Pemphigus Vulgaris; Peripheral
Vascular; Peripheral Vein; Peripheral
Vessel; Picornavirus; Pityriasis Versicolor;
Plasma Viscosity; Plasma Volume; Pneumonia
Virus; Polio Vaccine; Poliovirus; Polycythemia
Vera; Polyoma Virus; Polyvinyl; Portal
Vein; Postvasectomy; Postvoiding; Poxvirus;
Predictive Value; Pressure Velocity;
Pressure Volume; Process Variable; Progressive
Vaccinia; Pulmonary Valve; Pulmonary
Vein
P-V Pressure Volume
P&V Pyloroplasty And Vagotomy
PV Ventricular Pressure
PV-1, 2, 3 Human Polioviruses 1, 2, 3
Pv Proteus Vulgaris; Venous Pressure
PVA Paralyzed Veterans Of America; Peripheral

Venous Alimentation; Polyvinyl Acetate;
Polyvinyl Alcohol; Pressure Volume
Area
Pva Pulmonary Venous Atrial
PVA-C Polyvinyl Alcohol Cryogel
Pvac Polyvinyl Acetate
Pvad Polyvinyladenine
PVALB Parvalbumin
PVARP Postventricular Atrial Refractory Period
PVB Cis-Platinum, Vinblastine, Bleomycin;
Paravertebral Block; Pigmented Villonodular
Bundle; Premature Ventricular Beat
PVC Peripheral Venous Catheterization; Permanent
Visual Circuit; Persistent Vaginal Cornification;
Polyvinyl Chloride; Postvoiding
Cystogram; Predicted Vital Capacity; Premature
Ventricular Complex; Premature Ventricular
Contraction; Primary Visual Cortex;
Pulmonary Venous Capillaries; Pulmonary
PTHC Percutaneous Transhepatic Cholangiography
PTHL Parathyroid Hormone–Like
PTHLP Parathyroid Hormone–Like Protein
PTH/Pthrp Parathyroid Hormone/Parathyroid
Hormone–Related Peptide
PTHR Parathyroid Hormone Receptor
PTHRP, Pthrp Parathyroid Hormone–
Related Peptide; Parathyroid Hormone–Related
Protein
PTHS Parathyroid Hormone Secretion
PTHV Pathun Thani Virus
PTI Pancreatic Trypsin Inhibitor; Penetrating
Trauma Index; Persistent Tolerant Infection;
Pictorial Test Of Intelligence; Placental
Thrombin Inhibitor; Pulsatility Transmission
Index

PTK Phosphotyrosine Kinase; Phototherapeutic
Keratectomy; Protein Tyrosine Kinase
PTL Peritoneal Telencephalic
Leukoencephalomyopathy;
Pharyngotracheal Lumen; Plasma
Thyroxine Level; Posterior Tricuspid Leaflet;
Preterm Labor
Ptl Posterior Tricuspid Leaflet
PTLA Pharyngeal Tracheal Lumen Airway
PTLC Precipitation Thin Layer Chromatography
PTLD Posttransplantation Lymphoproliferative
Disorder; Prescribed Tumor Lethal Dose
PTLV Primate T-Lymphotropic Virus
PTLV 1, 2, 3 Primate T-Lymphotropic Viruses
1, 2, 3
PTM Posterior Trabecular Meshwork; Posttransfusion
Mononucleosis; Posttranslational
Modification; Posttraumatic Meningitis; Prothymosin;
Pulse Time Modulation
PTM Transmural Pressure
Ptm Pterygomaxillary
PTMA Percutaneous Transvenous Mitral
Annuloplasty; Phenyltrimethylammonium;
Posttransplantation Thrombotic Microangiopathy;
Prothymosin Alpha
PTMDF Pupils, Tension, Media, Disc, Fundus
PTMPY Per Thousand Members Per Year
PTMR Percutaneous Transluminal Myocardial
Revascularization
PTMS Parathymosin
PTN Pain Transmission Neuron; Pleiotrophin;
Posterior Tibial Nerve; Prevention Trials
Network; Proximal Tibial Nail; Public Telephone
Network
Ptnm Pathologic Classification Of Primary

Tumors, Regional Nodes, And Metastases
PTO Klemperer's Tuberculin [Ger. Perlsucht
Tuberculin Original]
Ptotal Total Pressure
PTP Pancreatic Thread Protein; Pediatric Telephone
Protocol; Percutaneous Transhepatic
Portography; Phosphotyrosine Phosphatase;
Physical Treatment Planning; Posterior Tibial
Pulse; Posttetanic Potential; Posttransfusion
Purpura; Pretest Probability; Previously Treated
Patient; Protein-Tyrosine Phosphatase;
Proximal Tubular Pressure
Ptp Transpulmonary Pressure
PTPA Phosphotyrosyl Phosphatase Activator
PTPC Protein Tyrosine Phosphatase C
PTPG Protein Tyrosine Phosphatase Gamma
PTPI Posttraumatic Pulmonary Insufficiency
Ptpinsp Inspiratory Pressure-Time Product
PTPM Posttraumatic Progressive Myelopathy
PTPN Protein Tyrosine Phosphatase, Nonreceptor
PTPRA Protein Tyrosine Phosphatase Receptor
Alpha
PTPRB Protein Tyrosine Phosphatase Receptor
Beta
PTPRF Protein Tyrosine Phosphatase Receptor
F
PTPRG Protein Tyrosine Phosphatase Receptor
Gamma
PTPS Postthrombophlebitis Syndrome; 6-
Pyruvoyl Tetrahydropterin Synthase
PTPT Protein Tyrosine Phosphatase, T-Cell
PT/PTT Prothrombin Time/Partial Thromboplastin
Time
PTQ Parent-Teacher Questionnaire
PTR Patellar Tendon Reflex; Patient Termination

Record; Patient To Return; Peripheral Total
Resistance; Plasma Transfusion Reaction;
Prothrombin
Time Ratio; Psychotic Trigger Reaction
Ptr Porcine Trypsin
Ptr Intratracheal Pressure
PTRA Percutaneous Transluminal Renal Angioplasty
PT Rep Patient Representative
PTRIA Polystyrene-Tube Radioimmunoassay
Ptrx Pelvic Traction
PTS Para-Toluenesulfonic [Acid]; Patient
Treatment File; Pediatric Trauma Score;
Postthrombotic
Syndrome; Posttraumatic Syndrome;
Posture Training Support, Weighted
[Vest]; Pressure And Tension Scale; Prior To
Surgery; 6-Pyruvoyl Tetrahydropterin Synthase
Pts, Pts Patients
PTSD Posttraumatic Stress Disorder
PTSM Plant, Technology, And Safety Management
PTSS Posttraumatic Stress Syndrome
PTT Partial Thromboplastin Time; Particle
Transport Time; Posterior Tibial Tendon; Protein
Truncation Test; Prothrombin Time; Pulmonary
Transit Time; Pulse Transit Time
Ptt Partial Thromboplastin Time
PTTI Penetrating Thoracic Trauma Index
354
Physical Therapy; Physical Training; Physiotherapy;
Pine Tar; Plasma Thromboplastin;
Pluridirectional Tomography; Pneumothorax;
Polynomial Transform; Polyvalent Tolerance;
Position Tracking; Posterior Tibial; Posttetanic;
Posttransfusion; Posttransplantation;

Posttraumatic; Preferred Term; Premature Termination;
Preoperative Therapy; Preterm; Preventive Therapy; Previously Treated; Primary Tumor; Propylthiouracil; Protamine; Prothrombin Time; Pseudotumor; Psychometric Test; Psychotherapy; Pulmonary Thrombosis; Pulmonary Tuberculosis; Pyramidal Tract; Temporal Plane
P&T Permanent And Total; Pharmacy And Therapeutics
Pt Patient; Platinum
Pt Pertussis Toxin; Postoperative Tumor Size
Pt0 No Evidence Of Primary Tumor
Pt1 No Visible Tumor Tissue
Pt2 Less Than 1.5 Cm Tumor Remains
Pt3 1.5 To 5.0 Cm Tumor Remains
Pt4 More Than 5.0 Cm Tumor Remains
Pt Part; Patient; Pint; Point
PTA Pancreatic Transplantation Alone; Parallel Tubular Arrays; Parathyroid Adenoma; Peak Twitch Amplitude; Percutaneous Transluminal Angioplasty; Peroxidase-Labeled Antibody; Persistent Truncus Arteriosus; Phosphotungstic Acid; Physical Therapy Assistant; Plasma Thromboplastin Antecedent; Posttraumatic Amnesia; Pretreatment Anxiety; Primitive Trigeminal Artery; Prior To Admission; Prior To Arrival; Prothrombin Activity
PTAB Pterygoalar Bar
PTAF Platelet Activating Factor
PTAFR Platelet Activating Factor Receptor
PTAH Phosphotungstic Acid Hematoxylin
PTAP Purified Diphtheria Toxoid Precipitated By Aluminum Phosphate

PTAT Pure Tone Average Threshold
PTB Patellar Tendon Bearing; Polypyrimidine
Tract Binding; Prior To Birth; Proximal
Tubal Blockage
Ptb Pulmonary Tuberculosis
PTBA Percutaneous Transluminal Balloon
Angioplasty
PTBBS Peripheral Type Benzodiazepine
Binding Site
PTBD Percutaneous Transhepatic Biliary
Drainage; Percutaneous Transluminal Balloon
Dilation
PTBE Pyretic Tick-Borne Encephalitis
PTBNA Protected Transbronchial Needle Aspirate
PTBPD Posttraumatic Borderline Personality
Disorder
PTBS Posttraumatic Brain Syndrome
PTBW Peak Torque To Body Weight
PTC Papillary Thyroid Carcinoma; Percutaneous
Transhepatic Cholangiography; Phase
Transfer Catalyst; Phenothiocarbazine;
Phenylthiocarbamide;
Phenylthiocarbamoyl; Plasma
Thromboplastin Component; Plugged
Telescopic Catheter; Posttetanic Count; Premature
Termination Codon; Premature Tricuspid
Closure; Prior To Conception; Prothrombin
Complex; Pseudotumor Cerebri
PTCA Percutaneous Transluminal Coronary
Angiography; Percutaneous Transluminal Coronary
Angioplasty; Pyrrole-2,3,5-Tricarboxylic
Acid
PT(C)A Percutaneous Transluminal [Coronary]
Angioplasty
Ptcco2 Transcutaneous Partial Pressure Of

Carbon Dioxide

PTCDA Perylene-Tetracarboxylic Dianhydride

PTCER Pulmonary Transcapillary Escape
Rate

PTCL Panniculitic T-Cell Lymphoma; Peripheral
T-Cell Lymphoma

Ptco2 Transcutaneous Oxygen Tension

PTCR Percutaneous Transluminal Coronary
Recanalization/Revascularization

PTCRA Percutaneous Transluminal Coronary
Rotational Ablation

PTD Percutaneous Transluminal Dilation;
Permanent Total Disability; Personality Trait
Disorder; Photothermal Deflection; Preterm
Delivery; Prior To Delivery

PTDS Posttraumatic Distress Syndrome

PTE Parathyroid Extract; Posttraumatic Epilepsy;
Pretibial Edema; Proximal Tibial Epiphysis;
Pulmonary Thromboembolism

PTEAM Particle Total Exposure Assessment
Methodology

PTED Pulmonary Thromboembolic Disease

Pteglu Pteroylglutamic Acid

Pter End Of Short Arm Of Chromosome

PTES Percutaneous Transcatheter Ethanol
Sclerotherapy

PTF Patient Treatment File; Plasma Thromboplastin
Factor; Posterior Talofibular; Preterm
Formula; Proximal Tubular Fragment

PTFA Prothrombin Time Fixing Agent

PTFE Polytetrafluoroethylene

PTFNA Percutaneous Transthoracic Fineneedle
Aspiration

PTFS Posttraumatic Fibromyalgia Syndrome

PTG Parathyroid Gland; Prostaglandin

PTGE Prostaglandin E
PTGER Prostaglandin E Receptor
PTH Parathormone; Parathyroid; Parathyroid
Hormone; Percutaneous Transhepatic
Drainage; Phenylthiohydantoin; Plasma
Thromboplastin
349
Prospective Randomized Evaluation; Proton
Relaxation Enhancement
Pre Preliminary; Preparation, Prepare; Pretreatment
PREA Pediatric Research Equity Act
Pre-AIDS Pre–Acquired Immune Deficiency
Syndrome
Pre-Amp Preliminary Amplifier
PRECEDE Predisposing, Reinforcing, And
Enabling Causes In Educational Diagnosis And
Evaluation
Precip Precipitate, Precipitated, Precipitation
PRECISE Prospective Randomized Evaluation
Of Carvedilol In Symptoms And Exercise
[Trial]
Pre-CRT Hb Prechemoradiotherapy Hemoglobin
PRED Prednisone
PREDICT Prospective Randomized Evaluation
Of Diltiazem CD Trial
PREFACE Pravastatin-Related Effects Following
Angioplasty On Coronary Endothelium
[Study]
Prefd Preferred
PREFER Patient Randomization To Either
Femoral Or Radial Catheterization [Trial]
Preg, Pregn Pregnancy, Pregnant
Prelim Preliminary
Prem Premature, Prematurity
Premace Prednisone, Methotrexate, Adriamycin,

Cyclophosphamide, Etoposide
PREMIS Prehospital Myocardial Infarction Study
Pre-Mrna Precursor Messenger Ribonucleic Acid
Preop, Pre-Op Preoperative
PREP Pattern Reversal Electrical Potential; Physician Review And Enhancement Program
Prep, Prepd Prepare, Prepared
Prer Peak Respiratory Exchange Ratio
Pres Resistive Pressure
PRESEP Pediatric Rural Emergency System And Education Project
Preserv Preservation, Preserve, Preserved
PRESERVE Prospective Randomized Enalapril Study Evaluating Regression Of Ventricular Enlargement
PRESS Percutaneous Retroperitoneal Splenorenal Shunt [Study]; Point-Resolved Spectroscopy
Press Pressure
PREV Pretoria Virus
Prev Prevention, Preventive; Previous
PREVENT Program In Ex Vivo Vein Graft Engineering Via Transfection; Proliferation Reduction Using Vascular Energy Trial; Prospective Randomized Evaluation Of The Vascular Effects Of Norvasc Trial
PREVMEDU Preventive Medicine Unit
PREZ Posterior Root Entry Zone
PRISMA Preferred Reporting Items For Systematic Reviews And Meta-Analyses
PRF Partial Reinforcement; Patient Report Form; Peak Repetition Frequency; Perforin; Plasma Recognition Factor; Pontine Reticular Formation; Postrepetition Frequency; Progressive

Renal Failure; Prolactin Releasing Factor;
Pulse Repetition Frequency
Prf Polyclonal Rheumatoid Factor
PRFF Peak Response, Fine Frequency
PRFLE Prospective Randomized Flosequinan
Longevity Evaluation
PRFM Platelet-Rich Fibrin Matrix; Premature
Rupture Of Fetal Membranes
PRG Phleborheography; Purge
PRGS Phosphoribosylglycineamide Synthetase
PRH Past Relevant History; Postrepetition
Frequency [Doppler]; Prolactin-Releasing Hormone
Prh Propositus Hypoglossi
PRHCIT Project For Rural Health Communication
And Information Technologies
PRHHP Puerto Rico Heart Health Program
PRI Pain Rating Index; Patient Review Instrument;
Phosphate Reabsorption Index;
Phosphoribose Isomerase; Placental Ribonuclease
Inhibitor
P-RIA Polyclonal Radioimmunoassay
PRIAS Packard Radioimmunoassay System
PRICE Protection, Relative Rest, Ice, Compression,
Elevation
PRICEMM Protection, Relative Rest, Ice,
Compression, Elevation, Modalities, Medication
PRICES Physician Modalities, Rehabilitation,
Injections, Cross-Training, Evaluation,
Salicylates; Protection, Rest, Ice, Compression,
Elevation, Support
PRIDE Parents Resource Institute For Drug
Education; Platelet Aggregation And Receptor
Occupancy With Integrilin-A Dynamic
Evaluation [Study]; Primary Implantable Defibrillator
[Study]

PRIH Prolactin Release–Inhibiting Hormone
PRIM Primase
PRIMA Primary Care Information Across Anglia
PRIME Preinversion Multiecho; Prematriculation Program In Medical Education; Promotion Of Reperfusion By Inhibition Of Thrombin During Myocardial Infarction
PPOCD Postpartum Obsessive-Compulsive Disorder
PPP Pain Perception Profile; Palatopharyngoplasty; Palmoplantar Pustulosis; Pearly Penile Papules; Pentose Phosphate Pathway; Peripheral Pulse Present; Photostimulable Phosphor Plate; Pickford Projective Pictures; Platelet-Poor Plasma; Pluripotent Progenitor; Point-To-Point Protocol; Polyphoretic Phosphate; Porcine Pancreatic Polypeptide; Portal Perfusion Pressure; Prospective Pravastatin Pooling [Project]; Protein Phosphatase; Purified Placental Protein
PPPA Protein Phosphatase Alpha
PPPBL Peripheral Pulses Palpable Both Legs
PPPD Pylorus-Preserving Pancreatoduodenectomy
PPPI Primary Private Practice Insurance
PPPMA Progressive Postpolio Muscle Atrophy
PPPP Porokeratosis Punctata Palmaris Et Plantaris
PPR Patient-Provider Relationship; Pentatricopeptide Repeat; Percentage Of Predicted Recovery; Photoparoxysmal Response; Physician-Patient Relationship; Physician Payment Reform; Posterior Primary Ramus; Price Precipitation Reaction

Ppr Paraprosthetic
PPRC Physician Payment Review Commission
PPRF Paramedian Pontine Reticular Formation;
Pontine Perireticular Formation; Postpartum
Renal Failure
PP1RG Protein Phosphatase Type 1, Regulatory
Subunit
PPRM Portable Patient Record Model
PPROM Preterm Premature Rupture Of Fetal
Membranes
PPRV Peste Des Petits Ruminants (Ovine
Rinderpest) Virus
PPRWP Poor Precordial R-Wave Progression
PPS Paris Prospective Study; Pentosan
Polysulfate Sodium; Personal Preference
Scale; Physician, Patient And Society; Polyvalent
Pneumococcal Polysaccharide; Popliteal
Pterygium Syndrome; Postpartum Sterilization;
Postperfusion Syndrome; Postpericardiotomy
Syndrome; Postpolio Syndrome;
Postpump Syndrome; Prescription Preparation
System; Primary Acquired Preleukemic
Syndrome; Prospective Payment System; Prospective
Pricing System; Protein Plasma Substitute;
Pulse Per Second
PPSC Play Performance Scale For Children
PPSH Pseudovaginal Perineoscrotal Hypospadias
PP1SR Protein Phosphatase Type 1, Sarcoplasmic
Reticulum
PPSTH Population Poststimulus Time Histogram
PPSV Pneumococcal Polysaccharide Vaccine;
Pneumococcal Vaccine Polyvalent
PPSV23 23-Valent Pneumococcal Polysaccharide
Vaccine
PPT Parietal Pleural Tissue; Partial Prothrombin

Time; Parts Per Thousand; Parts
Per Trillion; Peak-To-Peak Threshold;
Pedunculopontine
Tegmental; Pfeiffer-Palm-Teller
[Syndrome]; Physical Performance Test; Plant
Protease Test; Polyp Prevention Trial; Polypurine
Tract; Postpartum Thyroiditis; Posterior
Pelvic Tilt; Preprotachykinin; Pressure Pain
Threshold; Pulmonary Physical Therapy; Pulmonary
Platelet Trapping
Ppt Parts Per Thousand; Parts Per Trillion;
Precipitate, Precipitation; Prepared
Pptd Precipitated
PPTL Postpartum Tubal Ligation
PPTS Pyridinium P-Toluenesulfonate
PPV Parapoxvirus, Parapoxvirus; Pneumococcal
Polysaccharide Vaccine; Porcine Parvovirus;
Positive Predictive Value; Positive
Pressure Ventilation; Precarious Point Virus;
Progressive Pneumonia Virus; Pulmonary
Plasma Volume
Ppvr Regional Pulmonary Plasma Volume
PPVT Peabody Picture Vocabulary Test
PPVT-R Peabody Picture Vocabulary Test,
Revised
PPW Patient Protective Wrap
Ppw Pulmonary Wedge Pressure
POA-HA Preoptic Anterior Hypothalamic
Area
POB Penicillin, Oil, Beeswax; Phenoxybenzamine;
Place Of Birth
POBA Plain-Old Balloon Angioplasty
POBJ Physical Object
POC Particulate Organic Carbon; Persistent
Organohalogen Compound; Point Of Care;

Polyolefin Copolymer; Postoperative Care;
Probability Of Chance; Product Of Conception;
Proof Of Concept; Pro-Opiomelanocortin
POCD Postoperative Cognitive Dysfunction
POCS Prescription Order Communication
System; Projection Onto Convex Sets
POCT Point-Of-Care Testing
POD Peroxidase; Place Of Death; Podiatry;
Polycystic Ovary Disease; Pool Of Doctors;
Postoperative Day; Pouch Of Douglas; Promyelocytic
Leukemia Oncogenic Domain
POD1 First Postoperative Day
POD2 Second Postoperative Day
Podx Preoperative Diagnosis
POE Pediatric Orthopedic Examination;
Physician Order Entry; Point Of Entry;
Polyoxyethylene; Postoperative Endophthalmitis;
Proof Of Eligibility
POEA Polyoxyethylene Amine
POEMS Patient-Oriented Evidence That
Matters; Polyneuropathy, Organomegaly,
Endocrinopathy,
M Protein, Skin Changes [Syndrome]
POET Physician Order Entry Term
POF Pattern Of Failure; Position Of Function;
Premature Ovarian Failure; Primary Ovarian
Failure; Pyruvate Oxidation Factor
Pofe Portal Of Entry
POFX X-Linked Premature Ovarian Failure
POG Pediatric Oncology Group; Polymyositis
Ossificans Generalisata
Pog Pogonion
POGO Percentage Of Glottic Opening
Poh Hydroxide Ion Concentration In A Solution
POHI Physically Or Otherwise Health

Impaired
POHS Presumed Ocular Histoplasmosis Syndrome
Pohv Pongine Herpesvirus
Pohv 1, 2, 3 Pongine Herpesviruses 1, 2, 3
POI Personal Orientation Inventory; Piece
Of Information
Poi Pourcelot Index
Poik Poikilocyte, Poikilocytosis
POIS Parkland On-Line Information Systems
Pois Poison, Poisoned, Poisoning
POL Physician's Office Laboratory; Physicians'
Online; Pollution Abstracts; Polymerase
Pol Polymerase
Pol Polish, Polishing
POLA Polymerase Alpha
Pol-GIK Polish Glucose-Insulin-Kalium
[Study]
Polio Poliomyelitis
POLIP Polyneuropathy, Ophthalmoplegiam
Leukoencephalopathy, Intestinal Pseudoobstruction
[Syndrome]
Pol-MONICA Polish Monitoring Trends
And Determinants In Cardiovascular Diseases
[Study]
POLONIA Polish-American Local Lovenox
NIR Stent Assessment [Study]
Poly Polymorphonuclear
Poly-A, Poly(A) Polyadenylic Acid
Poly-C, Poly(C) Polycytidylic Acid
Poly(CPH) Poly[1,6-Bis(P-Carboxyphenoxy)
Hexane]
Poly-Da, Poly(Da) Polydeoxyadenylic Acid
Poly-G, Poly(G) Polyguanylic Acid
Poly-I, Poly(I) Polyinosinic Acid
Poly-IC, Poly-I:C Copolymer Of Polyinosinic

And Polycytidylic Acids

Polys Polymorphonuclear Leukocytes

Poly(SA) Poly(Sebacic Anhydride)

Poly-T, Poly(T) Polythymidylic Acid

Poly-U, Poly(U) Polyuridylic Acid

POM Pain On Motion; Prescription-Only
Medicine; Purulent Otitis Media

POMC Pro-Opiomelanocortin

POMONA Pregnancy And Postpartum, Osteoporosis,
Mastectomy Rehabilitation, Osteoarthritis,
Nerve Pain, Athletic Injuries

POMP Phase-Offset Multiplanar; Principal
Outer Material Protein

POMR Problem-Oriented Medical Record

POMS Problem-Oriented Medical Synopsis;
Profile Of Mood States

POMT Phenol O-Methyltransferase

PON Paraoxonase; Particulate Organic Nitrogen;
Pollution And Toxicology Database

Pond By Weight [Lat. Pondere]; Heavy [Lat.
Ponderosus]

P-One First Parental Generation

PONV Postoperative Nausea And Vomiting

POOV Poovoot Virus

POP Diphosphate Group; Pain On Palpation;
Paroxypropione; Pelvic Organ Prolapse; Persistent
Occipitoposterior; Pituitary Opioid
Peptide; Plasma Osmotic Pressure; Plaster Of
Paris; Point Of Presence; Polymyositis Ossificans
Progressiva; Post Office Protocol

Pop Popliteal; Population

POPG Population Group

POPLA Presurgical Orthopedics,
Gingivoperiosteoplasty,
And Lip Adhesion

POPLINE Population
343
PNAC Parenteral Nutrition–Associated Cholestasis
PNALD Parenteral Nutrition–Associated
Liver Disease
Pnavq Positive-Negative Ambivalent Quotient
PNB Perineal Needle Biopsy; Peripheral Nerve
Block; P-Nitrobiphenyl; Premature Nodal Beat
PNBA P-Nitrobenzoic Acid
PNBT P-Nitroblue Tetrazolium
PNC Pakistan Nursing Council; Penicillin;
Peripheral Nucleated Cell; Pneumotaxic Center;
Premature Nodal Contracture; Primitive
Neuroendothelial Cell
Pnc Pneumococcus
PNCA Proliferating Nuclear Cell Antigen
PNCB Pediatric Nursing Certification Board
PNCG Preconditioned Nonlinear Conjugate
Gradient
PND Paroxysmal Nocturnal Dyspnea; Partial
Neck Dissection; Postnasal Drainage; Postnasal
Drip; Postnatal Death; Prenatal Diagnosis;
Principal Neutralizing Determinant; Purulent
Nasal Drainage
Pndb Perceived Noise Decibel
PNDM Permanent Neonatal Diabetes Mellitus
PNDS Postnasal Drip Syndrome
PNE Peripheral Neuroepithelioma; Plasma
Norepinephrine; Pneumoencephalography;
Pseudomembranous Necrotizing Enterocolitis
PNEM Paraneoplastic Encephalomyelitis
PNET Peripheral Neuroepithelioma; Primitive
Neuroectodermal Tumor
PNEU, Pneu, Pneum Pneumonia
Pneumoadip Pneumococcal Vaccines

Accelerated Development And Introduction
Plan
PNF Proprioceptive Neuromuscular Facilitation
PNG Penicillin G
PNH Paroxysmal Nocturnal Hemoglobinuria;
Polynuclear Hydrocarbon
PNHA Physicians National Housestaff Association
PNI Peripheral Nerve Injury; Postnatal Infection;
Prognostic Nutritional Index
PNID Peer Nomination Inventory For Depression
PNK Polynucleotide Kinase; Pyridoxine Kinase
PNK(H) Pyridoxine Kinase, High
PNK(L) Pyridoxine Kinase, Low
PNL Peripheral Nerve Lesion; Polymorphonuclear
Neutrophilic Leukocyte
PNLA Percutaneous Needle Lung Aspiration
PNM Perinatal Mortality; Peripheral Dysostosis,
Nasal Hypoplasia, And Mental Retardation
[Syndrome]; Peripheral Nerve Myelin
PNMK Pyridine Nucleoside Monophosphate
Kinase
PNMR Postnatal Mortality Risk
PNMT Phenyl-Ethanolamine-N-Methyltransferase
PNN Polynomial Neural Network; Probabilistic
Neural Network
PNO Principal Nursing Officer
P-NO2 P-Nitrosochloramphenicol
PNP Pancreatic Polypeptide; Paraneoplastic
Pemphigus; Para-Nitrophenol; Peak Negative
Pressure; Pediatric Nurse Practitioner; Peripheral
Neuropathy; Pneumoperitoneum; Polyneuropathy;
Predictive Value Of Negative
Results; Psychogenic Nocturnal Polydipsia;
Purine Nucleoside Phosphorylase
P-NP Para-Nitrophenol

Pnpase Polynucleotide Phosphorylase
PNPB Positive–Negative Pressure Breathing
PNPG Alpha-P-Nitrophenylglycerol
PNPP Para-Nitrophenylphosphate
PNPR Positive–Negative Pressure Respiration
PNS Paranasal Sinuses; Paraneoplastic Syndrome;
Parasympathetic Nervous System;
Partial Nonprogressive Stroke; Perinephric
Stranding; Peripheral Nerve Stimulation; Peripheral
Nervous System; Posterior Nasal
Spine; Practical Nursing Student
PNSA Partial Negative Surface Area
PNT Partial Nodular Transformation; Patient;
Picture Naming Task
Pnt Patient
Pnthx Pneumothorax
PNU Protein Nitrogen Unit
PNUT Portable Nursing Unit Terminal
Pnvim Poly-N-Vinyl Imidazole
PNVX Pneumococcal Vaccine
Pnx Pneumothorax
Pnx Regional Lymph Node Tumor Metastases
Cannot Be Assessed
PNZ Posterior Necrotic Zone
PO By Mouth, Orally [Lat. Per Os]; Parietal
Operculum; Parietooccipital; Period Of Onset;
Perioperative; Posterior; Postoperative;
Power Output; Predominant Organism; Pulse
Oximetry
PO2, PO2, Po2 Partial Pressure Of Oxygen
Po Porion
Po Airway Occlusion Pressure; Open Probability;
Opening Pressure
P.O. By Mouth, Orally [Lat. Per Os]
P/O Postoperative

POA Pancreatic Oncofetal Antigen; Phalangeal
Osteoarthritis; Preoptic Area; Primary
Optic Atrophy
POADS Postaxial Acrofacial Dysostosis Syndrome
POAG Primary Open-Angle Glaucoma
German
P.A. - Posterior-Anterior, Strahlengang Beim Röntgen
(Rö-Thorax)
Pavk - Periphere Arterielle Verschlusskrankheit
PCP - Cave! 2 Mögliche Bedeutungen: 1.
Pneumocystes-Pneumonie, 2. Bisherige Abkürzung
Für Pneumocystes Carinii (Jetzt Umbenannt In
Pneumocystes Jirovecii)
PCR - Polymerase Chain Reaction,
Polymerasekettenreaktion
PCT - Procalcitonin
P.M. - Punctum Maximum
P.O. - Per Os
Post - Posterior
Ppm - Parts Per Million
Proc - 2 Bedeutungen: 1. Processus, 2. Procedere
(Weiteres Vorgehen)
Prox - Proximal
PSR - Patellarsehenreflex
PT - Physiotherapie
PTC - Percutane Transhepatische Cholangiografie
PTCA - Percutane Transluminare Coronare
Angiografie

Italian

P Fosforo

Pa

Pb Piombo

;Platino

PA

(Acronimo Italiano) Pressione Arteriosa

PAM

(Acronimo Italiano) Pressione Arteriosa Media

PAO

(Acronimo Italiano) Pressione Arteriosa Omerale

PAOD

(Acronimo Italiano) Pressione Arteriosa Omerale
Diastolica

PAOS

(Acronimo Italiano) Pressione Arteriosa Omerale
Sistolica

PAP

(Acronimo Inglese) Positive Airway Pressure
(Pressione Positiva Delle Vie Aeree)

PCA

Angioplastica Coronarica Percutanea

PE

(Acronimo Italiano) Potenziali Evocati

PEA

(Acronimo Inglese) Pulseless Electrical Activity
(Attività Elettrica Senza Polso)

PEEP

(Acronimo Inglese) Positive End-Expiratory Pressure
(Pressione Positiva Di Fine Espirazione)

PEG

(Acronimo Inglese)Percutaneous Endoscopic
Gastrostomy (Gastrostomia Endoscopica Percutanea)

PET

(Acronimo Inglese) Positron Emission Tomography
(Tomografia E Emissione Di Protoni)

PIC

(Acronimo Italiano) Pressione Intra Cranica

PICC

(Acronimo Inglese) Peripherally Inserted Central
Catheter (Catetere Centrale Inserito Perifericamente)

PICCO

(Acronimo Inglese Rianimazione) Pulse-Induced
Contour Cardiac Output

PM

(Acronimo Italiano) Pacemaker

PPC

(Acronimo Italiano) Pressione Di Perfusione
Cerebrale

PPD

(Acronimo Inglese) Protein Purified Derivative (Un
Test Per La Tubercolosi)

PPLO

(Acronimo Inglese) Pleuro Pneumonia Like Organism
(Infezione Opportunistica Legata All'aids)

PT

(Abbreviazione Esami Di Laboratorio) Tempo Di
Protrombina

PUM

(Acronimo Italiano) Potenziali Di Unità Motoria
[Parametro Della ELETTROMIOGRAFIA]

PVC

(Acronimo Italiano) Pressione Venosa Centrale

Pz

(Abbreviazione Italiano) Paziente

Po

(Simbolo Chimica) Polonio (Polonium In Inglese)

Pu

(Simbolo Chimica) Plutonio (Plutonium In Inglese)

Russian

	Пульс
PA	Заднепередний
PADP	Диастолическое Давление В Легочной Артерии
PAP	Давление В Легочной Артерии
PAS	Рааминосалициловая Кислота (ПАСК)
PASP	Систолическое Давление В Легочной Артерии
PAT	
PAWP	Давление Заклинивания В Легочной Артерии (ДЗЛА)
PBC	Первичный Биллиарный Цирроз
PCO	Поликистозные Яичники
PCOS	Синдром Поликистозных Яичников (СПЯ)
PCP	Пневмоцистная Пневмония
PCR	Полимеразная Цепная Реакция
PCWP	Давление Заклинивания В Капиллярах Легочной Артерии
PE	Осмотр, Физикальное Обследование
	Чрескожная Эндоскопическая Гастростомия
PERRLA	Зрачки Равные, Круглые, Реагирующие На Свет И Аккомодацию
PFT	(ФВД)
PGE	Prostaglandin Простагландин
Phos	Псевдогипопаратиреоидизм
PI	Астоящее Заболевание
PIP	Проксимальный Межфаланговый
PKU	Фенилкетонурия
PLA	Активатор Плазминогена

PML   Полинуклеарный Лейкоцит
PMP   Предыдущий (Предшествующий)
Менструальный Цикл
            Пароксизмальное Ночное Диспноэ,
Синдром Ночного Апноэ
            Пароксизмальная Ночная Гемоглобинурия
            Послеоперационный

Chinese

P Paragonimus 并殖吸虫属

P Pastrurella 巴斯德氏菌属

P Penicillin 青霉素

P Percussion 叩诊

P Pharmacy 药剂学; 药房

P Phlebotomus 白蛉属

P Phthirus 阴虱属

P Pico 皮可

P Planorbis 扁卷螺属

P Plasmodium 疟原虫属

P Pneumocystis 肺孢子虫属

P4 Progesterone 黄体酮

P Progesterone (Hormone) 孕酮; 黄体酮

P Propranolol 心得安

P Propylene 丙烯

P-12 Prostaphlin 苯甲异□唑青霉素钠; 新青霉素 II 钠

P Pulvis 〔拉〕粉剂

PA Pernicious Anemia 恶性贫血【注释】〔因缺乏吸收维生素 B12 所需的因子而导致的 VB12 缺乏症。高色素性贫血〕

PA Primary Anemia 原发性贫血

PA Pulmonary Artery 肺动脉

Pacon Pain Control 疼痛控制

Pacr Pancreas 胰腺

Pacrc Pancreatic 胰 的

Pacrcy Pancreatectomy 胰 切除术

Pacri Pancreatitis 胰腺炎

PAH Pulmonary Ar Tery Hypertension 肺动脉高压

PAH Pulmonary Ar Tery Hypotension 肺动脉低压

PAHO Pan American Health Organization 泛 美卫生组织

Paho Parathyroid Hormone 甲状旁腺激素

Pahy Par Tial Hysterectomy 子宫部分切除术

Pama Pacemaker ① 起搏器② 起搏点③定调质; 定向质

Paman Pain Management 疼痛处理

Pamx Pain Medication 疼痛药物; 疼痛药物治疗

PAN Periodic Alternating Nystagmus 周期交替性眼球震颤【注释】〔以 1～5 分钟的周期交替眼震方向, 然后静止数秒钟〕

PAN Ployar Teritis Nodosa 多 发性结节性动脉炎【注释】〔多发性的中、小肌肉动脉坏死和炎症, 症状表现多种多样, 进展急速。发病与免疫学机制有关〕

PAN Poly Acrylo Nitrile 多 聚内烯腈

PAN Polyar Teritis Nodosa 结 节性多发

性动脉炎

Pana Paranasal 鼻侧的; 鼻旁窦炎

PANDAS Pediatric Autoimmune Neuropsychiatric
Disorders Associated With
Streptococcal Infection 与 链球菌感染
有关的儿童免疫性神经障碍【注释】〔突然发作
的与链球菌感染有关
的儿童抽搐或强迫症, 这类神经系统表
现异常的病儿血中含有高效价的抗 A
型链球菌抗体〕

Pane Panendoscope 广 视野膀胱内镜

Paney Panendoscopy 全 上消化道内镜
检查(术)

Panu Parenteral Nutrition 肠 外营养

PAO2 Alveolar Oxygen Par Tial Pressure
肺泡氧分压

Pao2 Alveolar Oxygen Pressure 肺泡氧
压

PAO2 Partial Pressure Of Oxygen In Arterial
Blood 动 脉血氧分压

PAO Peak Acid Output 高 峰胃酸排出量【注释】
〔通过刺激显示最高酸度时的胃
酸分泌量, 用 Meq/ Hr 表示〕

PAO Periar Ticular Ossification 关 节周
围骨化

Pao Pulmonary Ar Tery Occlusion Pressure
肺 动脉闭塞压

Paoc Parieto-Occipital 顶 枕的

Pao(PAO) Peak Gastric Acid Output
最大胃酸排出量

PAP 3′-Phosphoadenosine-5′-Phosphate

3′磷酸腺苷 5′磷酸【注释】〔在适当接纳体存在下
从 PAPS

PAL 445 PAP

形成的化合物, PAPS + 接纳体→ PAP +
产物〕

Pap Papanicolaou Test Or Smear 巴氏试
验或涂片

PAP Peroxidase - Antiperoxidase Smear
Test 过氧化酶-抗过氧化酶涂片试验

PAP Peroxidase-Anti-Peroxidase (Staining)
过 氧化物酶- 抗过氧化酶(染色)

PAP Primary Atypical Pneumonia 原 发
性非典型性肺炎【注释】〔细菌感染导致的肺炎
称为典型

肺炎, 与此相对应, 由支原体以及一部
分病毒感染引起的肺炎叫 PAP〕

PAP Pulmonary Ar Terial Pressure 肺 动
脉压【注释】〔将特殊导管从右心插入, 沿血
流进入肺动脉测定。正常值: 收缩期平
均为 20mmhg , 舒张期平均为 8mmhg〕

Papar Paraparesis 后 躯轻瘫; 后肢轻
瘫; 轻截瘫

Pape Parietoperitoneum 腹膜壁层

Paped Papilledema 视神经乳头水肿

Paph Prostatic Acid Phosphatase 前 列
腺酸性磷酸酶

Papi Papilla ① 乳头②乳头状突起

Papiy Papillary 乳头的; 乳头状的

Papl Paraplegia 截 瘫

Paplc Paraplegic 截 瘫的

Paplo Papilloma 乳头状瘤

Paplots Papillomatosis 乳头(状) 瘤病

Paplous Papillomatous 乳 头(状) 瘤的

PAPP Pregnancy-Associated Plasma Protein 妊 娠相关血浆蛋白

PAPP(Papp) Pulmonary Arterial Perfusion Pressure 肺动脉灌注压

Pasc Paranoid Schizophrenia 妄 想型精 神分裂症

Pasy Pain Syndrome 疼痛综合征

PAT Pain Apperception Test 疼觉试验

PAT Paroxysmal Atrial Tachycardia 阵 发性房性心动过速【注释】〔多见于洋地黄中毒, 配合使用 利尿剂而引发的低 K 是其诱因〕

PAT Prism Adaptation Test 棱镜适应试 验

Patas Palpitations 心悸

Path Pathology / Pathologie 病 理学

Pathc Pathologic 病理的

Pathcl Pathological 病理学的; 病理的

Pathec Parathyroidectomy 甲 状旁腺切 除术

Path .Fx Pathological Fracture 病理性骨 折

Patht Pathologist 病理学家

Pathy Pathology 病理学

PB(Pb) Presbyopia 老视

PC Prostatic Carcinoma 前列腺癌

PC Protein C 蛋白 C; 补体蛋白 【注释】 〔一种重 要的具有抑制血凝作用

的血浆蛋白质, 因从离子交换层析的 C
组分中发现故而得此名。 PC 缺乏易形
成血栓〕

PCD Polycystic Disease 多囊性疾病

PCM Protein Calorie Malnutrition 蛋 白
热量营养不良【注释】 〔短肠综合征患者由于脂
肪吸收
障碍, 脂肪酸利用减少, 会加重 PCM〕

PCO Polycystic Ovary 多囊性卵巢

PCOD Polycystic Ovarian Disease 多 囊
性卵巢病

PCP Peripheral Coronary Pressure 外周
冠脉压

PCP Phencyclidine 苯 环利定; 苯环己

Pct Polycythemia 红细胞增多症

PD Potential Difference 电位差

PD Principal Diagnosis 主 要诊断

PD Prosthetic Dehiscence 假 体裂开

PD Protein Degradation 蛋白降解

PD Protein Deprived 蛋白丢失

PD Pulmonary Disease 肺 部疾病; 肺病

PD Pyloric Dilator 幽门扩张器

PD Pathology Diagnosis 病理学诊断

PDS Pediatric Surgery 小 儿外科

PE Preeclampsia 先 兆子痫

PE Pulmonary Edema 肺水肿

PE Pulmonary Embolism 肺栓塞

PE Pulmonary Embolus 肺动脉栓子

Pefuj Perfusion ①灌流; 灌注(法) ② 灌
注液

Pefx Pelvic Fracture 骨盆骨折

Pelpa Pelvic Pain 盆腔(疼) 痛

Pelre Pelvic Rest 骨盆支持架; 骨盆靠

Pelri Pelvic Rim 骨 盆缘

Pels Pelvis 肾 盂

Pelwa Pelvic Wall 盆壁

Pelwas Pelvic Washings 盆腔冲洗

Pevi Peripheral Vision 周 边视觉

Pevw Pulmonary Ext Ravascular Water
肺血管外积水

PF Pulmonary Function 肺功能

PGH Pituitary Glycoprotein Hormone
垂体糖蛋白激素

PGH Pituitary Gonadotropic Hormone
垂体促性腺激素

PH Parathyroid Hormone 甲 状旁腺激
素; 甲状旁腺素

Phx Pharynx 咽
=

PHYS Physiology 生理学

Phys Exam Physical Examination 体 格
检查

Phyth Physiotherapy 物理疗法; 理疗

Phyths Physiotherapist 理疗医师; 理疗
学家

PID Pelvic Inflammatory Disease 盆 腔
炎; 骨盆炎性疾病【注释】〔妇科用语, 笼统指由
卵巢、输卵
管及其周围炎症所引起的症状〕

PIDR Plasma Iron Disappearance Rate

血浆铁消失率(放射性)【注释】〔静脉注入的 59
Fe 被造血组织摄
取从而在血浆中消失, 消失速度反映造
血能力, 用血浆铁半数消失时间(T1/ 2)
来表示。正常值为 60～ 120 分钟〕

Pidx Pelvic Inflammatory Disease 盆 腔
炎症性疾病

PIE Postinfectious Encephalomyelitis
感染后脑脊髓炎

PIE Pulmonary Infilt Rate With
Eosinophilia 嗜酸细胞增多性肺浸润

PIE Pulmonary Interstitial Edema 肺间

PHT 460 PIE

质性水肿

PIE Pulmonary Interstitial Emphysema
间质性肺气肿

Pied Pitting Edema 凹陷性水肿

PIE Syndrome Pulmonary Infilt Ration
With Eosinophilia Syndrome 嗜 酸细胞
肺浸润综合征

PIF Permeability Increasing Factor 通
透性增加因子

PIF Prolactin Inhibiting Factor 催 乳激
素抑制因子

PIF Proliferation Inhibiting Factor 增
生抑制因子

Pifo Piriform 梨形的

PIFR Peak Inspiratory Flow Rate 吸 气
流速峰值(最大吸气流速)

Pig Polyclonal Immunoglobulin 多 克隆
免疫球蛋白

PIH Pregnancy Induced Hyper Tension
妊娠诱发高血压; 妊娠性高血压

PIH Pregnancy-Induced Hypertension
Syndrome 妊 娠性高血压综合征

Pihog Pinholing 穿 孔

PIIS Posterior Inferior Iliac Spine 髂 后
下棘

PIJAC Pet Industry Joint Advisory
Council (Canada) 宠 物工业联合咨询
委员会

PILO Pilocarpine 毛 果云香碱; 匹罗卡
品

PIM Penicillamine- Induced Myasthenia
青霉胺诱发肌无力

PIMMF Postinflammatory Medial
Meatal Fibrosis 炎 症后中鼻道纤维变性

PIN Posterior Interosseous Nerve 骨 间
背侧神经

Pind Pinned 插针的

Pinng Pinning ①连接销② 黏合③ 填塞

PIO Phenylisohydantoin 苯异妥英

PION Pion Π 介子

PION Posterior Ischemic Optic Neuropathy
后部缺血性视神经病变

PIP Paralytic Infantile Paralysis 瘫 痪
性小儿麻痹症

PIP Peak Inspiratory Pressure 峰 吸气
压力

PIP Phosphatidylinositol Phosphate 磷
脂酰肌醇磷酸

PIP Probable Intrauterine Pregnancy

可能的宫内妊娠

PIP Proximal Interphalangeal 近 位指
节间关节的

PIP Proximal Interphalangeal (Joint)
近端指(趾) 间关节

PIPC Piperacillin 哌 拉西林〔抗生素类
药〕

PIPES Piperazine-N , N′-Bis (2-Ethanesulfonic
Acid) 哌嗪(双) 乙磺酸【注释】 〔用于制备 Ph6 . 1
～ 7 . 5 范围的

缓冲液〕

PIPJ Proximal Interphalangeal Joint 近
位指节间关节

Pipo Pinpoint ① 针尖② 精确定位③非
常精细的; 非常精确的

Pipr Pinprick 针刺

PIPS Pattern Information Processing
System 模式信息处理系统

PIRF Postischemic Renal Failure 缺 血
后肾功能衰竭

Piro(S) Pituitary Rongeur(S) 垂 体咬骨
钳

PISA Proximal Isovelocity Surface Area
近位局部等速曲面【注释】 〔心血管术语〕

Pisis Pin Sites 插 针部位

PIT Patellar Inhibition Test 髌骨抑制试
验

Pit Ind Pitocin Induction 催 产素诱导

Pitu Pituitary ① 垂体② 垂体的③ 黏液
的

PIV Parainfluenza Virus 副流感病毒

PIE 461 PIV

PIVAG Pet Insurance Veterinary Advisory Group 宠物保险兽医咨询小组

PIVKA- II Protein Induced By Vitamin K Absence Or Antagonist-II 维生素 K 缺乏或对抗剂诱发蛋白质; 异常凝血酶原

PIVR Pulseless Idioventricular Rhythm 无脉动性心室自身节律

Pj Palpation 触诊

PJB Premature Junctional Beat 交界区早搏

PJT Paroxysmal Junctional Tachycardia 阵发性交界性心动过速

Pjt Premature Junctional Tachycardia 交接区心动过速性期前收缩

Pk Dissociation Constant 分离常数; 解离常数【注释】〔电解质的解离常数, 蛋白质和配体的结合常数则用 K 表示〕

Pk Pack 包裹法

PK Penet Rating Keratoplasty 全层角膜移植术

PK Pericardial Knock 心包叩击音

PK Pyruvate Kinase 丙酮酸激酶

PKC Paroxysmal Kinesigenic Choreoa - Thetosis 阵发性运动性舞蹈手足徐动症

PKC Phlyctenular Keratoconjunctivitis 泡性角膜结膜炎

PKD Polycystic Kidney Disease 多囊性肾病

PKD Proliferative Kidney Disease 增生性肾脏疾病

PKF Phagocytosis And Killing Function
吞噬和杀伤功能

PKG Phonocardiogram 心 音图

PKK Plasma Kallikrein 血 浆激肽释放
酶

PKN Parkinsonism 帕 金森氏病; 帕金
森氏综合征【注释】〔一种常见的锥体外系疾病,
特
点为肌强直、动作少和震颤〕

PK 〔R〕 Prausnitz-Kustner (Reaction)
P-K 氏反应【注释】〔检测变态反应患者血中抗体
的
方法。将受检者血清 0 .1ml 注射到健康
者皮内, 在注射后 24 ～ 48 小时期间,
将怀疑抗原注射到前次注射部位, 30
分后出现红斑即为阳性〕

PKU Phenylketonuria 苯 丙酮酸尿
(症) ; 苯丙酮尿症【注释】〔一种白痴病的表现。
苯丙氨酸
代谢障碍是其病因。尿中排出苯丙酮
酸〕

Pkur Phenylketonuria 苯 丙酮尿症(由
于肝苯丙氨酸羟化酶缺乏引起的疾病)

PKV Poliomyelitis Killed Vaccine 灭 活
脊髓灰质炎疫苗

PL Partial Laryngectomy 喉部分切除术

P .L . Perception Of Light 光 觉

PL Phospholipid 磷 脂【注释】〔正常值 150～
250mg/ Dl , 急性肝
炎、肝硬化时减少〕

PL Placebo 安慰剂; 无效(对照) 剂

PL Polymyxin 多黏菌素 〔微〕

Pl Posterolateral 后侧的

PL Prolactin 催乳激素

PL Prolymphocytic Leukemia 前 淋巴细
胞性白血病

PL Purkinje Layer 浦肯野氏细胞层

PLA Phospholipase A 磷脂酶 A

Plac Placenta ①胎盘②胎座 〔植物〕

PLAP Placental Alkaline Phosphatase
胎盘碱性磷酸酶

Platy Platysma 颈 阔肌 〔解〕 Pla Tysma
〔拉〕

PLB Primary Lymphoma Of Bone 原 发
性骨淋巴瘤

Plc Placenta ①胎盘②胎座 〔植物〕

PLC Primary Liver(Cell) Cancer 原发性
肝细胞癌

Plcajs Plications 褶 〔直翅目昆虫后翅〕

Plcb Placebo 无 效(对照) 剂

PLCC Primary Liver Cell Cancer 原 发性
PIV 462 PLC
肝细胞癌

Plce Pleurocentesis 胸 腔穿刺术

Plcl Placental 胎 盘的

Plco Platelet Count 血 小板计数

Plcs Placentas 胎盘

Plcy Pleocytosis 脑脊液(淋巴) 细胞增多

Plcyt Plasmacytoma 浆 细胞瘤

PLD Potentially Lethal Damage 潜 在致

死损伤

PLD Programmable Logic Device 可 编
辑逻辑器材

Plde Pleurodesis 胸 膜固定术

PLE Panlobular Emphysema 全 肺泡性
气肿; 全叶肺气肿

PLE Polymorphous Light Eruption 多
形性日光疹

PL-E Polymyxin E; Colistin 多 黏菌素
E ; 抗敌素; 黏杆菌素

PLE Protein-Losing Enteropathy 蛋 白
质丢失性肠病

Pled Pledget 小拭子

Pledd Pledgeted 脱脂的

PLEDS Periodic Lateral Epileptiform Discharges
周期性一侧(性) 癫痫样放电

Plef Pleural Effusion 胸 腔积液

Plefs Pleural Effusions 胸膜积液

PLEVA Pityriasis Lichenoides Et Varioliformis
Acuta 〔拉〕急性苔癣痘疹样糠
疹

Plfl Plantar Flexion 跖 屈

PLG Plasminogen 纤 维蛋白溶解酶原

PLGA Poly Lactic Glycolic Acid (Polymer)
聚 乙烯乳酸乙醇酸

PLGE Protein-Losing Gast Roenteropathy
胃 肠蛋白质丢失症【注释】 〔因胃肠道疾病导致
蛋白质从消
化道大量丢失而引起的症状。常表现
为低蛋白血症、水肿、腹水、少尿、贫血
等〕

PLH Partial Loss Of Hearing 部 分听力
丧失

PLH Pharyngeal Lymphoid Hyperplasia
咽淋巴样增生

PLL Polar Lepromatous Leprosy 极 性瘤
型麻风

PLL Prolymphocytic Leukemia 幼 淋巴
细胞性白血病

PLLSD Pseudolymphoma Of Lung In
Sjogren□s Disease Sjogren 病 肺假淋巴
瘤

PLN Probabilistic Logic Neuron 概 率逻
辑神经元

PLO Pharyngo-Laryngo-Oesophagectomy
咽喉食管切除术

Plo/ Vac Poliomyelitis Vaccine 脊 髓灰
质炎疫苗

Plph Plasmapheresis 血浆分离置换法

PL(Pl) Placebo 安慰剂; 无效(对照) 剂 【注释】
〔评价某种药物的作用时, 往往
同时给予对照组在外观上与待评药物
一样但无特定药理作用的无害制剂, 以
消除心理暗示的影响, 这类制剂即为安
慰剂〕

Plq Plaque 噬 斑(微)

Plqs Plaques 斑 块

PLR Pupillary Light Reflex 瞳孔光反射

Plri Pleuritic 胸 膜炎的

PLRIA Paired Label Radioimmunoassay
配对标记放射免疫测定

PLS Platelet Lysate Supernatant 血小板

溶解物上清液

PLS Pseudolymphoma Syndrome 假 淋巴瘤综合征

Plsu Plastic Surgery 整 形外科; 成形外科; 整复外科

Plsur Plantar Surface ①跖面② 趾面

Plsus Plastic Surgeons 整形外科医师

PLT Primed Lymphocyte Test 原 始淋巴细胞试验

PLT Primed Lymphocyte Typing 原 始淋巴细胞分型

Plc 463 PLT

PLT Psittacosis , Lymphogranulomatosis Inguinalis And Trachoma 鹦 鹉热、 腹股沟淋巴肉芽肿和沙眼【注释】 〔上述三种病的病原均为衣原体, 故用此三病英文名称的头一个大写字母组合在一起表示〕

Plth Pleural Thickening 胸膜增厚

Plti Pleural Tissue 胸 膜组织

PLT(Plt) Platelets 血小板; 小片

Pltr Plantar 跖的; 足底的; 趾的

Plts Platelets 血小板; 小片

PLV Poliomyelitis Live Vaccine 脊 髓灰质炎活疫苗【注释】 〔脊髓灰质炎疫苗有福尔马林灭活苗和弱毒活苗 2 种, 现多使用弱毒活疫苗, 在出生后 3 ～ 18 个月期间, 以 6 周以上间隔分 2 次口服〕

PLWA People (Or Person) Living With

Aids 靠辅助器生活的人

PLWS Prader-Labhar T-Willi Syndrome
肌张力、智力、性功能减退、肥胖综合征

PM Pacemaker 起 搏器; 起搏点; 心脏
起搏器

Pm Palmomental 掌颏

PM Papular Mucinosis 丘 疹性黏蛋白病

PM Petit Mal 癫痫短时发作【注释】〔特点是短时
间内意识突然丧
失〕

PM Pm 钷

PM Poliomyelitis 脊 髓灰质炎; 小儿麻
痹【注释】〔由脊髓灰质炎病毒引起的脊髓
性小儿麻痹, 又称为海-梅氏病。现通
过活疫苗免疫, 其发生率急剧减少〕

PM Polymyositis 多 发性肌炎【注释】〔表现为肌
收缩力低下、肌肉压
迫痛、呼吸肌麻痹等。检查可见深部腱
反射减弱, 活体病检显示肌肉炎症,
GOT、CPK、LDH 上升, CRP 呈阳性,
怀疑与胶原病有关〕

PM Premolar ① 前磨牙; 双尖牙②磨牙
前的

PM Pretibial Myxedema 胫骨前黏液水
肿

PM Preventative Medicine 预 防医学

PM Puerperal Myocardiopathy 产 后心
肌病

PM Pulmonary Macrophage 肺 巨噬细
胞

PMA Papillary-Marginal-Attached 乳头边缘性附着性〔齿龈炎指数〕【注释】〔流行病学术语, 用于齿龈炎的流行病学调查〕

PMA Progressive Muscular At Rophy 渐进性肌萎缩; 慢性脊髓前角灰质炎【注释】〔左右对称性渐进性肌萎缩, 无力, 运动功能障碍。分为脊髓型、末梢神经型、渐进性肌型、肌肉萎缩性侧索硬化型等〕

PMB Polymorphonuclear Basophilic Leukocyte 嗜碱性多形核白细胞

PMB Polymyxin B 多 黏菌素 B

PMC Premature Mitral Closure 二 尖瓣过早关闭

PMC Pseudomembranous Colitis 伪 膜性结肠炎; 假膜性结肠炎【注释】〔滥用抗生素导致肠内正常菌群失调而发生的一种结肠炎〕

PMCT Percutaneous Microcoagulation Therapy 经皮微波凝固疗法【注释】〔对肝癌等治疗时, 在超声波引导下确认肿瘤部位后刺入穿刺针, 然后拔去穿刺针内芯, 换上微波电极插入病变部位进行照射以破坏肿瘤的方法〕

PMD Primary Myocardial Disease 原发性心脏病【注释】〔排除冠状动脉硬化或已知的炎症性心脏病, 心脏本身有原发性缺陷的原因不明的心脏病。心内膜和心肌组

织活体检查是确诊的依据〕

PMD Private Medical Doctor 私人医生

PMD Progressive Muscular Dystrophy

PLT 464 PMD

渐进性肌营养不良; 渐进性萎缩【注释】〔以骨骼肌渐进性萎缩和肌力低

下为主要特点的遗传性、家族性、原发性肌变性病变〕

PM-DM Polymyositi And Dermatomyositi 多肌炎和皮肌炎

PMDS Primary Myelodysplasti Syndrome 原发性脊髓发育不良综合征

PME Polymorphonuclear Eosinophil Leukocytes 嗜酸性多形核白细胞

PME Post-Moningoencephalitic Epilepsy 脑膜脑炎后癫痫

PME Progressive Myoclonus Epilepsy 进行性癫痫性肌阵挛

PMF Primary Myelofibrosis 原发性骨髓纤维化

PMF Progressive Massive Fibrosis 渐进性块状纤维化

PMG Pneumomediastinogram 纵隔充气造影片

PMI Perioperative Myocardial Infarction 手术期间心肌梗塞

Pmi Point Of Maximal Impulse 最强心尖搏动点

PMI Point Of Maximal Impulse (On Chest Palpation) 最高搏动点

PMI Point Of Maximum Impact 最强撞

击点; 最强搏动点(心尖)

PMI Point Of Maximum Impulse 最 强
心尖搏动点

PMI Posterior Myocardial Infarction
后壁心肌梗塞

PMI Post-Myocardial Infarction (Syndrome
) 心肌梗死后综合征【注释】〔心肌梗死急性期症
状消失后出
现的发热和胸痛, 通常会认为是病情蔓
延或是肺梗塞, 但其症状持续时间长,
且反复发作, 同时合并胸膜炎、心肌炎,
故被命名为 PMI (1956 年)。此病是坏
死心肌抗体形成的结果, 甾体激素治疗
有效〕

PMI Proportional Mortality Indicator
死亡构成比; 相对死亡指标; 均衡死亡指
数【注释】〔在死亡总人口中 50 岁以上死者
所占的比例〕

PMI Pulmonary Mixing Index 肺 内气
体混合指数【注释】〔表示肺内气体分布的一个
指
标〕

PMIP Post-Myocardial Infarction Pericarditis
心 肌梗塞后心包炎

PMIS Post-Myocardial Infarction Syndrome
心 肌梗塞后综合征

PML Pharmacy Merchants List 药 房
经营目录

PML Progressive Multifocal Leukodystrophy
进 行性多病灶脑功能障碍; 进
行性多灶性脑白质营养不良

PML Progressive Multifocal Leukoencephalopathy 渐 进性多病灶性脑白质病【注释】〔一种脑渐进性脱髓鞘病, 与恶性肿瘤、网状内皮系统等导致免疫功能低下的疾病同时发生〕

PML Prolapse Of Mit Ral Leaflets 二尖瓣叶脱垂

PML Prolapse Of The Mitral Leaflet 二尖瓣叶脱垂

PMLGI Primary Malignant Lymphoma Of The Gastrointestinal T Ract 胃 肠道原发性恶性淋巴瘤

PM Lividity Postmorte Lividity 尸 斑

PMMA Polymethylmethracrylate 聚甲基丙烯酸甲酯

PM-MC Flap Pectoralis Major Mycocutaneus Flap 胸 大肌皮瓣

PMN Periodic Migrainous Neuralgia 周期性偏头痛性神经痛; 周期性神经性偏头痛

PMN Polymorphonuclear (Cell) 多 形核(细胞)

PMD 465 PMN

PMN Polymorphonuclear Leukocytes 多形核白细胞

Pmns Polymorphonuclear Lymphocytes 多形核淋巴细胞

PMO Postmenopausal Osteoporosis 绝经后骨质疏松症

PMP Past Menstrual Period 前 次月经期

PMP Persistent Mentoposterior Position
Of The Face Presentation 持续性颏后位
面先露

PMPC Pivmecillinam 匹美西林; 氧咪
青霉素双酯

PMR Palmomental Reflex 掌 颏反射(划
拇指或小指皮肤引起颏肌收缩)

PMR Percutaneous Myocardial Revascularization
经 皮心肌血管重建术

PMR Pimaricin 那他霉素

PMR Polymyalgia Rheumatica 风 湿性
多发性肌痛

PMR Propor Tional/ Propor Tionate Mortality
Ratio 均衡死亡率【注释】 〔死亡总人口中 50 岁
以上死者所
占的比例, 值高表示年轻死亡者少〕

PMR Protonic Magnetic Resonance 质
子磁共振

PMS Patient Monitoring System 病 人
监护系统

PMS Periodic Movements During Sleep
睡眠时周期性运动【注释】 〔睡眠中有节律的拇
指伸展、足
关节背屈, 有时还伴有膝及股关节的部
分屈伸〕

PMS Pregnant Mare Serum 孕马血清【注释】 〔特
指妊娠 2 ～ 3 个月的马血清,
内含来自子宫内膜的马绒毛膜促性腺
激素, 对马属动物之外的动物具有强烈
的 F SH 和 LH 双重活性, 用于同期发情
和超数排卵〕

PMS Premenst Rual Syndrome 经前期综合征

PMS Premenst Rual (Tension) Syndrome 月经前(紧张) 综合征

PMSC Pluipotent Myelold Stem Cell 多能髓样干细胞

PMSF Phenylmethylsulfonyl Fluoride 苯甲磺酰氟

PMSG Pregnant Mare Serum Gonadotropin 孕马血清促性腺激素

PMT Photomultiplier 光 电倍增管; 光电倍增器

PMT (S) Premenstrual Tension 〔Syndrome 〕经前紧张综合征【注释】〔周期性出现于月经来临之前,
表现为不安、头痛、易怒、抑郁等精神神经症状,并有浮肿、乳房疼痛等体征〕

PN Parenteral Nutrition 胃肠外营养

PN Pemphigus Nconatorum 〔拉〕新生儿天疱疮

PN Periar Teritis Nodosa 结 节性动脉周围炎; 结节性动脉外膜炎【注释】〔中小动脉壁的广泛部位的炎症
性变化,以产生小结节为特点,多死于肾功能衰竭〕

PN Peripheral Nerve 外周神经; 周围神经; 末梢神经

PN Phrenic Nerve 膈神经

Pn Pneumonia 肺 炎

Pn . Pneumothorax 气胸

PN Polyar Teritis Nodosa 结 节性多动脉
炎
PN Polyneuritis 多发性神经炎
P .N . Practical Nurse 经 验护士
PN Pyelonephritis 肾 盂肾炎
PNA Peanut Agglutinin 花 生凝集素
PNA Progressive Neurospinal Amyot Rophy
进行性脊髓神经性肌萎缩
PNB Pregnant Bleeding 妊娠出血
PNB Pulseless Non-Breathing 非呼吸性
无脉
Pnbx Prostate Needle Biopsy 前 列腺针
PMN 466 PNB
刺活检
Pnc Pneumonic 肺的; 肺炎的
PNC Pneumotaxic Center 呼 吸调整中
枢
Pncl Pneumococcal 肺 炎球菌的
Pnco Pneumococcus 肺炎球菌
Pncy Pneumocystis 肺孢子虫
PND Paroxysmal Nocturnal Dyspnea 阵
发性夜间呼吸困难【注释】〔主诉夜间突发呼吸
困难。如是
哮喘发作, 则从半夜开始并持续到天
亮, 并伴有喘鸣音。R_E_N 如是淤血性心功能
不全引起, 则易于在刚入睡或睡后 1 ～
2 个小时期间发生并被迫坐起呼吸〕
PND Post Nasal Drip (Discharge) 鼻 后
分泌物
PND Purulent Nasal Drainage 鼻脓性引

流

Pndr Postnasal Drip 后鼻滴流

Pndx Paroxysmal Nocturnal Dyspnea
阵发性夜间呼吸困难

PNE Pneumoencephalogram 脑 充气 X
线照片; 气脑造影照片

Pnecy Pneumonectomy 肺切除术

PNET Primitive Neuroectodermal Tumor
原始性神经外胚层肿瘤; 未分化神经外胚
层肿瘤

Pneu . Pneumonia 肺炎

Pneumoc Pneumococcus 肺 炎球菌属

PNF Proprioceptive Neuromuscular Facilitation
本 体感受性神经肌肉促通; 本
体感受性神经肌肉接通(作用) 【注释】 〔良好的
神经肌肉冲动的传导,
会很自然地协调相关肌肉群的活动达
到最佳效率, 这种现象在神经生理学上
称为 PNF〕

PNG Photoelect Ronystagmograph 光 电
眼球震颤描记器

PNH Paroxysmal Nocturnal Hemoglobinuria
阵 发性夜间血红蛋白尿; 阵发性
睡眠性血红蛋白尿【注释】 〔夜间突发性溶血, 排
出血色素
尿。为后天因素引起, 原因不明〕

PNHA Primary Non-Hepatic Autoimmune
Disease 原 发性非肝脏自身免疫
病

PNI Peripheral Nerve Injury 周 围神经
损伤

PNI Postnatal Infection 生 后感染

PNI Psychoneuroimmnnology 精 神神
经免疫学【注释】〔揭示神经系统与免疫系统的
关
系, 从新的角度阐明机体调节机制的一
门新兴学科〕

PNL Percutaneous Nephrolithotomy 经
皮肾取石术

PNL Peripheral Nerve Lesion 周 围神经
损伤

PNL Polymorphonuclear Neutrophilic
Leukocyte 多形核中性白细胞

PNMA Progressive Neural Muscular Atrophy
进行性神经性肌萎缩症

Pnmed Pneumomediastinum 纵 隔积气

Pnni Pneumonitis 肺 炎; 局限性肺炎

PNO Progressive Nuclear Ophthalmoplegia
进行性核性眼肌麻痹

PNP Peripheral Neuropathy 周 围神经
病

PNP Polyneuropathy 多 神经病

PNP Purine Nucleoside Phosphorylase
嘌呤核苷磷酸化酶

PNPB Positive-Negative Pressure
Breathing 正 负压呼吸法【注释】〔利用人工呼吸
机, 正压时吸气,
负压时呼气, 两者交替进行的呼吸法。
此法优点是能保持肺气量接近生理状
态〕

PNP Deficiency PNP (Purine-Nucleoside
Phosphorylase) Deficiency 嘌呤核苷磷

酸化酶缺乏

Pnpe Pneumoperitoneum 气腹; 腹腔积气

Pnc 467 Pnp

Pns Penis 阴 茎; 雄性交接器

PNS Percutaneous Nephrostomy 经 皮穿刺肾造瘘术

PNS Peripheral Nerve Stimulator 周 围神经刺激器

PNS Peripheral Nervous System (Same As SNP) 周围神经系统

PNST Peripheral Nerve Sheath Tumor 周围神经鞘瘤

PNT Paroxysmal Nodal Tachycardia 阵发性结性心动过速

PNT Pentamycin 戊霉素

Pnth(Pnth .) Pneumothorax 气胸

Pnths Pneumothoraces 气胸

Pnto Pneumatosis 积气

Pnton Pneumatic Tourniquet 充 气止血带

PNU Protein Nitrogen Unit 蛋白氮单位

PNU Protein Nit Rogen Units 蛋 白氮单位

Pnva Pneumovax 肺炎疫苗

PNX Pneumonectomy 肺切除术

PNX Pneumothorax 气 胸

PO2 Ar Terial Oxygen Pressure 动脉氧分压

PO2 Oxygen Pressure 氧气压力

PO2 Partial Pressure Of Oxygen 氧 分压

PO Pump-Oxygenator 泵 -氧发生器

POA Pancreatic Oncofetal Antigen 胰 腺
原癌胎抗原

POA Phalangeal Osteoar Thritis 指 (趾)
骨关节炎

POA Power Of At Torney 授权文书

POA Primary Optic Atrophy 原 发性视
神经萎缩

POAG Primary Open-Angl Glaucoma 原
发性开角型青光眼

Poan Postanesthesia 麻醉后

Poanpl Postangioplasty 血 管成型术后

PO-Anti-PO Peroxidase-Antiperoxidase
过氧物酶-抗过氧物酶

Poar Polyarthropathy 多关节病

Poart Popliteal Ar Tery □动脉〔解〕Ar T Eria

Popli Tea 〔拉〕

Poau Postauricular 耳 廓后的

POB Phenoxybenzamine 苯 氧苄胺【注释】〔一种
A 受体阻断剂, 用于治疗
高血压〕

POC Postoperative Care 术后护理

Poca Postcatheterization 插管术后

Poch Posterior Chamber 后房〔解〕Came

Ra Poste Rior 〔拉〕

Pochl Potassium Chloride 氯 化钾

Pocho Polychondritis 多软骨炎

Pock(S) Pocket (S) ① 袋; 囊②蜂窝胃

Pocl Par Tial-Occlusion Clamp 部 分阻塞
夹

Poco Postoperative Course 手术后病程

Pocotr Poor Concent Ration 集中力差

Pocy Polycystic 多囊的

POD Peroxidase 过氧化物酶

POD Polycystic Ovarian Disease 多囊卵巢病

Poden Poor Dentition 生齿差

Podit Podiatrist 手足医

Podx Preoperative Diagnosis 术前诊断

Poed Periorbital Edema 框周水肿

POEMS Polyneuropathy , Organomegaly , Endocrinopathy , M-Protein , Skin Change (Syndrome) 多神经病、器官巨大症、内分泌病、M 蛋白、皮肤病变(综合征)

POF Periphera Ossifying Fibroma 外周骨化性纤维瘤

Pofos Popliteal Fossa □ 窝〔解〕Fos Sa Poplit Ea〔拉〕

POG Polymysitis Ossifcans Generalisata 全身性多发性骨化肌炎

Pohen Postherpetic Neuralgia 带状疱疹后神经痛

Pns 468 Poh

POHS Presumed Ocular Histoplasmosis Syndrome 假定性眼组织胞浆菌病综合征

Pohy Polyhydramnios 羊水过多

Poig Pointing ① 指点; 指示② 出现脓头

Poik . Poikilocyte 异形红细胞

POL Physician On Line 值班医生

Pola Posterolateral 后 外侧的; 接近背中
部的

Polam Postlaminectomy 椎板切除后

Polay Posterolaterally 后 侧的

Polio . Poliomyelitis 脊 髓灰质炎

POLY Polymorphonuclear (Leukocyte)
多形核(白细胞)

Poly Polyuria 多尿(症) ; 尿频

Poly A Polyadenylic Acid 多聚腺苷酸

Poly U Polyuridylate Ribonucleotide 聚
尿苷酸核苷酸

POM Pain On Motion 活动性痛

POM Pneumococcal Otitic Media 肺 炎
球菌性中耳炎

POM Prescription Only Medicine 处 方
药物

POM Purulent Otitis Media 化 脓性中
耳炎

POMC Proopiomelanocortin 类鸦片肽、
促黑激素和促肾上腺皮质激素共同前体
物质【注释】 〔已发现, MSH 样肽物质为
ATCH 和 Blph 前身物, 由于这些前体
物均含有类鸦片、MSH 和 ACTH , 因
此, 获得该名称〕

POME Persistent Otitis Media With Effusion
持续性渗出性中耳炎

Pome Posteromedial 后 中的; 位于背正
中线的

Pomen Postmenopausal 经绝后的

POMPA Prednisone , Oncovin , MTX ,

6-MP , And Asparagine 强的松、长春新
碱、氨甲喋呤、6-巯基嘌呤和天冬酰胺(化
疗方案)

PO(M) R Problem Oriented (Medical)
Record 问题导向(医学) 记录(系统) 【注释】
〔1968 年由 Weed 提出的一项医
学教育和医疗改革措施。这个记录的
内容要求包括医生对病人诊治的主观
意见、解释、处置以及治疗过程, 还包括
治疗方案及对患者的教育等〕

Pomy Polymyositis 多肌炎

Pone Polyneuropathy 多神经病

Poob Postobst Ructive 梗阻后的

Poof Pop-Off 出 气冒口; 溢流冒口

POP Plasma Osmotic Pressure 血 浆渗
透压

Pop Popliteal 腿弯部的

Poph Polyphonic ①贪食; 食欲亢进; 食
欲增强②杂食

Pophy Porphyria 卟 啉症; 紫质症

Popl Popliteal 腿弯部的

Popp Peripheral Occluded Por Tal Pressure
周围阻塞性门静脉压

POP(P .O .P .) Plaster Of Paris 熟 石
膏; 塑模石膏

Porh Polymyalgia Rheumatica 风 湿性
多发性肌痛

PORP Par Tial Ossicular Replacement
Prothesis 部 分听骨链(重建) 赝复物

PORP(TORP) Par Tial (Total) Osscicular

Replacement Prosthesis 一 种人造耳小骨【注释】〔用于再建传音功能的鼓室成形术〕

Portl Portal ①门静脉② 门静脉的③肝门④ 肝门的

POS Point Of Service Plan 医 疗服务网点【注释】 〔HMO 的一种变化形式, 基本上与 HMO 体系相同, 但允许患者接受没有在该系统登记的医师诊治〕

POS Polycystic Ovary Syndrome 多 囊卵巢综合征

POH 469 POS

Pos Posterior ①后面的② 后裔③后部; 后躯

Poso Polysorb 多孔性聚合物微球; 有机物担体

POSTOP Postoperative 手术后的

Post-Sp Post-Synthetic Phase G2 期; 合成后期

Post-T Posterior Tibial 胫 骨后

Posur Postsurgical 手 术后的

POT Periostitis Ossificans Toxica 骨 化性骨膜炎毒

Poti Posterior Tibial 胫骨后

Pove Por Tal Vein 门 静脉

Pover Polycythemia Vera 真性红细胞增多症

POVMR Problem-Oriented Veterinary Medical Record 面向问题的兽医病历

POVS Principal Official Veterinary Surgeon

法定兽医外科医生原则

Powa Posterior Wall 后 壁〔解〕Par Ies
Poste Rior〔拉〕

P .OX-K Proteus Vulgari Antigen St Rain
普通变形杆菌抗原染色-K(斑疹伤寒血清
凝集反应)

POZ Posterior Optical Zone 后视带

Pp Parietal Pleura 胸膜壁层

Pp Partial Paralysis 部分瘫痪

PP Pasteurella Pestis〔拉〕鼠疫杆菌

PP Perfusion Pressure 灌流压

PP Periodic Paralysis 周期性麻痹

PP Peripheral Pulses 周围脉搏

PP Pinprick (Method) 针刺痛觉法【注释】〔脊椎
麻醉时为检查无痛范围,
用针沿皮节轻扎皮肤表面, 以此确认麻
醉效果〕

PP Plasmapheresis 血浆分离置换疗法【注释】〔离
心沉淀血球, 除去上清, 然
后加等量生理盐水, 将其再输回到血管
中。适用于多发性骨髓炎、多种免疫性
疾病、药物中毒、高胆固醇血症、重症肝
炎等〕

PP Pneumoperitoneum 气 腹

PP Post Partum 分娩后的; 产后的

PP Presynthetic Phase G1 期; 合成前
期

PP Progressive Paralysis 渐进性麻痹【注释】〔由
梅毒螺旋体引起的慢性灰质
脑炎, 表现为瘫痪和痴呆。梅毒感染后

5～ 20 年发病, 易感染年龄为 40 ～ 50
岁〕

PP Pancreatic Polypeptide 胰 多肽

PP Protoporphyria 原卟啉症

PP Protoporphyrin 原卟啉

PP Pulse Pressure 脉搏压

PP Purulent Pericarditis 化 脓性心包炎

PPA Phenylpropanolamine 苯 丙醇胺;
去甲麻黄碱〔升压药〕

PPA Pipemidic Acid 吡哌酸

PPA Postpar Tum Amenorrhea 产 后闭
经

Ppaw Pulmonary Ar Terial Wedge Pressure
肺 动脉楔压

PPB Positive Pressure Breathing 正 压
呼吸

PPBS Postprandial Blood Sugar 餐 后血
糖

PPC Progressive Patient Care 阶段性患
者管理方式【注释】〔根据病人的病情轻重所采
取的
对应性管理体系。主要包括 6 种方式,
分别为集中管理、一般管理、自我管理、
长期管理、病房管理和门诊管理〕

PPCA Platelet Prothrombin Conver Ting
Activity 血小板凝血酶原转化活性

PPCF Peripartum Cardiac Failure 围 产
期心力衰竭

PPCF Plasma Prothrombin Conversion

Factor 血浆凝血酶原转化因子【注释】〔即第 V 因子, 该因子的先天性
缺陷症为一种常染色体劣性遗传性出
血性疾病, 表现为鼻出血、皮下出血等〕

Pos 470 PPC

PPCM Postpartum Cardiomyopathy 产后心肌病

PPD Protein Purified Derivative 蛋白质净化衍生物

PPD Purified Protein Derivative 纯蛋白衍生物

PPE Permeability Pulmonary Edema 肺通透性水肿

PPE Plasma Protein Ext Ravasation 血浆蛋白外渗

PPE Posterior Pelvic Exenteration 后盆腔脏器剜除术

PPED Persistent Post-Enteritis Diarrhoea 肠炎后持续性腹浮

PPG Polymorphonuclear Cells Per Glomerulus 多形核细胞/ 肾小球

Ppgpp Guanosine Tetraphosphate 鸟苷四磷酸; 四磷酸鸟苷

PPH Posterior Pituitary Hormone 垂体后叶激素【注释】〔由垂体后叶分泌的激素群, 目前已发现 10 多种, 其中主要的为催产素和加压素〕

PPH Postpar Tum Hemorrhage 产后出血【注释】〔胎儿娩出后产妇产道异常流血(超过 500ml)〕

PPH Primary Pulmonary Hypertension

原发性肺动脉高血压【注释】〔原因不明的肺动
脉压上升, 随
病情发展可导致右心功能障碍〕

PPHN Persistent Pulmonary Hypertension
Of The New-Born 新生儿持续性肺
动脉高压

PPHUS Postpartum Hemolytic Uremic
Syndrome 产后溶血性尿毒症综合征

PPI Progressive Pulmonary Insufficiency
进行性肺动脉瓣闭锁不全

PPI Proton Pump Inhibitor 质子泵抑制
剂【注释】〔抑制胃酸分泌最后阶段的质子
泵功能, 比 H2 受体阻断剂具有更强抑
制胃酸分泌功能〕

PPKD Primary Pyruvate Kinase Deficiency
原发性丙酮酸激酶缺乏症

PPLO Pleuropneumonia-Like Organism
类胸膜肺炎菌

PPM Permanent Pacemaker 永久性起
搏器

PPM Posterior Papillary Muscle/ Musculus
Papillaris Posterior 〔拉〕后乳头肌
〔解〕【注释】〔心脏超声波检查用语〕

PPMA Post-Poliomyelitis Progressive
Muscular Atrophy 脊髓灰质炎后迟发
性渐进性肌萎缩【注释】〔幼儿期或少年期患过
急性脊髓
灰质炎而留有一定程度的麻痹后遗症,
其功能后来虽然获得一定程度恢复, 但
是, 到了中年期后突然出现肌力下降、
肌肉关节疼痛、易疲劳性等症状。1950

年前后有过大流行, 近年又有增加趋
势〕

PPN Partial Parenteral Nut Rition 部 分
肠外营养

PPN Peripheral Parenteral Nut Rition 周
围肠外营养

PPO Preferred Provider Organization
优惠医疗服务机制【注释】 〔一种 HMO 的变化形
式。同意
提供优惠服务的医疗机构与医师签订
合约, 对加入其保险的会员提供比
HMO 范围更广的优惠服务〕

PPOM Persistent Purulent Otitis Media
持续性化脓性中耳炎

PPP Palatopharyngoplasty 腭 咽成形术

PPP Pustulosis Palmaris Et Plantaris 掌
跖脓疱病【注释】 〔发生于手掌和足底的脓疱性
病
变, 由于反复发作, 易误诊为汗疱状白
癣。有轻度骚痒, 尚没有探明是真菌还
是细菌是其病因〕

PPC 471 PPP

PP-Pc Phenoxyproply Penicillin 苯 氧
丙基青霉素

PPPC Propicillin 苯氧丙基青霉素

PPR Peste De (S) Petit (S) Ruminants
小反刍动物瘟疫

PPRM Preterm Premature Rupture Of
The Membrane 未足月胎膜早破

PPRPE Preserved Para-Ar Teriolar Retinal
Pigment Epithelium 动脉旁视网膜色素

保护上皮

PPRWP Poor Precordial R-Wave Progression
心 前导联缺少 R 波连续〔心电
图〕

PPS Pain Producing Substance 致 痛物
质【注释】〔指在适当浓度下可引起疼痛的
化学物质。常见的有胺类(组胺、5 羟
色胺、乙酰胆碱) 、肽类(舒缓激肽、P 物
质、加压素) 、脂肪酸(前列腺素) 等〕

PPS Pepsin 胃蛋白酶

PPS Postperfusion Syndrome 灌注后综
合征

PPS Pure Pulmonary Stenosis 纯型肺动
脉瓣狭窄【注释】〔心脏超声波检查用语〕

PPSH Pseudovaginal Peritoneoscrostal
Hypospadias 假阴道会阴阴囊尿道下裂

PPU Peripheral Processor Unit 外 围处
理设备

PPV Pars Plana Vitrectomy 玻 璃体扁
平部切除术

PPV Pneumococcal Polysaccharide Vaccine
肺 炎球菌多糖疫苗

PPV Progressive Pneumonia Virus 进 行
性肺炎病毒

PPZ Perphenazine 奋乃静; 羟哌氯丙嗪

PQ Paraquat 百 草枯〔除莠剂〕【注释】〔一种农
药(除草剂) , 中毒患者
常致命, 难以抢救。原来浓度为 24% ,
现改为 5% , 与其他除草剂配伍出售〕

Pq Plaque 噬 斑(微)

PQ Primaquine 伯氨喹; 伯氨喹啉

PQE Protein Quality Evaluation 蛋白质质量评价

PQ(Pq) Uncalcified Pleural Plaque 未钙化胸膜斑

PR Perennial Rhinitis 常年性鼻炎

PR Peripheral Resistance 末梢阻力; 外周阻力【注释】〔在血液循环过程中, 细小动脉壁的平滑肌发生收缩而调节血流量, 由此产生的血流阻力称之为末梢阻力或外周阻力。而细小动脉又称之为阻力血管〕

PR Phenol Red 酚磺酞

PR Pregnancy Rate 受胎率; 妊娠率

PR Propranolol 心得安; 萘心安

PR Pulse Rate 脉搏率

PRA Plasma Renine Activity 血浆凝乳酶活性; 血浆肾素活性【注释】〔凝乳酶是从肾小球分泌的一种
升压激素, 作用于血管紧张素原, 使之转变为血管紧张素 I , 再进一步转变为血管紧张素 II 。除这种直接作用外, 还刺激醛固酮分泌, 促进 Na 的重吸收。因此, 通过测定它的活性, 可以间接地测定血管紧张素 I 的生成能力。以此与高血压及醛固酮血症相鉴别。正常值为 0 .1 ～0 .2ng/ Ml/ Hr〕

PRA Progressive Retinal Atrophy 进行性视网膜萎缩

PRBC Packed Red Blood Cells 红细胞压

积; 血细胞压积

Prbe Premature Beats 期 前收缩

PRC Packed Red Cells 红 细胞压积

PRC Pesticide Residues Committee 农药残留物委员会

PRCA Pure Red Cell Anemia 单 纯红细胞性贫血

Prcan Prostate Cancer 前 列腺癌

Prcau(S) Precaution(S) 预 防法; 预防措施

PPP 472 Prc

Prcla Preeclampsia 子 痫前期; 惊厥前期

Prco Precordium 心 前区

Prcol Precordial 心窝的; 心前区的

PRD Postradiation Dysplasia 照 射后发育不良

PRD Prednisone 去氢可的松

PRDC Porcine Respiratory Disease Complex 猪 复杂的呼吸疾病

Prdo Predominant ① 特优生物; 特优种 ②占优势的; 支配其他的

Prdro Prodrome 前驱症状

Prdrol Prodromal 前驱的

PRE Photoreacting Enzyme 光 反应酶

PRE Progressive Resistance Exercise 渐进性抗阻训练【注释】〔利用机械逐渐增加阻力, 以此增加肌力和耐力的方法〕

Pregt Pregnant 怀 孕的; 妊娠的

Prem Premature ①早产仔畜②早熟的

Premed Premedicate 前 驱用药; 术前
(用) 药

Premedd Premedicated 术 前用药的

Premedg Premedicating 术前用药

Premedj Premedication 麻醉前用药

Premedjs Premedications 术前用药

Premty Prematurity 早 熟

Premy Prematurely 期 前收缩的

Preoc Preoccupied 全神贯注的; 被先占
的

PRE-OP(Preop) Preoperative 手 术前
的

Preopy Preoperatively 手术前的

Prep Preparation ①制备; 准备② 制剂;
制品③标本

Prepd Prepared 准 备好的; 精制的

Prepg Preparing 预梳

Prepj (S) Preparation(S) 制 剂; 准备

Presg Pressing 压成声盘; 压型毛坯; 压
制; 压制唱片; 迫切的; 按压法; 施压

Prete Pre- Effector-T-Cell 前 T 效应细
胞

PRF Prolactin Releasing Factor 催 乳素
释放因子

PRF Prolactin-Releasing Factor 催 乳素
释放因子; 催乳激素释放因子

Prfa(S) Precipitating Factor(S) 诱 发因
子

PRH Preretinal Hemorrhage 视 网膜前

出血

PRI Phosphoribose Isomerase 磷 酸核
糖异构酶

PRIF Prolactin Release Inhibitory Factor
催乳素释放抑制因子

Primip Primipara 初 产妇

PRIM&R Public Responsibility In
Medicine And Research 在 医学和研究
方面的公共责任

PR Int An Electrocardiogram Interval PR
间期〔心电图〕

PRIST Paper Radioimmunosorbent Test
纸放射免疫吸附试验

PRK Photorefractive Keratectomy 屈
光性角膜切削术【注释】〔一种角膜切除术。通
过切除角
膜光区而改变屈光的屈光矫正术〕

PRL Prolactin 催乳激素【注释】〔由垂体前叶分
泌, 通过维持黄
体的激素分泌而促进乳汁分泌。正常
值为 30ng/ Ml 以下〕

Prl Prolene 聚 丙烯纺织纤维

Prla Prolapse 脱 垂; 脱出

Prlad Prolapsed 脱 垂的

Prlif Proliferate 增 生; 增殖

Prlifj Proliferation 蔓延

Prlifv Proliferative 增 生的; 增殖的

PRM Paromomycin 巴龙霉素(微)

PRM Primidone 扑 米酮; 扑痫酮〔抗癫
痫药〕

Prmat Premature 未 成熟的

Prmaty Prematurely 期前收缩的

Prc 473 Prm

PRM-TC Rolitetracycline 罗利环素【注释】〔抗生素类药, 化学名为 Npyrrolidinomethlyl-

Tet R Acycline〕

Prnat Pronator 旋前肌

Prnatd Pronated 旋前的

Prnatj Pronation 内 转

Prnod Prurigo Nodularis 结节性痒疹

PRN, P .R .N . Pro Re Nata , As Occasion Arises (As Needed) , As Often As Necessary; Whenever Necessary 〔拉〕需要时; 必要时

PRO Proline (Aminoacid) 脯氨酸

Pro Protein 蛋白质; 蛋白; 朊

Procol Proctocolectomy 直 肠与结肠切除术

Proll Prolymphocytic Leukemia 前 淋巴细胞性白血病

PROM Passive Range Of Motion 被动活动度

PROM Premature Rupture Of Membrane (S) 胎膜早破; 前期破水【注释】〔分娩开始前羊膜破裂, 约占分娩总人数的 10% ～20 %〕

PROM Programmable Read-Only Memory 可编程只读存储器

PROMIS Problem Orientated Medical Information System 面 向问题的医学信息系统

Prooh Hydroxyproline 羟脯氨酸

Prop . Propranolol 心 得安

PROPLA Prophospholipase A 磷 脂酶 A

PRO(Pro) Prothrombin 凝血酶原

Pro Time Prothrombin Time 凝 血酶原 时间

PROTO-O Protoporphyrinogen Oxidase 卟啉原氧化酶

Protrg Protruding 插筋

PRP Panretinal Photocoagulation 广 泛 视网膜光凝术

PRP Platelet-Rich Plasma 多 血小板血 浆【注释】〔指含很多血小板的血浆。采血 后加入抗凝剂, 约 1000rpm 离心 10 分 钟, 可以获得上层含有很多血小板的血 浆〕

PRP Pneumoretroperitoneum 腹 膜后 积气造影法【注释】〔由肛门与尾骨尖之间注入 空 气、氧气或氮气等气体, 利用 X 线摄影 弄清肾脏及肾上腺形状的方法。临床 上检查肾脏肿瘤时采用〕

PRP Pressure Rate Product 血压心率乘 积值【注释】〔用血压× 心率的积表示血液循 环动态变化〕

PRP Problem Reporting Program (Of Medical Device & Laboratory Product) 问题通报计划(医疗器械事故) 【注释】〔1973 年 美国制订的制度, 与 MDR 不同, 具有较大的随意性〕

PRP Progressive Rubella Panencephalitis

进行性风疹全脑炎

Prphs Prophylaxis 预防; 预防法

Prphy Primary Physician 初期治疗医师

PR(PI) Pulmonic Regurgitation 肺动脉瓣回流【注释】〔指由于功能性或器质性原因, 在舒张期血液从肺动脉向右心室回流〕

Prpois Pressure Points 压迫点

PRPPS Phosphoribosy Pyrophosphate Synthetase 磷酸核糖焦磷激酸合成酶

PR (Pr) Prion (Protein) 朊病毒(蛋白质)

PRPS Overactivity Phosphoribosy Pyrophosphate Synthetase Overactivity
磷酸核糖焦磷酸合成酶活性亢进

Prpz Prone Position 俯卧位

Prri Pruritus 瘙痒

PRRS Porcine Reproductive And Respira-
PRM 474 PRR
Tory Syndrome 猪生殖呼吸综合征

PRS Pierre Robin Syndrome 皮 -罗二氏综合征; 小颌畸形综合征; 舌下垂综合征

Prsco Proctoscope 直肠镜

Prsic Proctosigmoidoscope 直 肠乙状结肠镜

Prsiy Proctosigmoidoscopy 直 肠乙状结肠镜检查

Prstc Prostatic 前列腺的

Prstec Prostatectomy 前列腺切除术

Prsti Prostatitis 前列腺炎

Prstm Prostatism 前 列腺病态; 前列腺

疾病

Prsy Presyncope 晕厥前

Prsyl Presyncopal 晕厥前的

Prtad Precipitated 沉淀碳酸钡

Prtase Phosphoribosyltransferase 磷
酸核糖转移酶

Prth Prosthesis ①修复术②假体

Prthc Prosthetic ① 假体的②修复的

Prti Proctitis 直肠炎

Prtim Prothrombin Time 凝血酶原时间

PRU Peripheral Resistance Unit 外周阻
力单位

Pruc Pruritic 瘙痒的; 痒的

Prur Proteinuria 蛋白尿(症)

Prut Prolapsed Uterus 子宫脱垂

PRV Pseudorabies Virus 假狂犬病病毒

PRVC Pressure Regulated Volume Cont
Rol Ventilation 压力调节式换气【注释】〔根据萨
博 300 式人工肺工作原
理的换气方式。由开始测到的换气压
力, 自动设定每次予想换气量的压力〕

P&S Paracentesis And Suction 穿刺和
抽吸

PS Paradoxical Sleep 反常睡眠; 睡眠倒
错

PS Pediatric Surgery 小儿外科

PS Peeling Superficial 剥离浅表

PS Permeability Surface 表面通透性

PS Phosphatidyl Serine 磷脂酰丝氨酸

PS Phrenic (Nerve) Stimulation 膈(神

经) 刺激

PS Physical Status 术前全身状态【注释】〔根据术前患者的全身状态, 将

手术危险度分为 5 类, 以此综合判断危

险性。是由美国麻醉学会(ASA) 进行的

分类, 紧急手术时皆用 E (Eme Rgency ,

紧急) 来表示〕

PS Physiological Saline 生理盐水

PS Plastic Surgery 整 形外科; 成形外

科; 整复外科

PS Polysaccharides 多 糖

PS Protein S S 蛋白【注释】〔一种新的维生素 K

依赖性蛋白

质, 作为 C 蛋白的辅助因子发挥抗凝作

用〕

Ps Pseudomonas 假 单胞菌; 绿脓假单

胞菌【注释】〔革兰氏阴性杆菌, 通常称为绿

脓杆菌〕

PS Pulmonary Stenosis 肺 动脉瓣狭窄;

肺动脉狭窄【注释】〔一种先天性心脏病〕

PS Pyloric Stenosis 幽门狭窄

PSA Poultry Science Association 家 禽

科学学会

PSA Problem Statement Analyzer 问 题

描述分析器

PSA Prostata Specific Antigen 前 列腺

特异抗原【注释】〔一种肿瘤标记物。取一滴血

液

滴于滤纸上, 自然干燥后即可测定, 用

于癌症早期普查〕

PSAGN Postst Reptococcal Acute
Glomerulonephritis 链 球菌感染后急性
肾小球肾炎

PSAGN Post-Streptococcus (Infection)
Acute Glomerulonephritis 溶 血性链球
菌感染后急性肾炎【注释】〔一种 IC 肾炎, 发病
早期血清补

PRS 475 PSA
体含量低, 肾小球基底膜上皮上可观察
到 IC〕

Psan Pseudoaneurysm 假动脉瘤

Psar Pseudoarthrosis 假关节

Psax Prostatic Specific Antigen 前 列腺
特异抗原

PSBR Pennsylvania Society For Biomedical
Research 宾 夕法尼亚州生物医学
研究会

PSC Posterior Subcapsular Cataract 后
囊下白内障

PSC Postsynaptic Current 突 触后电流

PSC Potential Sensitive Channel 电位敏
感性通道

PSC Primary Sclerosing Cholangitis 原
发性硬化性胆管炎【注释】〔以胆管弥漫性炎症
和纤维化及
伴有胆汁郁积为特征。它是导致肝硬
化的原因不明性疾病〕

Pscap Pseudocapsule 假包膜; 假被膜

Pscl Pseudoclaudication 假性跛行

Psco Psychotic 精神病的

Pscos Psychosis 精 神病

Pscy Pseudocyst 假性囊肿

PSD Pesticides Safety Directorate 农
药安全董事会

PSD Psychosomatic Disease 身心疾病 【注释】
〔从身心医学角度, 将身心作为
整体来考虑的疾病。狭义指由心的因
素产生的疾病(高血压、胃溃疡等), 广
义指与精神因素有关的身体疾病〕

Psdy Psychodynamic 心理动力的

Psdys Psychodynamics 精神动力学

PSE Photosensitive Eczema 光敏湿疹

PSE Present State Examination 精神现
状检查; 精神现状检查表 【注释】 〔以精神分裂症、
燥狂、神经病等
为主要对象, 由 140 项提问构成〕

Psfa Psychological Factors 心理因素

Psfes Psychotic Features 精神病特征

PSG Presystolic Gallop 收缩期前奔马律

PSGB Primate Society Of Great Britain
大英灵长类动物学会

Psge Psychogeriat Ric 老年精神病学的

Psgen Psychogenic 精神性的; 心因性的

Psges Psychogeriat Rics 老年精神病学

PSGN Poststreptococcal Glomerulonephritis
链球菌感染后肾小球肾炎

Psgo Pseudogout 假痛风; 软骨钙质沉
着病

PSH Postspinal (Anesthesia) Headache
脊椎麻醉后头痛 【注释】 〔用所谓的 Blood Patc H
法治疗有

效〕

Pshas Pseudohallucinations 假性幻觉

PSI Passive Suicidal Ideation 被动自杀观念

PSI Pharmaceutical Society Of Ireland 爱尔兰药物学会

PSI Presynaptic Inhibition 突触前抑制

PSIC Primate Supply Information Clearinghouse 灵长类动物提供信息情报交换所

Psil Psychiat Ric Illness 精神疾病

PSL Parasternal Line 胸骨旁线〔解〕

Lin Ea Pa Rastern Alis〔拉〕

PSM Presystolic Murmur 收缩前期杂音【注释】〔在第1心音之前出现, 为舒张期杂音的一种, 是由心房收缩导致〕

PSM Psychosomatic Medicine 身心医学【注释】〔指重视身心关系, 以身心一体化为主题的诊疗研究领域〕

PSMA Progressive Spinal Muscular At Rophy 进行性脊髓性肌萎缩

Psma Psychosomatic 心身的

Psme Pseudomembrane 伪膜

Psmen Pseudomeningocele 假性脑脊膜膨出

Psmeos Pseudomembranous 假膜的

Psmes Pseudomembranes 假膜

Psa 476 Psm

Psmo Pseudomonas 绿脓假单胞菌

Psno Pseudonormalization 假性正常化

PSO Physostigmine Salicylate Ophthalmic

毒扁豆碱水杨酸眼炎患者

Psor Psoriasis 牛皮癣; 银屑病

Psorc Psoriatic ① 牛皮癣的 ② 牛皮癣患者

P/ Sore Pressure Sore 褥疮

PSOS Polycystic Sclerotic Ovary Syndrome 多囊硬化性卵巢综合征

PSP Pancreatic Stone Protein 胰石蛋白【注释】〔与慢性胰腺炎相关的蛋白〕

PSP Phenolsulfonphthalein (Test) 酚磺酞; 酚红排泄试验【注释】〔一种观察肾小管功能的肾色素
排泄试验〕

PSP Postsynaptic Potential 突触后电位

Psph Pseudophakia 假晶状体

Psphc Pseudophakic 假晶状体的

PS(Ps) Pseudomonas 假单胞菌属

PSP Test Phenolsulfonphthalein Test 酚磺酞试验; 酚红试验

PSR Pain Sensitivity Range 疼痛敏感域 (范围)

PSR Patellar Tendon Reflex (Patellar-Sehnen-Reflex) 膝腱反射【注释】〔一种深部神经肌肉反射, 中枢
神经障碍时该反射亢进〕

PSR Proliferative Sickle (Cell) Retinopa - Thy 增生性镰状(细胞性) 视网膜病

Psre Psychomotor Retardation 精神运动性阻抑

PSS Painful Shoulder Syndrome 肩痛综

合征

PSS Physiologic Saline Solution 生 理盐
水溶液

PSS Porcine Stress Syndrome 猪 刺激综
合征; 猪应激综合征【注释】〔用猪制作的恶性高
热动物模
型〕

PSS Progressive Supranuclear Palsy 渐
进性核上性麻痹

PSS Progressive Systemic Scleroderma
渐进性全身性硬皮病

PSS Progressive Systemic Sclerosis 渐
进性系统性硬皮病【注释】〔以皮肤硬化病变为
特征, 关节、
肌肉、肌腱等的慢性泛发性结缔组织
病, 是一种胶原性疾病〕

PSSA Penicillin-Streptomycin Solution A
青霉素- 链霉素溶液 A

Psse(S) Pseudoseizure (S) 假 性癫痫发
作

PST Paroxysmal Supraventricular Tachycardia
阵发性室上性心动过速

PST Penicillin , St Reptomycin , And Tetracycline
青 霉素、链霉素和四环素

PST Perceptual Span Test 知 觉广度测
验

PST Postural Stress Test 姿 势性应力试
验

PST Protamine Sulfate Test 硫 酸鱼精蛋
白试验

PST Protein-Sparing Therapy 低 蛋白质

疗法

PSTI Pancreatic Secretory Trypsin Inhibitor
胰源性胰蛋白酶抑制剂【注释】〔作为重症胰腺炎、侵袭性炎症
和肿瘤标记物而被广泛应用〕

PSTI Protein Secretory Trypsin Inhibitor
蛋白分泌腺蛋白酶抑制物

Pstr Psychot Ropic 治疗精神病的

Pstu Pseudotumor 假瘤

Pstx Psychotherapy 心理疗法; 精神疗法

Pstxt Psychotherapist 精神疗法师

PSV Pressure Suppor T Ventilation 压力支持通气【注释】〔为帮助患者自主呼吸的一种辅
助性机械人工呼吸法。自吸气开始时开始, 于吸气流速最小时结束〕

Psm 477 PSV

PSVE Progressive Subcortical Vascular
Encephalopathy 进行性皮质下血管性脑病

PSVT Paroxysmal Supraventricular
Tachycardia 阵发性室上性心动过速【注释】〔虽然阵发性房性心动过速和阵
发性房室接合部心动过速可通过 P 波形态加以区别, 但当两者无法鉴别时,
笼统称之为 PSTV〕

Psw Pelvic Side Wall 骨盆侧壁

PSW Psychiatric Social Worker 精神病社会服务者; 精神病社会工作者【注释】〔通过生活方面的照料, 帮助精

神病患者解决各种问题的工作机构或个人〕

PSWC Periodic Sharp Wave Complexes 间歇性尖锐复合波

Psy Psychiat Ry 精 神病学

Psyc Psychiat Ric 精 神病学的

Psych Psychiat Ry / Psychiatrie 精 神病学/ 精神病学医生

PSYCHINFO Psychological Information 心 理学信息库〔美〕

Psychopath . Psychopathic 病 态人格的; 精神变态的

Psych Testing Psychological Testing 心 理测试

Psycl ,Psycly Psychiatrically 精 神病学地

Psyhx Psychiatric History 精 神病史

Psyol Psychological 心 理学的

Psyoly Psychologically 心 理学的

Psyt Psychiat Rist 精 神科医师; 精神病学家

PT Paroxysmal Tachycardia 发 作性心动过速【注释】〔突然心率加快又突然消失, 短者可持续数秒, 长者可持续 2 ～3 天〕

PT Par Tial- Thickness (Burn) 部 分皮肤层(烧伤)

PT Patch Test 斑 贴试验

PT Pericardial Tamponade 心 包填塞; 心包压塞

PT Physical Therapist 理疗师【注释】〔有时医学处置暂停的患者为使

其回到社会, 有必要对其脏器功能, 特
别是四肢、呼吸功能进行恢复性训练,
从事这种训练指导的康复专业技术人
员称为理疗师〕

PT Physiotherapy (Physical Therapy)
理疗【注释】〔与作业疗法共同构成康复医学
的 2 大疗法, 理疗包括运动疗法、动作
训练、水疗、热疗、按摩等〕

PT Posterior Tibial Pulse 胫 骨后动脉搏
动

PT Premature Termination 早 期终止
(妊娠)

PT Primary Thrombocytosis 原 发性血
小板增多症

PT Prothrombin Time 凝血酶原时间【注释】 〔血
液凝固异常的检查方法, 正
常值为 12～ 15 秒〕

PT Proximal Tubulopathy 近 端肾小管
病

PT Pulmonary Thrombosis 肺栓塞

PT Pulmonary Tuberculosis 肺结核

PT Pyramidal T Ract 锥体束

PTA Parathyroid Adenoma 甲 状旁腺腺
瘤

PTA Parent -Teacher Association 家
长教师联谊会

PTA Percutaneous T Ransluminal Angioplasty
经 皮腔内血管成形术【注释】 〔在动脉硬化等狭
窄动脉内插入
前端配有气囊的导管, 给位于狭窄处的

气囊充气,压挤扩展血管内腔使血流通畅的治疗方法。近年除用于手足等处的大动脉之外还用于肾动脉和冠状动脉〕

PTA Peritonsillar Abscess 扁 桃体周围脓肿

PSV 478 PTA

PTA Peritubal Adhesion 输卵管周粘连

PTA Plasma Thromboplastin Antecedent (FactorXI) 血 浆凝血激酶前体【注释】 〔即XI 因子,为一种接触因子,

参与内源性凝血过程,该因子缺乏症又称为 C 型血友病〕

PTA Postt Raumatic Amnesia 外 伤性遗忘症; 创伤后遗忘症

PTA Post- Traumatic Ar Thritis 创 伤后关节炎; 外伤性关节炎

PTA Primary Tubular Acidosis 原 发性肾小管性酸中毒

PTA Pure Tone Average 纯 音听阈均值

PTA (Factor XI) Plasma Thromboplastin Antecedent 血 浆凝血激酶前体(XI 因子)

Ptao T Ransmural Aor Tic Pressure 透壁主动脉压

PTAP Purified Toxoid Aluminium Phosphate 精制类毒素磷酸铝【注释】 〔一种预防注射用的白喉类毒素〕

PTB Par Tial- Thickness Burn 部 分皮层

烧伤; 非全层皮肤烧伤

PTB Prothrombin 凝血酶原

PTB Pulmonary Tuberculosis 肺结核

PTBA Percutaneous T Ransluminal Balloon Angioplasty 经 皮腔内气囊血管成 形术 【注释】 〔针对闭塞性末梢动脉硬化而实 施的经皮血管成形术〕

PTBD Percutaneous Transhepatic Biliary Drainage 经 皮经肝胆管引流术

PTC Papillary Thyroid Carcinoma 乳 头 状甲状腺癌

PTC Percutaneous Transhepatic Cholangiogram 经皮经肝胆管造影照片

PTC Percutaneous Transhepatic Cholangiography 经 皮经肝胆管造影术 【注释】 〔是将造影剂经皮 直接注入肝内 胆管的造影法〕

PTC Pheochromocytoma , Thyroid Carcinoma (Syndrome) (Multiple Endocrine Neoplasia , Type 2) 嗜 铬细胞瘤、甲状 腺瘤(综合征) 〔多发性内分泌肿瘤, II 型〕

PTC Plasma Thromboplastin Component 血浆凝血激酶成分 【注释】 〔指血浆凝固因子IX , 该因子缺 乏症又称为 B 型血友病〕

PTCA Percutaneous T Ranshepatic Cholangiogram 经皮经肝胆管造影照片

PTCA Percutaneous T Ransluminal Coronary Angioplasty 经 皮腔内冠状动脉成 形术 【注释】 〔用球囊导管挤压扩张冠状动

脉。紧急危重病人可在 PCPS 辅助下实
施。最近多使用无球囊的不锈钢管〕

PTCAS Percutaneous Transluminal Coronary
Angioscopy 经 皮腔内冠状动脉窥
镜法【注释】 〔不同于冠脉造影法, 是一种可
准确掌握病变部位的病理学诊断法。
可以观察再疏通手术的效果及采取预
防措施后的血管内腔状态〕

PTCB Percutaneous T Ranshepatic Cholangiobiopsy
经 皮肝穿刺胆管活检术

PTCCS Percutaneous T Ranshepatic Cholecystoscopy
经皮经肝胆囊镜检查(术)

PTCD Percutaneous Transhepatic Cholangial
Drainage 经 皮经肝胆管引流术

PTCD Percutaneous Transhepatic Cholangiodrainage
经皮经肝胆管引流术【注释】 〔胆结石或肿瘤堵
塞胆道可引发
黄疸, 此时从体表经由肝脏通入专用引
流管到肝胆管内, 使郁积的胆汁排出体
外。使用这种引流管还可去除胆结石
及进行激光照射等〕

PTCR Percutaneous Transluminal Coronary
Recanalization 经 皮腔内冠状动脉
开通(血栓溶解) 疗法【注释】 〔在冠状动脉内形
成血栓后血流

PTA 479 PTC
急剧减少。在早期, 可以将导管插入冠
状动脉内, 将溶血栓剂(激酶) 直接送到
血栓形成部位而使血栓溶解, 再开通血
管〕

PTCS Percutaneous Cardiopulmonary

System 经皮人造心肺系统【注释】〔心功能不全
或心源性休克导致
泵障碍时所采用的一种新型辅助循环
疗法, 为一种简易型人造心肺。它是经
皮导管使动脉-静脉搭桥术简易化〕

PTCS Percutaneous Transhepatic Cholangioscopy
经皮经肝胆管镜检查(术)

PTD Percutaneous Thrombolytic Device
经皮血栓溶解装置

Ptdcho Phosphatidylcholine 磷 脂酰胆
碱; 卵磷脂

Ptdeth Phosphatidylethanolamine 磷
脂酰乙醇胺

Ptdins Phosphatidylinositol 磷 脂酰肌
醇

PTE Pretibial Edema 胫骨前水肿

PTE Pulmonary Thromboembolism 肺
血栓栓塞症

PTF Plasma Thromboplastic Factor 血
浆凝血酶激酶因子; 血浆血小板因子【注释】 〔即
第Ⅷ 因子, 该因子缺乏症又
称为 A 型血友病〕

PTF Post- Tetanic Facilitation 破 伤风刺
激后增强【注释】 〔在 1 秒时间内, 对末梢神经施
以 20～ 50 次的电刺激时, 破伤风引起
的痉挛会迅速减弱。而当终止刺激后,
再遇到单一刺激时, 破伤风性痉挛会短
时间增强〕

PTF-A Plasma Thromboplastin Factor A
血 浆促凝血酶原激酶因子 A

PTFR Polymorphisme De Taille Des Fragments De Restriction 限制性片段长度多态

PTG Plethysmogram 体积描记图

PTGC Percutaneous T Ranshepatic Gallbladder Catheterization 经皮经肝胆囊插管

PTH Parathyroid Hormone 甲状旁腺素; 甲状旁腺激素【注释】〔由甲状旁腺分泌的, 参与钙、磷代谢的激素。正常值为 0 . 3 ～ 1 .2ng/ Ml〕

PTH Post- Transfusion Hepatitis 输血后肝炎; 输血性肝炎

PTH Prothionamide 丙硫异烟胺〔抗结核药〕

PTH-C Parathyroid Hormoni-C (- Terminal) 甲状旁腺激素-C(- 末端)

PTH(Pth) Primary Thrombocythemia 原发性血小板增多

Pthrp PTH-Related Proteins 甲状旁腺素相关蛋白

PTI Pictorial Test Of Intelligence 绘画智力测验

PTIA Pet Trade And Industry Association 宠物交易和工业学会

PTL Proliferative T Lymphocyte 增生性 T 淋巴细胞

PTLD Post Transplantation Lymphoproliferative Disorder 移植后淋巴结增生性病变【注释】〔外科移植手术后, 因使用了免

疫抑制剂而导致的感染所引起的淋巴
结增生性病变〕

PTLV Prime T-Lymphot Ropic Viruses
灵长类 T 细胞白血病病毒【注释】〔是指 HTLV
和 STLV 的总称,
包括 PTLV- Ⅰ 及 PTLV- Ⅱ〕

PTM Pretibial Myxoedema 胫骨前黏液
性水肿

PTOL Prior To Onset Of Labor 产 程开始
前

PTP Press Through Package 压 板包装【注释】〔将
药粒放在两片板材之间, 施
压后将药粒包装起来, 药粒突出于正
面, 所用板材为高强度透明塑料, 底面

PTC 480 PTP
板材为特殊用纸, 易于挤破而便于取出
药粒。此种包装保存性能好, 卫生美
观, 携带方便。目前许多药剂均采用此
种包装〕

PTR Patellar Tendon Reflex 膝 反射

PTS Permanent Threshold Shif T (Noise
Induced) 永久性阈移

PTS Post- Thoracotomy Pain Syndrome
开胸术后疼痛综合征【注释】〔因手术操作时损
伤肋间神经而
引起的神经原性疼痛。不易治愈〕

PTSD Post- T Raumatic St Ress Disorder
心灵创伤后应激性精神障碍; 外伤后紧张
综合征【注释】〔病人遭受心灵创伤后出现的一
种主诉为全身不适、异常痛苦的精神障
碍〕

PTSR Post-T Raumatic Stress Reaction
心灵创伤后应激反应【注释】〔超过通常范围, 通
过几乎所有
的重创经历为契机而发现的精神方面
的反应〕

PTT Phenol Turbidity Test 酚 浊度试验

PTT Protein Tolerance Test 蛋白耐受试
验

PTT Par Tial Thromboplastin Time 部 分
促凝血酶原激酶时间【注释】〔为一种血液凝固
异常检查法。
最近采用能够快速得到检查结果的活
化部分凝血酶时间(APT T) 方法〕

Pttx Par Tial Thromboplastin Time 部 分
凝血致活酶时间

PTU Propyl Thiouracil 丙 硫脲嘧啶【注释】〔一种
抗甲状腺亢进药, 具有抑
制甲状腺素合成的作用〕

PTU Propylthiouracil 丙 硫氧嘧啶〔抗甲
状腺药〕

PTV Patient T Rigger Ventilation 患者扳
机式同步呼吸【注释】〔一种人工呼吸器。利用
患者的
微弱呼吸作为扳机, 控制人工呼吸器与
患者的呼吸同步〕

P Tx Pelvic T Raction 骨 盆牵引

PTX Parathyroidectomy 甲 状旁腺切除
术

P .Tx Pelvic Traction 骨盆牵引

PTX Pneumothorax 气胸

Ptxes Pneumothoraces 气胸

PU Per Urethra 经尿道; 经尿道

PU Pyloric Ulcer 幽门溃疡

Puar Pulmonary Artery 肺动脉

Puat Pulmonary Atresia 肺动脉瓣闭锁

Pubi Punch Biopsy 钻取活组织检查

PUBS Percutaneous Umbilical Blood
Sampling 经皮脐带采血【注释】〔胎血采集方法〕

Pucon Pulmonary Consultation 肺动脉
收缩压

PUD Peptic Ulcer Disease 消化性溃疡
病

Pud Pulmonary Disease 肺部疾病

Pudi Purulent Discharge 浓脓

Pudie Pureed Diet 泥状饮食

Pudr Purulent Drainage 脓性排出物

Pudx Peptic Ulcer Disease 消化性溃疡
病

Pued Pulmonary Edema 肺水肿

Puem Pulmonary Embolus 肺动脉栓子

Puemb Pulmonary Emboli 肺动脉栓子

PUF Peak Urinary Flow Rate 最大尿流
速

Pufi Pulmonary Fibrosis 肺纤维化

Puf J Pulmonary Function 肺功能

Pufl Purulent Fluid 脓液

PUH Pregnancy Urine Hormone 孕尿激
素

Puhn Pulmonary Hyper Tension 肺动脉

高血压; 肺动脉血压过高

Pulv Pulverized , Powder 研 磨成粉的;
粉剂

PULV (Pulv .) Pulveres 〔拉〕散剂

Puly Pulmonary 肺 的; 肺部的

PTR 481 Pul

PUN Plasma Urea Nit Rogen 血浆尿素氮

Pup Pupil 瞳 孔 〔解〕

Pupa Pulsus Paradoxus 奇 脉; 逆脉

PUPP(P) Pruritic Urticarial Papules And
Plaques (Of Pregnancy) 妊 娠搔痒性风
团性丘疹和斑块

Pupr Puboprostatic 耻骨前列腺的

Pups Pupils 瞳 孔

PU(Pu) Peptic Ulcer 消化性溃疡

Pura Pubic Ramus 耻 骨支

Pura Urethral Pressure 尿 道压力

Purat Pulse Rate 脉搏率
脉振

Pusaj Pulsation 搏 动

Pusajs Pulsations 跳动; 搏动

Pusal Pulsatile 搏动的

Puves Pulmonary Veins 肺静脉 〔解〕

PV Papilloma Virus 乳头瘤病毒

PV Plasma Volume 血浆容量

PV Poliomyelitis Virus 脊髓灰质炎病毒

PV Polycythemia Vera 真性红细胞增多
症【注释】〔一种以慢性经过、原因不明的
骨髓增生性疾病。伴有脾肿大, 多因血
栓或出血而致死。又称奥- 瓦二氏病〕

PV Portal Vein 门静脉

PV Pulmonary Valve 肺动脉瓣【注释】〔心脏超
声波检查用语〕

PV Pulmonary Vein 肺静脉

P&V Pyloroplasty And Vagotomy 幽门
成形术和迷走神经切断术

Pyul Pyloric Ulcer 幽门溃疡

Pyy Polypectomy 息肉切除术

Pyys Polypectomies 息肉切除术
肺动脉狭窄【注释】〔一种先天性心脏病〕

PS Pyloric Stenosis 幽门狭窄

PSA Poultry Science Association 家禽
科学学会

PSA Problem Statement Analyzer 问题
描述分析器

PSA Prostata Specific Antigen 前列腺
特异抗原【注释】〔一种肿瘤标记物。取一滴血
液
滴于滤纸上,自然干燥后即可测定,用
于癌症早期普查〕

PSAGN Postst Reptococcal Acute
Glomerulonephritis 链球菌感染后急性
肾小球肾炎

PSAGN Post-Streptococcus (Infection)
Acute Glomerulonephritis 溶血性链球
菌感染后急性肾炎【注释】〔一种 IC 肾炎, 发病
早期血清补

PRS 475 PSA
体含量低, 肾小球基底膜上皮上可观察
到 IC〕

Psan Pseudoaneurysm 假动脉瘤

Psar Pseudoarthrosis 假关节

Psax Prostatic Specific Antigen 前列腺

精神动力学

光敏湿疹

多囊硬化性卵巢综合征

PSP Pancreatic Stone Protein 胰石蛋白【注释】
〔与慢性胰腺炎相关的蛋白〕

PSP Phenolsulfonphthalein (Test) 酚
磺酞; 酚红排泄试验【注释】〔一种观察肾小管功
能的肾色素
排泄试验〕

PSP Postsynaptic Potential 突触后电位

Psph Pseudophakia 假晶状体

Psphc Pseudophakic 假晶状体的

PS(Ps) Pseudomonas 假单胞菌属

PSP Test Phenolsulfonphthalein Test 酚
磺酞试验; 酚红试验

PSR Pain Sensitivity Range 疼痛敏感域
(范围)

PSR Patellar Tendon Reflex (Patellar-
Sehnen-Reflex) 膝腱反射【注释】〔一种深部神经
肌肉反射, 中枢
神经障碍时该反射亢进〕

PSR Proliferative Sickle (Cell) Retinopa -
Thy 增生性镰状(细胞性) 视网膜病

Psre Psychomotor Retardation 精神运
动性阻抑

PSS Painful Shoulder Syndrome 肩痛综
合征

PSS Physiologic Saline Solution 生理盐
水溶液

PSS Porcine Stress Syndrome 猪刺激综
合征; 猪应激综合征【注释】〔用猪制作的恶性高
热动物模
型〕

PSS Progressive Supranuclear Palsy 渐
进性核上性麻痹

PSS Progressive Systemic Scleroderma
渐进性全身性硬皮病

PSS Progressive Systemic Sclerosis 渐
进性系统性硬皮病【注释】〔以皮肤硬化病变为
特征, 关节、
肌肉、肌腱等的慢性泛发性结缔组织
病, 是一种胶原性疾病〕

PSSA Penicillin-Streptomycin Solution A
青霉素- 链霉素溶液 A

Psse(S) Pseudoseizure (S) 假性癫痫发
作

PST Paroxysmal Supraventricular Tachycardia
阵发性室上性心动过速

PST Penicillin , St Reptomycin , And Tetracycline
青霉素、链霉素和四环素

PST Perceptual Span Test 知觉广度测
验

PST Postural Stress Test 姿势性应力试
验

PST Protamine Sulfate Test 硫酸鱼精蛋
白试验

PST Protein-Sparing Therapy 低蛋白质
疗法

PSTI Pancreatic Secretory Trypsin Inhibitor
胰 源性胰蛋白酶抑制剂【注释】〔作为重症胰腺
炎、侵袭性炎症
和肿瘤标记物而被广泛应用〕
PSTI Protein Secretory Trypsin Inhibitor
蛋白分泌腺蛋白酶抑制物
Pstr Psychot Ropic 治 疗精神病的
Pstu Pseudotumor 假瘤
Pstx Psychotherapy 心 理疗法; 精神疗
法
Pstxt Psychotherapist 精神疗法师
PSV Pressure Suppor T Ventilation 压 力
支持通气【注释】〔为帮助患者自主呼吸的一种
辅
助性机械人工呼吸法。自吸气开始时
开始, 于吸气流速最小时结束〕
Psm 477 PSV
PSVE Progressive Subcortical Vascular
Encephalopathy 进 行性皮质下血管性
脑病
PSVT Paroxysmal Supraventricular
Tachycardia 阵发性室上性心动过速【注释】〔虽
然阵发性房性心动过速和阵
发性房室接合部心动过速可通过 P 波
形态加以区别, 但当两者无法鉴别时,
笼统称之为 PSTV〕
Psw Pelvic Side Wall 骨盆侧壁
PSW Psychiatric Social Worker 精 神病
社会服务者; 精神病社会工作者【注释】〔通过生
活方面的照料, 帮助精
神病患者解决各种问题的工作机构或

个人〕

PSWC Periodic Sharp Wave Complexes 间歇性尖锐复合波

Psy Psychiat Ry 精 神病学

Psyc Psychiat Ric 精 神病学的

Psych Psychiat Ry / Psychiatrie 精 神病学/ 精神病学医生

PSYCHINFO Psychological Information 心 理学信息库〔美〕

Psychopath . Psychopathic 病 态人格的; 精神变态的

Psych Testing Psychological Testing 心 理测试

Psycl ,Psycly Psychiatrically 精 神病学地

Psyhx Psychiatric History 精 神病史

Psyol Psychological 心 理学的

Psyoly Psychologically 心 理学的

Psyt Psychiat Rist 精 神科医师; 精神病学家

PT Paroxysmal Tachycardia 发 作性心动过速【注释】〔突然心率加快又突然消失, 短者可持续数秒, 长者可持续 2 ～3 天〕

PT Par Tial- Thickness (Burn) 部 分皮肤层(烧伤)

PT Patch Test 斑 贴试验

PT Pericardial Tamponade 心 包填塞; 心包压塞

PT Physical Therapist 理疗师【注释】〔有时医学处置暂停的患者为使其回到社会, 有必要对其脏器功能, 特

别是四肢、呼吸功能进行恢复性训练,
从事这种训练指导的康复专业技术人
员称为理疗师〕

PT Physiotherapy (Physical Therapy)
理疗【注释】〔与作业疗法共同构成康复医学
的 2 大疗法, 理疗包括运动疗法、动作
训练、水疗、热疗、按摩等〕

PT Posterior Tibial Pulse 胫 骨后动脉搏
动

PT Premature Termination 早 期终止
(妊娠)

PT Primary Thrombocytosis 原 发性血
小板增多症

PT Prothrombin Time 凝血酶原时间【注释】 〔血
液凝固异常的检查方法, 正
常值为 12～ 15 秒〕

PT Proximal Tubulopathy 近 端肾小管
病

PT Pulmonary Thrombosis 肺栓塞

PT Pulmonary Tuberculosis 肺结核

PT Pyramidal T Ract 锥体束

PTA Parathyroid Adenoma 甲 状旁腺腺
瘤

PTA Parent -Teacher Association 家
长教师联谊会

PTA Percutaneous T Ransluminal Angioplasty
经 皮腔内血管成形术【注释】 〔在动脉硬化等狭
窄动脉内插入
前端配有气囊的导管, 给位于狭窄处的
气囊充气, 压挤扩展血管内腔使血流通

畅的治疗方法。近年除用于手足等处
的大动脉之外还用于肾动脉和冠状动
脉〕

PTA Peritonsillar Abscess 扁桃体周围
脓肿

PSV 478 PTA

PTA Peritubal Adhesion 输卵管周粘连

PTA Plasma Thromboplastin Antecedent
(FactorXI) 血浆凝血激酶前体【注释】 〔即XI 因
子, 为一种接触因子,
参与内源性凝血过程, 该因子缺乏症又
称为 C 型血友病〕

PTA Postt Raumatic Amnesia 外 伤性遗
忘症; 创伤后遗忘症

PTA Post- Traumatic Ar Thritis 创 伤后关
节炎; 外伤性关节炎

PTA Primary Tubular Acidosis 原 发性
肾小管性酸中毒

PTA Pure Tone Average 纯 音听阈均值

PTA (Factor XI) Plasma Thromboplastin
Antecedent 血 浆凝血激酶前体(XI
因子)

Ptao T Ransmural Aor Tic Pressure 透壁主
动脉压

PTAP Purified Toxoid Aluminium Phosphate
精制类毒素磷酸铝【注释】 〔一种预防注射用的
白喉类毒
素〕

PTB Par Tial- Thickness Burn 部 分皮层
烧伤; 非全层皮肤烧伤

PTB Prothrombin 凝血酶原

PTB Pulmonary Tuberculosis 肺结核

PTBA Percutaneous T Ransluminal Balloon Angioplasty 经皮腔内气囊血管成形术【注释】〔针对闭塞性末梢动脉硬化而实施的经皮血管成形术〕

PTBD Percutaneous Transhepatic Biliary Drainage 经皮经肝胆管引流术

PTC Papillary Thyroid Carcinoma 乳头状甲状腺癌

PTC Percutaneous Transhepatic Cholangiogram 经皮经肝胆管造影照片

PTC Percutaneous Transhepatic Cholangiography 经皮经肝胆管造影术【注释】〔是将造影剂经皮直接注入肝内胆管的造影法〕

PTC Pheochromocytoma , Thyroid Carcinoma (Syndrome) (Multiple Endocrine Neoplasia , Type 2) 嗜铬细胞瘤、甲状腺瘤(综合征)〔多发性内分泌肿瘤,Ⅱ型〕

PTC Plasma Thromboplastin Component 血浆凝血激酶成分【注释】〔指血浆凝固因子Ⅸ,该因子缺乏症又称为 B 型血友病〕

PTCA Percutaneous T Ranshepatic Cholangiogram 经皮经肝胆管造影照片

PTCA Percutaneous T Ransluminal Coronary Angioplasty 经皮腔内冠状动脉成形术【注释】〔用球囊导管挤压扩张冠状动脉。紧急危重病人可在 PCPS 辅助下实

施。最近多使用无球囊的不锈钢管〕

PTCAS Percutaneous Transluminal Coronary
Angioscopy 经皮腔内冠状动脉窥
镜法【注释】〔不同于冠脉造影法, 是一种可
准确掌握病变部位的病理学诊断法。
可以观察再疏通手术的效果及采取预
防措施后的血管内腔状态〕

PTCB Percutaneous T Ranshepatic Cholangiobiopsy
经皮肝穿刺胆管活检术

PTCCS Percutaneous T Ranshepatic Cholecystoscopy
经皮经肝胆囊镜检查(术)

PTCD Percutaneous Transhepatic Cholangial
Drainage 经皮经肝胆管引流术

PTCD Percutaneous Transhepatic Cholangiodrainage
经皮经肝胆管引流术【注释】〔胆结石或肿瘤堵
塞胆道可引发
黄疸, 此时从体表经由肝脏通入专用引
流管到肝胆管内, 使郁积的胆汁排出体
外。使用这种引流管还可去除胆结石
及进行激光照射等〕

PTCR Percutaneous Transluminal Coronary
Recanalization 经皮腔内冠状动脉
开通(血栓溶解)疗法【注释】〔在冠状动脉内形
成血栓后血流

PTA 479 PTC
急剧减少。在早期, 可以将导管插入冠
状动脉内, 将溶血栓剂(激酶)直接送到
血栓形成部位而使血栓溶解, 再开通血
管〕

PTCS Percutaneous Cardiopulmonary

System 经 皮人造心肺系统【注释】〔心功能不全
或心源性休克导致
泵障碍时所采用的一种新型辅助循环
疗法,为一种简易型人造心肺。它是经
皮导管使动脉-静脉搭桥术简易化〕

PTCS Percutaneous Transhepatic Cholangioscopy
经皮经肝胆管镜检查(术)

PTD Percutaneous Thrombolytic Device
经皮血栓溶解装置

Ptdcho Phosphatidylcholine 磷 脂酰胆
碱; 卵磷脂

Ptdeth Phosphatidylethanolamine 磷
脂酰乙醇胺

Ptdins Phosphatidylinositol 磷 脂酰肌
醇

PTE Pretibial Edema 胫骨前水肿

PTE Pulmonary Thromboembolism 肺
血栓栓塞症

PTF Plasma Thromboplastic Factor 血
浆凝血酶激酶因子; 血浆血小板因子【注释】〔即
第VIII 因子, 该因子缺乏症又
称为 A 型血友病〕

PTF Post- Tetanic Facilitation 破 伤风刺
激后增强【注释】〔在 1 秒时间内, 对末梢神经施
以 20～ 50 次的电刺激时, 破伤风引起
的痉挛会迅速减弱。而当终止刺激后,
再遇到单一刺激时, 破伤风性痉挛会短
时间增强〕

PTF-A Plasma Thromboplastin Factor A
血 浆促凝血酶原激酶因子 A

PTFR Polymorphisme De Taille Des Fragments De Restriction 限制性片段长度多态

PTG Plethysmogram 体积描记图

PTGC Percutaneous T Ranshepatic Gallbladder Catheterization 经皮经肝胆囊插管

PTH Parathyroid Hormone 甲状旁腺素; 甲状旁腺激素【注释】〔由甲状旁腺分泌的, 参与钙、磷代谢的激素。正常值为 0 . 3 ～ 1 .2ng/ Ml〕

PTH Post- Transfusion Hepatitis 输血后肝炎; 输血性肝炎

PTH Prothionamide 丙硫异烟胺〔抗结核药〕

PTH-C Parathyroid Hormoni-C (- Terminal) 甲状旁腺激素-C(- 末端)

PTH(Pth) Primary Thrombocythemia 原发性血小板增多

Pthrp PTH-Related Proteins 甲状旁腺素相关蛋白

PTI Pictorial Test Of Intelligence 绘画智力测验

PTIA Pet Trade And Industry Association 宠物交易和工业学会

PTL Proliferative T Lymphocyte 增生性 T 淋巴细胞

PTLD Post Transplantation Lymphoproliferative Disorder 移植后淋巴结增生性病变【注释】〔外科移植手术后, 因使用了免

疫抑制剂而导致的感染所引起的淋巴
结增生性病变〕

PTLV Prime T-Lymphot Ropic Viruses
灵长类 T 细胞白血病病毒【注释】〔是指 HTLV
和 STLV 的总称,
包括 PTLV-Ⅰ及 PTLV-Ⅱ〕

PTM Pretibial Myxoedema 胫骨前黏液
性水肿

PTOL Prior To Onset Of Labor 产 程开始
前

PTP Press Through Package 压 板包装【注释】〔将
药粒放在两片板材之间, 施
压后将药粒包装起来, 药粒突出于正
面, 所用板材为高强度透明塑料, 底面

PTC 480 PTP
板材为特殊用纸, 易于挤破而便于取出
药粒。此种包装保存性能好, 卫生美
观, 携带方便。目前许多药剂均采用此
种包装〕

PTR Patellar Tendon Reflex 膝 反射

PTS Permanent Threshold Shif T (Noise
Induced) 永久性阈移

PTS Post- Thoracotomy Pain Syndrome
开胸术后疼痛综合征【注释】〔因手术操作时损
伤肋间神经而
引起的神经原性疼痛。不易治愈〕

PTSD Post- T Raumatic St Ress Disorder
心灵创伤后应激性精神障碍; 外伤后紧张
综合征【注释】〔病人遭受心灵创伤后出现的一
种主诉为全身不适、异常痛苦的精神障
碍〕

PTSR Post-T Raumatic Stress Reaction
心灵创伤后应激反应【注释】〔超过通常范围, 通过几乎所有
的重创经历为契机而发现的精神方面
的反应〕

PTT Phenol Turbidity Test 酚 浊度试验

PTT Protein Tolerance Test 蛋白耐受试
验

PTT Par Tial Thromboplastin Time 部 分
促凝血酶原激酶时间【注释】〔为一种血液凝固
异常检查法。
最近采用能够快速得到检查结果的活
化部分凝血酶时间(APT T) 方法〕

Pttx Par Tial Thromboplastin Time 部 分
凝血致活酶时间

PTU Propyl Thiouracil 丙 硫脲嘧啶【注释】〔一种
抗甲状腺亢进药, 具有抑
制甲状腺素合成的作用〕

PTU Propylthiouracil 丙 硫氧嘧啶 〔抗甲
状腺药〕

PTV Patient T Rigger Ventilation 患者扳
机式同步呼吸【注释】〔一种人工呼吸器。利用
患者的
微弱呼吸作为扳机, 控制人工呼吸器与
患者的呼吸同步〕

P Tx Pelvic T Raction 骨 盆牵引

PTX Parathyroidectomy 甲 状旁腺切除
术

P .Tx Pelvic Traction 骨盆牵引

PTX Pneumothorax 气胸

Ptxes Pneumothoraces 气胸

PU Per Urethra 经尿道; 经尿道

PU Pyloric Ulcer 幽门溃疡

Puar Pulmonary Artery 肺动脉

Puat Pulmonary Atresia 肺动脉瓣闭锁

Pubi Punch Biopsy 钻取活组织检查

PUBS Percutaneous Umbilical Blood
Sampling 经皮脐带采血【注释】〔胎血采集方法〕

Pucon Pulmonary Consultation 肺动脉
收缩压

PUD Peptic Ulcer Disease 消化性溃疡
病

Pud Pulmonary Disease 肺部疾病

Pudi Purulent Discharge 浓脓

Pudie Pureed Diet 泥状饮食

Pudr Purulent Drainage 脓性排出物

Pudx Peptic Ulcer Disease 消化性溃疡
病

Pued Pulmonary Edema 肺水肿

Puem Pulmonary Embolus 肺动脉栓子

Puemb Pulmonary Emboli 肺动脉栓子

PUF Peak Urinary Flow Rate 最大尿流
速

Pufi Pulmonary Fibrosis 肺纤维化

Puf J Pulmonary Function 肺功能

Pufl Purulent Fluid 脓液

PUH Pregnancy Urine Hormone 孕尿激
素

Puhn Pulmonary Hyper Tension 肺动脉

高血压; 肺动脉血压过高

Pulv Pulverized , Powder 研 磨成粉的; 粉剂

PULV (Pulv .) Pulveres 〔拉〕散剂

Puly Pulmonary 肺 的; 肺部的

PTR 481 Pul

PUN Plasma Urea Nit Rogen 血浆尿素氮

Pup Pupil 瞳 孔 〔解〕

Pupa Pulsus Paradoxus 奇 脉; 逆脉

PUPP(P) Pruritic Urticarial Papules And Plaques (Of Pregnancy) 妊 娠搔痒性风团性丘疹和斑块

Pupr Puboprostatic 耻骨前列腺的

Pups Pupils 瞳 孔

PU(Pu) Peptic Ulcer 消化性溃疡

Pura Pubic Ramus 耻 骨支

Pura Urethral Pressure 尿 道压力

Purat Pulse Rate 脉搏率

Puru Purulent 脓 性的; 化脓的

Puruc Purulence ① 脓性; 化脓② 脓; 脓液

Purxs Pupillary Reflexes 瞳孔反射

Pusa Pulsate 搏动

Pusag Pulsating 搏 动的; 脉冲; 脉动; 脉振

Pusaj Pulsation 搏 动

Pusajs Pulsations 跳动; 搏动

Pusal Pulsatile 搏动的

Pusp Purulent Sputum 脓性痰

Pusta Pulmonary Status 肺功能状态

Pustes Pulsed Steroids 脉冲式类固醇

Puti Pulsatile 搏动的

Puto Pulmonary Toilet 肺创口洗涤

Putu Pubic Tubercle 耻骨结节〔解〕

PUV Pelvic Urethral Valve 骨盆尿道瓣

PUVA Psolaren Ultraviolet A (Therapy)
补骨脂素和紫外线 A 照射(光化学疗
法)【注释】〔一种将诱晒剂与长波紫外光结
合在一起的光化学疗法, 用于治疗皮肤
病〕

Puvas Pulmonary Vascular 肺血管的

Puve Pubovesical 耻骨膀胱的

Puves Pulmonary Veins 肺静脉〔解〕

PV Papilloma Virus 乳头瘤病毒

PV Plasma Volume 血浆容量

PV Poliomyelitis Virus 脊髓灰质炎病毒

PV Polycythemia Vera 真性红细胞增多
症【注释】〔一种以慢性经过、原因不明的
骨髓增生性疾病。伴有脾肿大, 多因血
栓或出血而致死。又称奥- 瓦二氏病〕

PV Portal Vein 门静脉

P/ V Pressure-To-Volume Ratio 压力与
体积比率

PV Pulmonary Valve 肺动脉瓣【注释】〔心脏超
声波检查用语〕

PV Pulmonary Vein 肺静脉

P&V Pyloroplasty And Vagotomy 幽门
成形术和迷走神经切断术

PVA Paralyzed Veterans Of America 美
国瘫痪退伍军人

PVA Population Viability Analysis 种群
生存力分析(动)

PVA Pulmonic Valve At Resia 肺 动脉瓣
闭锁

PVC Polyvinyl Chloride 聚氯乙烯

PVC Premature Ventricular Contraction
(Same As VPB) 室 性期前收缩; 室性
早搏

PVC Pulmonary Venous Congestion 肺
静脉充血

PVCM Paradoxical Vocal Cord Motion
反常的声带运动声带反常运动

Pvco Pulmonary Vascular Congestion 肺
血管充血

Pvco2 Venous Carbon Dioxide Pressure
静脉二氧化碳压

PVD Peripheral Vascular Disease 末 梢
血管病

Pvdx Peripheral Vascular Disease 末 梢
血管病

PVE Premature Ventricular Extrasystole
室性期前收缩室性早搏

PVE Prosthetic Valve Endocarditis 人
工瓣膜心内膜炎

Pves Vesical Pressure 膀胱压力

PUN 482 Pve

PVF Por Tal Venous Flow 门 静脉血流
(量)

PVF Primary Ventricular Fibrillation 原
发性室性纤维性颤动

PVG Pneumovent Riculogram (Phy) 脑

室充气摄影【注释】〔将气体注入脑室内后进行 X 线

摄影的脑病诊断方法。通过这种检查, 可诊断畸形、脑肿瘤、大脑水肿等〕

PVH Prolonged Viral Hepatitis 延迟性 病毒性肝炎

PVI Primary Valvular Incompetence 原 发性瓣膜闭锁不全

PVNO Poly-2-Vinylpyridine-N-Oxide 克矽平; 聚-2-乙烯吡啶-N- 氧化物〔治矽 肺药〕

PVNS Pigmented Villonodular Synovitis 色素性绒毛结节性滑膜炎

Pvo Partal Venous Oxygen Pressure 静 脉氧分压

Pvo2 Portal Vein Occlusion 门静脉闭塞

PVP Peripheral Venous Pressure 外 周 静脉压

PVP Polyvinylpyrrolidone 聚 乙烯吡咯 烷酮【注释】〔以前作为代用血浆使用, 现已 淘汰〕

PVP Portal Vein Perfusion 门静脉灌注

PVP Portalvein Pressure 门 脉压【注释】〔门脉压 的正常范围为 18 ～

180mmh2o, 超过此值称为门脉压亢 进〕

PVR Paroxysmal Ventricular Rhythm 阵发性室性节律

PVR Peripheral (Vascular) Resistance 外周(血管) 阻力

Pvr Postvoiding Residual 排尿后残余

PVR Progressive Vit Reous Ret Raction 进
行性玻璃体牵引

PVR Proliferative Vit Reoretinopathy 增
生性玻璃体视网膜病变【注释】〔指合并于视网
膜脱落的眼内细
胞增生〕

PVR Prosthetic Valve Replacement 人
工瓣膜置换

PVR Pulmonary Vascular Resistance 肺
血管阻力【注释】〔血液从右心室射出到达左心
房
为止的肺血管内所受阻力的总和〕

PVS Pig Veterinary Society 猪 兽医学
会

PVS Premature Ventricular Systole 室
性期前收缩

PVS Programmed Ventricular Stimulation
程 序性心室刺激

PVS Pulmonary Valvular Stenosis 肺 动
脉瓣狭窄

PVS Pulmonary Vein Stenosis 肺静脉狭
窄

PVSM Pulmonary Vascular Smooth Muscle
肺 血管平滑肌

PVT Paroxysmal Vent Ricular Tachycardia
阵发性室性心动过速【注释】〔起源于心室, RP
间隔缩短、不
齐, QRS-T 变形, QRS 峰尖与 T 波方
向相反, 波幅变宽, 有时与 T 波融合〕

PVY Potato Virus Y 马铃薯 Y 病毒

PW Peristaltic Wave 蠕动波

PW Posterior Wall 后壁〔解〕Par Ies Post
Er Ior〔拉〕

Pwas P-Waves P 波

PWC Payne Whitney Clinic 佩 恩惠特
尼诊所

PWD Precipitated Withdrawal Diarrhea
突然撤药性腹泻

PWI Posterior Wall Infarct 后壁(心肌)
梗塞

PWM Pokeweed Mitogen 美 州商陆丝
裂素; 商陆有丝分裂原【注释】〔从美州商陆中提
取的一种植物
凝集素。在 T 细胞存在的条件下, 促进
B 细胞分化为产生抗体的细胞〕

PWP Pulmonary Capillary Wedge Pressure
肺 毛细血管楔压

PVF 483 PWP

PWP Pulmonary Wedge Pressure 肺 动
脉楔压

PWS Port-Wine Stains 葡 萄酒色痣; 焰
色痣

Pwtd End-Diastolic Thickness Of Posterior
Wall 舒 张末期后壁厚度【注释】〔可用超声心动
图测量, 正常值
为 8 .8 ±1 .3mm〕

Pwts End-Systolic Thickness Of Posterior
Wall 收 缩末期后壁厚度【注释】〔可用超声心动
图测量, 正常值
为 15 .7± 2 .4mm〕

PWV Pulse Wave Velocity 脉 搏波传播
速度【注释】〔脉膊波传播速度比血液流速

快, 大动脉为 3～5m/ 秒, 中动脉为 7～
10m/ 秒, 小动脉为 15～35m/ 秒〕

Px Pneumothorax 气 胸

Px Prednisone 去 氢可的松

PXE Pseudoxanthoma Elasticum 弹 性
(纤维) 假黄瘤

Pych Pyloric Channel 幽门管

Pyd Polypoid 息肉状的

Pydh Pyruvate Dehydrogenase 丙 酮酸
脱氢酶

PYE Peptone Yeast Ext Ract (Medium)
蛋白胨酵母提取物(培养基)

PYG Peptone Yeast (Extract) Glucose (A -
Gar/ Broth) 蛋 白胨-酵母(提取物) -葡萄
糖(琼脂/ 肉汤培养基)

PYGM Peptone-Yeast Glucose Maltose
(Agar/ Broth) 蛋 白胨- 酵母-葡萄糖-麦
芽糖(琼脂/ 肉汤培养基)

Pygr Pyelogram 肾盂 X 线照片

Pyl Pylorus 幽 门; 幽门口 Ostium Pyloricum
〔拉〕

Pylc Pyloric 幽门的

Pyne Pyelonephritis 肾 盂肾炎

Pyo Bacillus Pyocyaneus 绿 脓杆菌【注释】 〔革兰
氏阴性厌氧菌, 产生绿色
色素以及荧光色素。 具有很强的对消
毒剂和抗菌剂的抵抗能力〕

Pypl Pyloroplasty 幽 门成形术

Pypo Polyposis 息肉病; 多发性息肉

Pys Polyps 息 肉

Pyst Pyloric Stenosis 幽门狭窄

Pyul Pyloric Ulcer 幽门溃疡

Pyy Polypectomy 息肉切除术

Pyys Polypectomies 息肉切除术

PZ Perphenazine 奋乃静; 羟哌氯丙嗪

PZA Pyrazinamide 吡嗪酰胺【注释】〔为一种结核病复发时所使用的
治疗药〕

PZI Protamine Zinc Insulin 鱼精蛋白锌胰岛素【注释】〔一种长效胰岛素〕

Pznr Positioner 矫正固位器

PWP 484 Pzn

Japanese

略語	日本語の意味	スペル
P	圧	Pressure
	後の	Posterior
	位置	Position
	確率	Probability
	計画	Plan
	血漿	Plasma
	出産歴、経産回数	Parity
	受動的	Passive
	精神医学	Psychiatry
	精神病	Psychosis
	蛋白	Protein
	瞳孔	Pupil(Of The Eye)
	脈、脈拍	Pulse
PA	悪性貧血	Pernicious Anemia
	後前方向	Posteroanterior
	心房圧	Atrial Pressure
	肺動脈	Pulmonary Artery
	肺動脈閉鎖	Pulmonary Atresia
P&A	打診と聴診	Percussion And Ausculation
PAB	肺動脈絞扼術	Pulmonary Artery Banding
PAC	心房期外収縮	Premature Atrial Contractions
PACE	コミュニケーション能力測定法	Promoting Aphasics' Communication Effectiveness
PACO2、Paco2	肺胞気二酸化炭素分圧	Partial Pressure Of Alveolar Carbon Dioxide

Paco2, Paco2　　　動脈血二酸化炭素分圧
　　　Partial Pressure Of Arterial Carbon Dioxide
PACS　（医用）画像管理システム　　　Picture
Archiving And Communication System
PACU 麻酔後回復室　　　Post Anesthesia Care
Unit
PADP 肺動脈拡張終（末）期圧　Pulmonary
Arterial Diastolic Pressure
PAF　発作性心房細動　　　Paroxymal Atrial
Fibrillation
PAG　骨盤内血管撮影（法）　　　Pelvic
Angiography
　　　肺動脈造影（法）　Pulmonary
Arteriongraphy
PAH　妊娠高血圧症　　　Pregnancy Associated
Hypertension
　　　肺高血圧（症）　　　Pulmonary Arterial
Hypertension
Pal　動悸　Palpitation
PAO2 肺胞気酸素分圧　　　Partial Pressure Of
Oxygen In Alveoli
Pao2　動脈血酸素分圧　　　Partial Pressure Of
Arterial Oxygen
PAOP 肺動脈閉塞圧　　　Pulmonary Artery
Occlusion Pressure
PAP　肺動脈圧　　Pulmonary Artery Pressure
PAP, Pap　パパニコロー染色法
　　　Papanicolaou Staining
PAPVC　　　部分肺静脈還流異常（症）
　　　Partial Anomalous Pulmonary Venous
Connection

PAPVD　　部分肺静脈還流異常（症）
Partial Anomalous Pulmonary Venous
Drainage

PAPVR　　部分肺静脈還流異常（症）
Partial Anomalous Pulmonary Venous Return

PAR　肺小動脈抵抗　　　Pulmonary Arteriolar
Resistance

Para　対麻痺　　　Paraplegia

Parox　発作の、痙攣の　　　Paroxysmal

PASG ショックパンツ　　　Pneumatic Antishock
Garment

PAT　血小板凝集試験　　　Platelet Aggregation
Test

発作性心房頻拍　　　Paroxysmal Atrial
Tachycardia

Paw　気道内圧　　Airway Pressure

PAWP肺動脈楔入圧　　　Pulmonary Artery
Wedge Pressure

PB　期外収縮　　Premature Beat

PB，ＰＢ　　大気圧　　　Barometric Pressure

Pb　鉛　　Plumbum

PBF　肺血流量　　Pulmonary Blood Flow

PC　褐色細胞腫　Pheochromocytoma

収縮性心膜炎　　　Pericarditis Constrictiva

濃厚血小板血漿　　Platelet Concentrate

肺毛細管　　Pulmonary Capillary

ペニシリン　Penicillin

PC，Pca　　前立腺癌　　Prostatic Carcinoma

PC(A) 後交通動脈　Posterior Communicating

PCA　患者による除痛管理　　Patient
Controlled Analgesia

後大脳動脈　Posterior Cerebral Artery

PCF　咽頭結膜熱　Pharyngoconjunctival Fever

PCG　心音図　　　Phonocardiogram

PC-HLA　　濃厚血小板 HLA　　Platelet Concentrate HLA

PC-IOL　　　後房レンズ　Posterior Chamber Intraocular Lens

PCL　後十字靱帯　Posterior Cruciate Ligament

PCN　経皮的腎瘻造設術　Percutaneous Nephrostomy

PCO　一酸化炭素分圧　　Carbon Monoxide Pressure

PCO2 二酸化炭素分圧　　Partial Pressure Of Carbon Dioxide

Pcom(A)　　後交通動脈　Posterior Communicating(Artery)

PCP　肺毛細血管圧　　　Pulmonary Capillary Pressure

PCPS 経皮的簡易人工肺　Percutaneous Dardiopulmonary Support

　　　部分的心肺補助装置　　　Partial Cardiopulmonary Support

PCS　門脈下大静脈吻合(術)　　Portacaval Shunt

PCU　緩和ケア病棟　　　Palliative Care Unit

PCV　圧調節式人工換気　Pressure Controlled Ventilation

PCWP 肺毛細血管楔入圧　Pulmonary Capillary Wedge Pressure

PD　　冠状動脈後下行枝　Posterior Descending Coronary Artery

　　　膵頭十二指腸切除(術)　　　Pancreatico-Duodenectomy

　　　腹膜透析　　Peritonael Dialysis

PDA　動脈管開存(症)　Patant Ductus Arteriosus

PDR　増殖型糖尿病網膜症　Proliferative Diabetic Retinopathy

PDS　胎盤機能不全症候群　Placental Dysfunction Syndrome

PE　血漿交換　Plasma Exchange

　　心嚢液貯留　Pericardial Effusion

　　肺気腫　Pulmonary Emphysema

　　肺塞栓(症)　Pulmonary Embolism

PECO2　呼気二酸化炭素分圧　Mixed Expired CO2 Tension

PEEP　呼気終末期陽圧呼吸　Positive End-Expiratory Pressure

PEF　最大呼気流量　Peak Expiratory Flow

PEFR　最大呼気速度　Peak Expiratory Flow Rate

PEG　気脳造影(法) Pneumoencephalography

PEP/(V)ET　心室駆出前期/駆出時間比　Preejection Period/Ventricular Ejection Time

PER　最大駆出率　Peak Ejection Rate

Pes　食道内圧　Esophageal Pressure

PET　陽電子放出形 CT、ポジトロンエミッション CT Positron Emission(Computerized)Tomography

PFO　卵円孔開存　Patent Foramen Ovale

PFR　最大充満速度　Peak Filling Rate

　　最大流速　Peak Flow Rate

PFT　肺機能検査　Pulmonary Function Test

PG　プロシタグランジン　Prostaglandin

PH　既往歴　Past History

　　個人歴　Personal History

　　肺高血圧(症)　Pulmonary Hypertension

　　被殻出血　Putaminal Hemorrhage

PHC　光凝固　　　　　Photocoagulation
Phc　セメント充填　　　　Phosphate Cemant
Filling
PI　　現病歴　　　　Present Illness
　　　肺動脈弁閉鎖不全(症)　　　Pulmonary
Insufficiency
PIB　部分回腸バイパス術　　　　Partial Ileal
Bypass
PICA　後下小脳動脈　　　　Posterior Inferior
Cerebellar Artery
PICU　周産期集中治療室　Perinatal Intensive Care
Unit
　　　小児科集中治療室　Pediatric Intensive Care
Unit
　　　精神科集中治療室　Psychiatric Intensive
Care Unit
PID　骨盤内炎症性疾患　Pelvic Inflammatory
Disease
PIH　妊娠性高血圧　　　　Pregnancy Induced
Hypertension
PIO2　吸入気酸素分圧　　Inspiratory O2 Pressure
PIP　最大吸気圧　Peak Inspiretory Pressure
PK　　膵癌　Pankreaskrebs
PKK　膵頭部癌
PKN　パーキンソン症候群　　　Parkinsonism
PKU　フェニルケトン尿症　　　Phenylketonuria
PL　　後側壁枝　　Poterolateal Artery(Branch)
Plat　血小板　　　　Platelet
PLE　胸膜　Pleura
PLF　後側方固定(術)　　Posterolateral Fusion
PLIF　後方経路腰椎椎体間固定(術)　　　Posterior
Lumbar Interbody Fusion

PLT　血小板　　　Platelet

PM　ペースメーカー　　Pacemaker

Pm　平均血圧　　Mean Blood Pressure

Pmax　最高圧　　Maximum Pressure

PMD　原発性心筋(症)　　Primary Myocardial
Disease

　　　　　進行性筋ジストロフィー　Prograssive
Muscular Dystrophy

PM/DM　　　多発性筋炎/皮膚筋炎
　　　　Polymyositis/Dermatomyositis Complex

PMI　術中心筋梗塞　　Perioperative
Myocardial Infaection

　　　　心筋梗塞後症候群　Post-Myocardial
Infarction(Syndrome)

PML　僧帽弁後尖　Posterior Mitral Leaflet

PMS　閉経期後症候群　　Postmenopausal
Syndrome

PN　腎盂腎炎　　Pyelonephritis

PNI　癌神経周囲浸潤　　Perineural Invasion

PNPB　陽陰圧呼吸法　　Positive Negative
Pressure Breathing

PNPV　(自動)陽陰圧呼吸装置　　Positive Negative
Pressure Ventilator

PNS　副交感神経系　　Parasympathetic
Nervous System

Pnx　気胸　Pneumothorax

PO　術後　Post Operative

　　　人工心肺装置　　Pump-Oxygenator

PO，Po　　　口から(摂取する)、経口的

PO2　酸素分圧　Partial Pressure Of Oxygen

POD　術後日　Post Operetive Day

POS　問題指向型システム　　　Problem-Oriented System

Post　後の、後方へ　　　Posterior

PP　灌流圧　　　Perfusion Pressure

　　　脈圧　Pulse Pressure

　　　幽門形成術　Pyloroplasty

Pp　血漿蛋白　　　Plasma Protein

Ppa　肺動脈圧　　　Pulmonary Arterial Pressure

PPB　陽圧呼吸　　　Positive Pressure Breathing

PPC　心嚢気腫　　　Pneumopericardium

PPF　血漿蛋白分画　　　Plasma Protein Fraction

PPG　幽門輪保存胃切除(術)　　　Pylorus Preserving Gastrectomy

PPH　原発性肺高血圧(症) Primary Pulmonary Hypertension

　　　分娩後出血　Postpartum Hemorrhage

PPHD　蛋白漏出性血液透析(法)　　　Protein-Permeating Hemodialysis

PPHDF　　　蛋白漏出性透析濾過(法)　　　Protein-Permeating Hemodiafiltration

PPHN　新生児遷延性肺高血圧症　　　Persistent Pulmonery Hypertension Of The Newborn

PPI　プロトンポンプ阻害薬　　　Proton Pump Inhibitor

Ppl　胸腔内圧　　　Intrapleural Pressure

PPPD　全胃幽門輪温存膵頭十二指腸切除(術)　　　Pylorus-Preserving Pancreatoduodenectomy

PPT　血漿プロトロンビン時間　Plasma Prothrombin Time

PPV　陽圧換気　　　Positive Pressure Ventilation

PQ　房室伝導時間　　　Atrio-Ventricular Conduction(Time)

パラコート　Paraquat

PR　骨盤動揺　Pelvic Rock

肺動脈弁逆流(症)　Pulmonary Regurgitation

部分寛解　Partial Remission

部分反応　Partial Response

末梢抵抗　Peripheral Resistance

脈拍数　Pulse Rate

Preg　妊娠　Pregnancy

Pre-Medi　前投薬　Preanesthetic Medication

PROM前期破水　Premature Rupture Of The
Membranes

PS　収縮期圧　Pressure Systolic

肺動脈弁狭窄(症)　Pulmonary Stenosis

パンクレオザイミン・セクレチン試験

Pancreozymin Secretin(Test)

PSG　睡眠脳波検査　Polysomnogram

PSH　脊髄麻酔後頭痛　Post Spinal Headache

PSI　肺動脈狭窄閉鎖不全　Pulmonic Steno-
Insufficiency

PSP　フェノールスルホンフタレイン

Phenolsulfonphthalein(Phenol Red)

PSR　肺動脈弁狭窄兼閉鎖不全症

Pulmonary Stenosis And Regurgitation

PSS　生理食塩水　Physiological Saline Solution

PST　パンクレオザイミン・セクレチン試験

Pancreozymin-Secretin Test

発作性上室性頻拍　Paroxysmal
Supraventricular Tachycardia

PSV　圧補助換気法　Pressure Spport
Ventilation

PSVT 発作性上室性頻拍　Paroxysmal
Supraventricular Tachycardio
PT　　錐体路　　　Pyramidal Tract
　　　プロトロンビン時間　　　Prothrombin
Time
Pt, Pt 患者　Patient
PTA　経皮的血管拡張(術) Percutaneous
Transluminal Angiodilatation
　　　経皮的血管形成(術)□　　Percutaneous
Transluminal Angioplasty
PTCA 経皮的冠状動脈形成(術)　Percutaneous
Transluminal Coronary Angioplasty
PTCD 経皮的肝胆道ドレナージ　Percutaneous
Transhepatic Cholangioldrainage
Ptco2 経皮酸素分圧　　　Partial Pressure Of
Transcutaneous Oxygen
PTCR 経皮的冠状動脈血栓溶解療法
　　　　Percutaneous Translumonal Coronary
Recanalization
PTE　肺動脈血栓塞栓(症) Puimonary
Thromboembolism
PTGBD　　　経皮経肝胆嚢ドレナージ
　　　　Percutaneous Transhepatic Gallbladder
Drainage
PTH　輸血後肝炎　Posy-Transfusion Hepatitis
PTLS　副甲状腺ホルモン様物質　Parathormonelike
Subtrance
PTMC 経皮的経静脈的僧帽弁交連切開(術)
　　　　Percutaneous Transluminal Mitral
Commissurotomy
PTN　錐体路ニューロン　Pyramidal Tract Neuron

PTO　経皮経肝(食道静脈瘤)塞栓(術)
Percutaneous Transhepatic Obliteration(Of
Gastroesophageal Varices)
PTP　経皮経肝的門脈造影(法)　Percutaneous
Transhepatic Portography
PTR　膝蓋腱反射　Patellar Tendon Reflex
PTSD 外傷後ストレス病　Post-Traumatic Stress
Disorder
PTX　気胸　Pneumothorax
PV　　肺静脈　　　Pulmonary Vein
　　　門脈　Portal Vein
P-V　腹腔静脈シャント　Peritoneo-Venous(Shunt)
PVC　心室期外収縮　　　Premature Ventricular
Contraction
Pvco2 混合静脈二酸化炭素分圧　Mixed Venous
Carbon Dioxide Pressure
PVE　人工弁心内膜炎　　Prosthetic Valve
Endocarsitis
PVG　気脳室造影(法)　　Pneumoventriculography
PVH　脳室周囲出血　　　Periventricular
Hemoyyhage
PVN　末梢静脈栄養　　　Peripheral Venous
Nutrition
PVO　肺静脈閉塞　Pulmonary Venous Obstruction
Pvo2　混合静脈酸素分圧　Mixed Venous Oxygen
PVOD 肺血管閉塞性病変　Pulmonary Vascular
Obstructive Disease
PVR　肺血管抵抗　Pulmonary Vascular Resistance
　　　末梢血管抵抗　　　Peripheral Vascular
Resistance
PVT　発作性心室頻拍　　Paroxysmal Ventricular
Tachycardia

PX	身体検査	Physical Examination
Px	既往歴	Past History
	気胸	Pneumothorax
	予後	Prognosis

Q

French

English

QUAL Qualitative Attribute
Qual Qualitative, Qualitaty
QUAL-PACS Quality Of Patient Care System
Qualys Quality-Adjusted Life-Years
QUAN Quantitative Attribute
Quant Quantitative, Quantitaty
Quar Quarantine
QUART Quadrantectomy, Axillary Dissection,
Radiotherapy
QUASAR Quinapril Anti-Ischemia And
Symptoms Of Angina Reduction [Trial]
QUEST Quality, Utilization, Effectiveness,
Statistically Tabulated
QU.E.S.T. Quality Of Life, Effectiveness,
Safety, And Tolerability
QUESTAR Query Estimation And Refinement
QUESTT Question The Child, Use Pain Rating
Scale, Evaluate Behavior And Physiologic
Changes, Secure Parents' Involvement, Take
Cause Of Pain Into Account, Take Action And
Evaluate Results [Mnemonic]
QUEXTA Quantitative Exercise Testing And
Angiography [Study]
QUICHA Quantitative Inhalation Challenge
Apparatus
QUIET Quinapril Ischemic Event Trial
Quic Quality Interagency Coordinating

Task Force
QUIN Quinolinic Acid
Quint Fifth
QUIS Questionnaire On User Interface Satisfaction
Quot Quotient
Quotid Daily, Quotidian [Lat. Quotidie]
QUPV Quailpox Virus
QUS Quantitative Ultrasound
Qv Which See [Lat. Quod Vide]
QWB Quality Of Well-Being
QYBV Qalyub Virus
QYD Qi And Yin Deficiency
QS As Much As Suffices [Lat. Quantum Satis
Or Quantum Sufficit]; Quad Set [Exercise];
Quality-Switched; Question Screening; Quiet
Sleep
Qs, Qs Systemic Blood Flow
Q.S. As Much As Suffices [Lat. Quantum Satis
Or Quantum Sufficit]
QSAR Quantitative Structure-Activity Relationship
QSART Quantitative Sudomotor Axon Reflex
Testing
QSFR Quantitative Structure-Function Relationship
QSM Quality Assurance And Safety Of Medicine
QSPR Quantitative Structure-Property Relationship
QSPV Quasi-Static Pressure Volume
QSQT Shunted Blood/Total Blood Flow [Ratio]
Qs/Qt Shunt Fraction
QSR Quality System Regulation
QSS Quantitative Sacroiliac Scintigraphy
QSSR Quantitative Structure-Stability Relationship
QST Quantitative Sensory Test
QSU Questionnaire Of Smoking Urges
QT Cardiac Output; Quick Test
Q-T Time Interval From The Beginning Of The

QRS Complex To The End Of The T Wave
[ECG]
Qt Quantity; Quart; Quiet
Qtc, Q-Tc Q-T Interval Corrected For Heart
Rate
Qter End Of Long Arm Of Chromosome
QTL Quantitative Trait Locus
Q-TWIST Quality-Adjusted Time Without
Symptoms Of Disease Or Subjective Toxic Effects
Of Treatment
Quad Quadratic
Quad Quadrant; Quadriceps; Quadriplegic
QUADS Quinapril Australian Dosing Study
QUAL Qualitative Attribute
Qual Qualitative, Qualitaty
QUAL-PACS Quality Of Patient Care System
Qualys Quality-Adjusted Life-Years
QUAN Quantitative Attribute
Quant Quantitative, Quantitaty
Quar Quarantine
QUART Quadrantectomy, Axillary Dissection,
Radiotherapy
QUASAR Quinapril Anti-Ischemia And
Symptoms Of Angina Reduction [Trial]
QUEST Quality, Utilization, Effectiveness,
Statistically Tabulated
QU.E.S.T. Quality Of Life, Effectiveness,
Safety, And Tolerability
QUESTAR Query Estimation And Refinement
QUESTT Question The Child, Use Pain Rating
Scale, Evaluate Behavior And Physiologic
Changes, Secure Parents' Involvement, Take
Cause Of Pain Into Account, Take Action And
Evaluate Results [Mnemonic]
QUEXTA Quantitative Exercise Testing And

Angiography [Study]
QUICHA Quantitative Inhalation Challenge
Apparatus
QUIET Quinapril Ischemic Event Trial
Quic Quality Interagency Coordinating
Task Force
QUIN Quinolinic Acid
Quint Fifth
QUIS Questionnaire On User Interface Satisfaction
Quot Quotient
Quotid Daily, Quotidian [Lat. Quotidie]
QUPV Quailpox Virus
QUS Quantitative Ultrasound
Qv Which See [Lat. Quod Vide]
QWB Quality Of Well-Being
QYBV Qalyub Virus
QYD Qi And Yin Deficiency

German

QS - Qualitätssicherung
Qual - Qualitativ

Chinese

Q Cardiac Output 心 搏出量; 心搏排血
量; 心排血量; 心输出量

Q-Band Q 带

QC Quinine And Colchicine 奎宁和秋水
仙碱

Qd Quinidine 奎尼丁〔抗心律失常药〕

QFB Querfingerbreite 横指【注释】〔腹部触诊时,
以检查者手指并
列的数目来表示肝脏肿大程度〕

QKOA Quarantine Kennel Owners Association
养狗者检疫学会

QLLC Qualified Logical-Link Control 限
定逻辑连接控制

Qlt Quality ① 羊毛细度; 羊毛品质支数
②品质; 质量; 性质

QMN Quar Tan Malaria Nephropathy 三
日疟肾病

QOUH Quality Of Ulcer Healing 溃 疡治
愈度【注释】〔溃疡的形态学上愈合程度, 即
为形态学上观察确认的溃疡面愈合程
度。应需要和内窥镜所见的结果与功
能情况综合做出评价〕

QP Quadrant Pain 象 限痛

QP Quanti-Pirquet Reaction 定 量皮尔
盖氏反应; 定量结核菌素划痕反应

Qpc Quality Of Patient Care 病 人护理质
量

QPT Quantitative Protamine Tit Ration

Test 定量鱼精蛋白滴定试验

Q-RB Interval EKG Time-Wave Interval
Q-RB 间 期; 心电图时间-波间期

QRC Quick Reaction Capability 快 速反
应能力

QS Quiet Sleep 安静睡眠

Qsan Anatomical Pulmonary Shunt 肺
解剖分流量

Q-Sign Unresponsive Person With Mouth
Open And Tongue Hanging Out Q 征
〔无反应者, 口张开, 舌伸出〕

Qs / Qt Intrapulmonary Shunt Fraction
(Right- To- Left Shunt Ratio) 肺 内短路血
流量比率【注释】 〔回流到右心的血液经肺动脉
输
送到肺泡处交换气体后变为动脉血, 但
由于肺部病变, 一部分血液不能进行气
体交换, 它所占的比率即为 Qs/ Qt , 又
叫做静脉短路率。在正常情况下也有
3 %～ 5%的短路血量〕

Qt Quart 夸 脱 〔容量单位〕

QT Quick Test 奎 克氏试验

Qupl Quadriplegia 四 肢麻痹; 四肢瘫

Quplc Quadriplegic ① 四肢麻痹的② 四
肢麻痹患者

Japanese

略語　日本語の意味　　　スペル

Q　　Q 熱（Q は疑問の意味）　Q Fever

QOL　生命の質、生活の質　　Quality Of Life

Qp/Qs 肺体血流比　Pulmonary Blood
Flow/Systemic Blood Flow Ratio

QT　　クイック試験　　　Quick Test

Quad　四肢麻痺　　Quadriplegic

　　　大腿四頭筋　Quadriceps(ラ)

R
French

RA Rétrécissement Aortique

RAA Rhumatisme Articulaire Aigu

RAC Rétrécissement Aortique Calcifié, Recherche
D'anomalie Chromosomique

RCF Rythme Cardiaque Foetal

RCIU Retard De Croissance Intra-Utérin (US=IUGR)

RD Rétinopathie Diabétique

REP Résection Endoscopique De Prostate

RGO Reflux Gastro-Oesophagien

RHJ Reflux Hépato-Jugulaire

RIVA Rythme Idio-Ventriculaire Accéléré

RM Rétrécissement Mitral

RP Radiographie Pulmonaire

RPCA Résistance À La Protéine C Activée

RPDE Rupture De La Poche Des Eaux

RPM Rupture Prématurée Des Membranes
(US=PROM)

RXP Radiographie Pulmonaire

English

RVSO Right Ventricular Stroke Output

RVSP Right Ventricular Systolic Pressure

RVSV Right Ventricular Stroke Volume

RVSW Right Ventricular Stroke Work

RVSWI Right Ventricular Stroke Work Index

RVT Radical Vaginal Trachelectomy; Renal
Vein Thrombosis

RVTE Recurring Venous Thromboembolism

RV/TLC Residual Volume/Total Lung Capacity

RVU Relative Value Unit

RVV Right Ventricular Volume; Rubella
Vaccine–Like Virus; Russell's Viper Venom

Rvv Recombinant Vaccinia Virus

RVVO Right Ventricular Volume Overload

RVVT Russell's Viper Venom Time

RVW Right Ventricular Wall

RVWT Right Ventricle Wall Thickness

RW Radiologic Warfare; Ragweed; Respiratory
Work; Romano-Ward [Syndrome]; Round
Window

R-W Rideal-Walker [Coefficient]; Romano-
Ward [Syndrome]

R/W Return To Work

RWAGE Ragweed Antigen E

RWC Receiving Water Concentration; Regional
Weaning Center

RWI Recreational Water Illness

RWIS Restraint And Water Immersion
Stress

RWJF Robert Wood Johnson Foundation

RWM Regional Wall Motion
RWMA Regional Wall Motion Abnormality
RWP Ragweed Pollen; R-Wave Progression
RWS Radiology Work Station; Ragweed Sensitivity
RWT Random Walk Theory; Relative Wall
Thickness
RWV Rotating Wall Vessel
RX Rapid Exchange; Reaction; Residual Tumor
Not Assessed
Rx Drug; Medication; Pharmacy; Prescribe,
Prescription; Prescription Drug; Take [Lat.
Recipe]; Therapy; Treatment
Rx&D Canada's Research-Based Pharmaceutical
Companies
RXLI Recessive X-Linked Ichthyosis
RXN Reaction
RXR Retinoid X Receptor
RXRA Retinoid X Receptor Alpha
RXRE Retinoic X Response Element
RXRG Retinoid X Receptor Gamma
RXT Right Exotropia
R-Y Roux-En-Y
RYD Ryanodine
RYR, Ryr Ryanodine Receptor
RVEDV Right Ventricular End-Diastolic Volume
RVEDVI Right Ventricular End-Diastolic Volume
Index
RVEF Right Ventricular Ejection Fraction;
Right Ventricular End Flow
RVESV Right Ventricular End-Systolic Volume
RVET Right Ventricular Ejection Time
RVF Renal Vascular Failure; Residual Volume
Fraction; Rift Valley Fever; Right Ventricular
Failure; Right Visual Field
RVFP Right Ventricular Filling Pressure

RVFV Rift Valley Fever Virus

RVG Radionuclide Ventriculogram Or
Ventriculography;
Right Ventral Gluteus; Right
Visceral Ganglion

RVH Renal Vascular Hypertension, Renovascular
Hypertension; Right Ventricular Hypertrophy

RVHD Rheumatic Valvular Heart Disease

RVHR Renovascular Hypertensive Rat

RVI Relative Value Index; Right Ventricle Infarction

RVID Ventricular Internal Dimension

RVIT Right Ventricular Inflow Tract

RV-IVRT Right Ventricular Isovolumic Relaxation
Time

RVL Right Vastus Lateralis

RVLG Right Ventrolateral Gluteal

RVLM Rostral Ventrolateral Medulla

RVM Right Ventricular Mass; Right Ventricular
Mean

RVMM Rostral Ventromedial Medulla

RVN Radionuclide Ventriculogram

RVO Regional Veterinary Officer; Relaxed
Vaginal Outlet; Right Ventricular Outflow

RVOT Right Ventricular Outflow Tract

RVOTO Right Ventricular Outflow Tract Obstruction

RVP Red Veterinary Petrolatum; Resting Venous
Pressure; Right Ventricular Pressure

RVPEP Right Ventricular Preejection Period

RVPFR Right Ventricular Peak Filling Rate

RVP/LVP Right Ventricular Pressure/Left
Ventricular Pressure Ratio

RVPRA Renal Vein Plasma Renin Activity

RVR Reduced Vascular Response; Renal Vascular
Resistance; Repetitive Ventricular Response;
Resistance To Venous Return

RVRA Renal Vein/Venous Renin Activity
RVRC Renal Vein Renin Concentration
RVS Rectal Visceral Sensitivity; Rectovaginal
Space; Relative Value Scale; Relative Value Study;
Reported Visual Sensation; Retrovaginal Space
RUMP Remnants Of Uncertain Malignant Potential
Rump Ribulose Monophosphate Pathway
RUOQ Right Upper Outer Quadrant
RUP Right Upper Pole
Ru1,5P Ribulose-1,5-Biphosphate
Ru5P Ribulose-5-Phosphate
Rupt Ruptured
RUPV Right Upper Pulmonary Vein
RUQ Right Upper Quadrant
RUR Resin Uptake Ratio
RURTI Recurrent Upper Respiratory Tract Infection
RUS Radioulnar Synostosis; Real-Time
Ultrasonography
RUSB Right Upper Sternal Border
RUT Rapid Urease Test
RUTH Raloxifene Use For The Heart [Study]
RUV Residual Urine Volume
RUX Right Upper Extremity
RUZ Right Upper Zone
RV Ranavirus; Random Variable; Rat Virus;
Rauscher Virus; Rectovaginal; Regurgitant Volume;
Reinforcement Value; Renal Vein; Reovirus;
Residual Volume; Respiratory Volume;
Retroventral; Retroversion; Retrovesical; Retrovirus;
Return Visit; Rhabdovirus; Rheumatoid
Vasculitis; Rhinovirus; Right Ventricle, Right
Ventricular; Rotavirus; Rotavirus Vaccine; Rubella
Vaccine; Rubella Virus; Russell's Viper
R/V, R&V Record And Verify
RV Radius Of View

Rv Venous Resistance

RVA Rabies Vaccine, Activated; Recombinant
Virus Assay; Reentrant Ventricular Arrhythmia;
Right Ventricle Activation; Right Ventricular
Apex; Right Vertebral Artery

RV-A To -G Rotaviruses A To G

RVAD Right Ventricular Assist Device

RVAW Right Ventricle Anterior Wall

RVB Red Venous Blood

RVBF Reversed Vertebral Blood Flow

RVC Reason For Visit Classification; Rectovaginal
Constriction

RVD Regulatory Volume Decrease; Relative
Vertebral Density; Relative Vessel Diameter;
Relative Volume Decrease; Right Ventricular
Dimension; Right Ventricular Dysplasia

RVDC Right Ventricular Diastolic Collapse

RVDO Right Ventricular Diastolic Overload

RVDV Right Ventricular Diastolic Volume

RVE Right Ventricular Enlargement

RVECP Right Ventricular Endocardial Potential

RVED Right Ventricular End-Diastolic

RVEDD Right Ventricular End-Diastolic Diameter

RVEDP Right Ventricular End-Diastolic Pressure

Rtnf Recombinant Tumor Necrosis Factor

RTO Return To Office; Right Toe-Off

RTOG Radiation Therapy Oncology Group

RTP Radiation/Radiotherapy Treatment Planning;
Renal Transplantation Patient; Reverse
Transcriptase Producing

Rtpa, Rtpa, Rt-PA Recombinant Tissue
Plasminogen Activator

RT-PACS Radiotherapy Picture Archival And
Communication System

RT-PCR Reverse Transcriptase Polymerase

Chain Reaction

RTPV Radiation Therapy Planning And Verification;
RT Parvovirus

RTR Recreational Therapist, Registered;
Red Blood Cell Turnover Rate; Retention Time
Ratio

RT(R)(ARRT) Registered Technologist (Radiography)
Certified By The American Registry
Of Radiologic Technologists

RT-RH Reverse Transcriptase–Ribonuclease H

RTRR Return To Recovery Room

RTS Rapid Throughput Screening; Real-Time
Scan; Rett Syndrome; Revised Trauma Score;
Right Toe Strike; Rothmund-Thomson Syndrome;
Rubinstein-Taybi Syndrome

RTSS Rest Technetium-99m Sestamibi Scan

RTT Round-Trip Time

RT(T)(ARRT) Radiologic Technologist (Ra

RT(R)(ARRT) Registered Technologist (Radiography)
Certified By The American Registry
Of Radiologic Technologists

RT-RH Reverse Transcriptase–Ribonuclease H

RTRR Return To Recovery Room

RTS Rapid Throughput Screening; Real-Time
Scan; Rett Syndrome; Revised Trauma Score;
Right Toe Strike; Rothmund-Thomson Syndrome;
Rubinstein-Taybi Syndrome

RTSS Rest Technetium-99m Sestamibi Scan

RTT Round-Trip Time

RT(T)(ARRT) Radiologic Technologist (Radiation
Therapy) Certified By The American
Registry Of Radiologic Technologists

RTTP Radiation Therapy Treatment Planning

RTU Real-Time Ultrasonography; Relative
Time Unit; Renal Transplantation Unit

RT3U Resin Triiodothyronine Uptake
RTUI Respiratory Therapy Utilization Index
RTV Recurrent Tracheoesophageal Fistula;
Resistance To Voltage; Rhinotracheitis Virus;
Ritonavir; Room Temperature Vulcanization
RTW Return To Work
RTX Resiniferatoxin; Robustotoxin
RU Radioulnar; Rat Unit; Reading Unit; Residual
Urine; Resin Uptake; Resistance Unit; Retrograde
Urogram; Right Upper; Roentgen Unit
RU-1 Human Embryonic Lung Fibroblasts
RU-486 Mifepristone
Ru Radiation Unit
RUA Reduced Under Anesthesia
RUBV Rubella Virus
RUC Rapid Update Cycle
RUCAM Roussel Uclaf Causality Assessment
Method
RUD Recurrent Ulcer Of The Duodenal Bulb;
Repeating Unit Domain
RUE Right Upper Extremity
RUG Resource Utilization Group; Retrograde
Urethrography
RUL Right Upper Eyelid; Right Upper Lateral;
Right Upper Limb; Right Upper Lobe
RPVC Resource Provider Of Virtual Center
RPVP Right Posterior Ventricular Preexcitation
RQ Recovery Quotient; [Hazardous Substance]
Reportable Quantities [List]; Reportable
Quantity; Respiratory Quotient; Riskadjusted
Quantity
RQDS Revised Quantified Denver Scale Of
Communication
RQL Rejectable Quality Level
RR Radiation Reaction; Radiation Response;

Rate Ratio; Rational Recovery; Recovery Room;
Recurrence Risk; Reference Reagent; Regulatory
Region; Relative Resistance; Relative Response;
Relative Risk; Renin Release; Resistant Relapse;
Respiratory Rate; Respiratory Reserve; Response
Rate; Results Reporting; Retinal Reflex; Rheumatoid
Rosette; Ribonucleotide Reductase; Risk
Ratio; Riva-Rocci [Sphygmomanometer];
Ross River [Virus]; Ruthenium Red
R&R Rate And Rhythm; Rest And Recuperation;
Rotablator And Restenosis
Rr Respiratory Rate
RRA Radioreceptor Assay; Registered Record
Administrator
RRAC Research Realignment Advisory
Committee
RRBAT Relative Rigid Body Accuracy Test
RRC Residency
RPIPP Reverse-Phase Ion Pair Partition
RPK Ribosephosphate Kinase
RPL Recurrent Pregnancy Loss; Right Precordial
Lead
RPLAD Retroperitoneal Lymphadenectomy
RPLC Reverse-Phase Liquid Chromatography
RPLD Repair Of Potentially Lethal Damage
RPLES Reversible Posterior Leukoencephalopathy
Syndrome
RPLND Retroperitoneal Lymph Node Dissection
RPM Rapid Pharmaceutical Management;
Rapid Processing Mode; Revolutions Per Minute;
Robust Point Matching
Rpm Rapid Processing Mode; Revolutions Per
Minute
RPMD Rheumatic Pain-Modulation Disorder
RPMI Roswell Park Memorial Institute

RPMS Relapsing-Progressive Multiple Sclerosis;
Resource And Patient Management System
RPN Registered Practical Nurse
RPO Right Posterior Oblique
RPP Heart Rate–Systolic Blood Pressure
Product; Rate-Pressure Product; Retropubic
Prostatectomy
RPPA Reverse-Phase Protein Microarray
RPPI Role Perception Picture Inventory
RPPR Red Cell Precursor Production Rate
RPR Rapid Plasmin Reagin; Reiter Protein
Proliferans; Retrograde Pyelogram; Retroperitoneal;
Reverse Phase; Rheumatoid Polyarthritis;
Ribonucleoprotein; Ribose Phosphate;
Ribosomal Protein; Roswell Park [Database]
R5P Ribose-5-Phosphate
R/P Respiratory Pulse
Rp Peripheral Resistance
Rp Pulmonary Resistance
RPA Radial Photon Absorptiometry; Replication
Protein A; Resultant Physiologic
Acceleration; Retinitis Punctata Albescens;
Retroperitoneal Approach; Reverse Passive
Anaphylaxis; Right Pulmonary Artery
R-PA Reteplase
Rpaf Receptor For Platelet Activating Factor
RPAHPET Royal Prince Albert Hospital
Positron Emission Tomography [Study]
Rpase Ribonucleic Acid Polymerase
RPC Reactive Perforating Collagenosis; Relapsing
Polychondritis; Relative Proliferative
Capacity; Remote Procedure Call; Restorative
Proctocolectomy
RPCA Reverse Passive Cutaneous Anaphylaxis
RPCF, RPCFT Reiter Protein Complement

Fixation Test
RPCGN Rapidly Progressive Crescenting
Glomerulonephritis
RPCH Rural Primary Care Hospital
RPD Removable Partial Denture
R-PDQ Revised Prescreening Developmental
Questionnaire
RPE Rapid Palatal Expansion; Rate Of Perceived
Exertion; Recurrent Pulmonary Embolism;
Retinal Pigment Epithelium; Ribulose
5-Phosphate 3-Epimerase
RPEP Rabies Post Exposure Prophylaxis
RPET Rapid Partial Exchange Transfusion
RPF Relaxed Pelvic Floor; Renal Plasma Flow;
Retroperitoneal Fibrosis
Rpfs Radiographic Progression-Free Survival
RPG Radiation Protection Guide; Retrograde
Pyelogram; Rheoplethysmography; Right
Paracolic Gutter
RPGMEC Regional Postgraduate Medical
Education Committee
RPGN Rapidly Progressive Glomerulonephritis
RPGR Retinitis Pigmentosa Guanosine
Triphosphatase
Regulator [Gene]
Rph Registered Pharmacist
RPHA Reversed Passive Hemagglutination
RPHAMCFA Reversed Passive Hemagglutination
By Miniature Centrifugal Fast Analysis
RP-HPLC, Rphplc Reverse-Phase High-Performance
Liquid Chromatography
RPI Regional Perfusion Index; Relative Percentage
Index; Reticulocyte Production
ROMAS Romanian Multicenter Study
ROM CP Range Of Motion Complete And

Pain Free

ROMI Rating Of Medication Influence; Rule
Out Myocardial Infarct

ROMIO Rule Out Myocardial Infarct Observation
[Study]

ROMS Radiation Oncology Management
System

ROOF Retro-Orbital Orbicular Fat

ROP Removal Of Pins Or Plates; Removal Of
Plaster; Retinopathy Of Prematurity; Right
Occipitoposterior

RO PACS Radiation Oncology Picture Archiving
And Communication System

ROPE Respiratory-Ordered Phase Encoding

ROPS Rollover Protective Structure

ROR Reactive Oxygen Radical; Risk Odds Ratio

Ror Rorschach [Test]

ROS Reactive Oxygen Species; Reflectance
Optical Shield; Relative Outcome Score; Review
Of Systems; Rod Outer Segment

Ros Rostral Sulcus

ROSC Restoration Of Spontaneous Circulation;
Return Of Spontaneous Circulation

ROSETTA Routine Vs. Selective Exercise
Treadmill Test After Angioplasty [Trial]

ROSP Rod Outer Segment Protein

ROSS Radiotherapy Oncology Support System;
Review Of Subjective Symptoms

ROSTER Rotational Atherectomy V. Balloon
Angioplasty For In-Stent Restenosis
[Trial]

ROT Real Oxygen Transport; Remedial Occupational
Therapy; Right Occipito-Transverse

Rot Rotating, Rotation

ROTA Rotablator Atherectomy

ROTACS Rotational Angioplasty Catheter
System
ROTASTENT Rotational Atherectomy With
Adjunctive Stenting [Trial]
ROU Recurrent Oral Ulcer
Rout Outflow Resistance
ROW Rendu-Osler-Weber [Syndrome]; Rest
Of The World
ROXIS Roxithromycin In Ischemic Syndromes
[Study]
RP Radial Pulse; Radical Prostatectomy;
Radiographic
Planimetry; Radiopharmaceutical;
Rapid Processing; Rapid Prototyping; Raynaud
Phenomenon; Reactive Protein; Readiness Potential;
Recessive Partitioning; Recreation And
Pastime; Rectal Prolapse; Re-Entrant Pathway;
Refractory Period; Regulatory
Protein; Relapsing
Polychondritis; Relative Power Or Potency;
Reperfusion; Replication Protein; Resident Physician;
Respiratory Rate; Responsible Party; Rest
Pain; Resting Position; Resting Potential; Resting
Pressure; Retinitis Pigmentosa; Retinitis
370
RHA Regional Health Authority; Relative
Highest Avidity; Right Hepatic Artery
Rha Rheumatoid Arthritis
Rhag Rh-Associated Glycoprotein
RHB Regional Hospital Board; Right Heart Bypass
RHBF Reactive Hyperemia Blood Flow
Rh-BMP Recombinant Human Bone Morphogenetic
Protein
Rhbs Regional Hospital Boards

RHC Rad Homolog In Cerevisiae; Resin
Hemoperfusion
Column; Respiration Has Ceased;
Right Heart Catheterization; Right Hypochondrium;
Rural Health Center
RHCSA Regional Hospitals Consultants And
Specialists Association
RHD Radiologic Health Data; Relative Hepatic
Dullness; Renal Hypertensive Disease; Rheumatic
Heart Disease
Rhd Rhesus Factor And D Antigen
RHDV Rabbit Hemorrhagic Disease Virus
RHDV-AST89 Rabbit Hemorrhagic Disease
Virus AST89
RHDV-BS89 Rabbit Hemorrhagic Disease
Virus BS89
RHDV-FRG Rabbit Hemorrhagic Disease
Virus FRG
RHDV-V351 Rabbit Hemorrhagic Disease
Virus V351
RHDV-SD Rabbit Hemorrhagic Disease Virus
SD
Rhdnase Recombinant Human Deoxyribonuclease
RHE Retino-Hepato-Endocrine [Syndrome]
RHEED Reflection High-Energy Electron Diffraction
Rheo Rheology
Rhepo Recombinant Human Erythropoietin
Rheu, Rheum Rheumatic, Rheumatoid
RHF Restricted Hartree-Fock [Level]; Right
Heart Failure
Rh F Rheumatic Fever
Rhfsh Recombinant Human Follicle Stimulating
Hormone
Rhfviii Recombinant Human Factor 8
RHG Right-Hand Grip

Rhg-CSF Recombinant Human Granulocyte
Colony-Stimulating Factor
Rhgh Recombinant Human Growth Hormone
Rhgm-CSF Recombinant Human Granulocyte–
Macrophage Colony-Stimulating Factor
RHI Rhesus Factor Immunoglobulin; Rural
Health Initiative
RHIA Registered Health Information Administrator
Rhig Rh [Rhesus] Factor Immunoglobulin
Rhigf Recombinant Human Insulin-Like
Rept Let It Be Repeated
Req Request, Requested
RER Renal Excretion Rate; Replication Error;
Respiratory Exchange Ratio; Rough Endoplasmic
Reticulum
RER+ Replication Error Positive
RERC Rehabilitation Engineering Research
Center
RERF Radiation Effects Research Foundation
RES Radionuclide Esophageal Scintigraphy;
Real Environment Sensing; Reproducibility
Echocardiography Study; Reticuloendothelial
System; Rotterdam Elderly Study
Res Research; Resection; Resident; Residue;
Resistance
RESAC Real-Time Expert System For Advice
And Control
RESCUE Randomized Evaluation Of Salvage
Angioplasty With Combined Utilization
Of Endpoints [Trial]
RESET Real Safety And Efficacy Of A
3-Month Dual Antiplatelet Therapy Following
Zotarolimus-Eluting Stents Implantation
[Trial]
Res Gen Research Genetics [Database]

RESIST Restenosis After Intravascular Ultrasound-
Guided Stenting [Study]
RESNA Rehabilitation Engineering Society
Of North America
RESOLVD, RESOLVED Randomized Evaluation
Of Strategies For Left Ventricular Dysfunction
[Study]
Resp Respiration, Respiratory; Response
Resp Ther Respiratory Therapy
REST Raynaud Phenomenon, Esophageal
Motor Dysfunction, Sclerodactyly, And
Telangiectasia

German

R. - Ramus
Rad. - Radix, Wurzel
RCA - Rechte Koronararterie
RCX - Ramus Circumflexus Der Koronargefäße
RIVA - Ramus Interventricularis Anterior Der
Koronargefäße
RKI - Robert-Koch-Institut
RKI Homepage
RKM - Röntgenkontrastmittel
RLS - Reizleitungsstörung
Rö - Röntgen
RR - Blutdruck (Nach Riva/Rocci)
RT - Rechtstyp Im EKG
RV - Rechter Ventrikel, Rechtsventrikulär

Italian

R
RBC Globuli Rossi (Red Blood Cell ()
Rcprianimazione Cardio Polmonare
RMN Risonanza Magnetica Nucleare
RSBI Respiro Rapido E Superficiale, Rapid Shallow
Breathing
Rx Radiografia

Russian

R, RR

Respiratory Rate (Per Min)

Частота Дыхания (В Мнуту)

RA

(1) Rheumatoid Arthritis

Ревматоидный Артрит

(2) Right Atrium

Правое Предсердие

RAP

Right Atrial Pressure

Давление В Правом Предсердии

RBBB

Right Bundle Branch Block

Блокада Правой Ножки Пучка Гисса [ЭКГ]

RBC

Red Blood Cells

Эритроциты

RDS

Respiratory Distress Syndrome

Респираторный Дистресс Синдром

Readm

Readmission

Повторная Госпитализация

RF

Rheumatoid Factor

Ревматоидный Фактор

Rh

Rhesus Blood Factor

Резус-Фактор

RL

Ringer's Lactate
Лактат Рингера
RIND
Reversible Ischemic Neurologic Deficit
Обратимый Ишемический Неврологический
Дефицит
RLL
Right Lower Lobe
Правая Нижняя Доля [Легкого]
RLQ
Right Lower Quadrant
Правый Нижний Квадрант
RML
Right Middle Lobe
Правая Средняя Доля [Легкого]
RNA
Ribonucleic Acid
Рибонуклеиновая Кислота
R/0, R/O
Rule Out
Исключить [Заболевание, Состояние]
RPGN
Rapidly Progressive Glomerulonephritis
Быстропрогрессирующий Гломерулонефрит
RPI
Reticulocyte Production Index
Индекс Продукции Ретикулоцитов
RSR
Regular Sinus Rhythm
Регулярный Синусовый Ритм [ЭКГ]
RTA
Renal Tubular Acidosis
Почечный Канальцевый Ацидоз
RTC
Return To Clinic

Возвращение В Клинику
RUL
Right Upper Lobe
Правая Верхняя Доля [Легкого]
RUQ
Right Upper Quadrant
Правый Верхний Квадрант
RV
(1) Right Ventricle
Правый Желудочек [Сердца]
(2) Residual Volume
Остаточный Объем
RVH
(1) Renovascular Hypertension
Реноваскулярная Гипертензия
(2) Right Ventricular Hypertrophy
Гипертрофия Правого Желудочка [Сердца]
Rx
(1) Therapy
Терапия [Лечение]
(2) Treatment
Лечение
(3) Prescription
Рецепт

Chinese

R Behnken□s Unit 本肯氏单位 〔X 线〕

R-1625 Haloperidol 氟 哌啶醇

R3 Poor Risk 中 度危险 〔麻醉第三期〕

R Rad 拉 德 〔辐射剂量单位〕

R Rectum 直肠

R Reductase 还 原酶

R Respiration (Rate) 呼 吸速度

R Respiratory Exchange Ratio 呼 吸商;
换气比值【注释】〔为二氧化碳呼出量与氧气摄入
量之间的比值, 亦即 VCO2/ VO2〕

R Rhodospirillum 红螺菌属

R Rickettsia 立克次氏体属

R . Rinne Test 林尼氏(音叉) 试验

R Roentgen 伦 琴【注释】〔表示射线量的单位〕

R Roentgen Unit 伦琴单位

RA Radioactive 放 射性的; 放射的

RA Recurrent Aphtha 复 发性口疮

RA Refractory Anemia 顽固性贫血

RA Renin Angiotensin 肾素血管紧张素

RA Rheumatic Arthritis 风湿性关节炎

RA Rheumatoid Arthritis 类 风湿性关节
炎; 萎缩性关节炎; 变形性关节炎【注释】〔呈慢
性经过, 以非化脓性多发
性关节炎为主要症状的原因不明的全
身性炎症性疾病, 女性多发。多在清晨
刚睡醒时出现指(趾) 小关节痛。被认
为是一种自身免疫性疾病。可检出类
风湿因子, 有人认为该因子与组织病变
有关。但其病因尚未探明。也有人认
为此病与 EB 病毒感染有关〕

RA Right Atrium 右心房

RAA Renin Angiotensin Aldosterone 肾
素血管紧张素醛固酮(系统)

Raar Radial Ar Tery 桡动脉〔解〕

RABI Royal Agricultural Benevolent
Institution 皇家农学院(英)

Rab/ Ser Rabies Antiserum 狂 犬病抗血清

Rab/ Vac Rabies Vaccine 狂犬病疫苗

RA Cell Ragocyct Cell 类风湿细胞

Rad Rad 拉德【注释】〔辐射剂量单位。近年用 SI 单位

的" 戈瑞(Gy)"表示。1r Ad = 1 × 10 - 2 Gy〕

Rad . Radiculitis 脊神经根炎

RAD Right Axis Deviation 心电轴右偏

RADAR Risk Assessment Of Drug- Analysis And Response 药 品分析和反应的危险评估; RADAR 活动【注释】〔围绕药品的毒副作用和疗效、价格成本等进行的分析评估,以此推动药品的合理使用和维护患者利益〕

RADS Reactive Airway Disease Syndrome 反应性气道病综合征

RADS Reactive Airways Dysfunction Syndrome 反 应性呼气道功能不全综合征【注释】〔例如在职业哮喘病中所见到的刺激性哮喘。以往无呼吸系统病史,偶然接触刺激源后, 24 小时内出现症状并持续 3 个月以上即可诊断为 RADS〕

Radse Reactive Airway Disease 反 应性气道疾病

Radt Radiologist 放 射学工作者; 放射学家; 放射科医师

Rae Right At Rial Enlargement 右 心房增大

RAEB Refractory Anaemia With Excess

Blasts 原始细胞过多性难治性贫血

RAEB-T Transformed RAEB 转化型原
始细胞过多性难治性贫血

RAF Rheumatoid Arthritis Factor 类 风
湿性关节炎因子

RAG Radioautogram 放 射性同位素

RAG Radioisotope Angiography 放 射性
同位素血管造影术【注释】 〔由肘静脉快速注入 RI 标记的
示踪剂, 利用置于靶部位体表处的闪烁
照相机连续摄影使该部血流可视化或
者进行定量分析〕

Ragg Rheumatoid Agglutinator 类 风湿
性凝集物(凝集素)

Ragr Radiograph X 射线照片

Ragrc Radiographic 放射照相的

Ragrs Radiographs X 光照片

RAGT Radioactivity Antiglobulin Test
放射抗球蛋白试验

RAH, Rah Right At Rial Hyper Trophy 右
心房肥大

Raio Radioactive Iodine 放射性碘

RAIU Radioactive Iodine Uptake 放 射
性碘摄取率(放射性碘摄取)

RALES Randomized Aldactone Evalua -
Tion Study 随机化安体舒通评价研究【注释】 〔一
种将 ACH 阻滞剂、 肾小管袢
型利尿剂与安体舒通合用的一种评价
安体舒通利尿效果的探索性试验〕

Ralo Radiculopathy 神 经根病

Ralv Rat Leukemia Virus 大鼠白血病病毒

RAM Rapid Alternating Movements 快速交替运动

Rama Radical Mastectomy 根治性乳房切除术

Rams Rapid Alternating Movements 快速交替运动

RANA Registered Animal Nursing Auxiliary 注册动物护理辅助人员

RANA Rheumatoid Arthritis- Associated Nuclear Antigen 类风湿性关节炎相关核抗原

RANA Rheumatoid Associated Nuclear Antigen 类风湿相关核抗原

Rane Radial Nerve 桡神经〔解〕

Raon Radiation Oncology 放射肿瘤学

RAP Recurrent Abdominal Pain 复发性腹痛

RAP Retinal Arterial Pressure 视网膜动脉压

RAP Rheumatoid Ar Thritis Precipitin 类风湿性关节炎沉淀素

RAP Right Atrial Pressure 右心房压力

Raph Raynaud□s Phenomenon 雷诺(氏)现象〔间歇性双侧手指或脚趾缺血性发作, 有时也见于耳和鼻, 四肢间歇性苍白或绀色〕

RAPM Refractory Anemia With Par Tial Myeloblastosis 难治性贫血伴发部分成髓细胞过多症

Rapr Radical Prostatectomy 根治性前列
腺切除术

Raps Resident Assessment Protocols 住
院护理指南

RAR Retinoic Acid Receptor 视黄酸受体

RARE Rapid Acquisition With Relaxation
Enhancement 快速摄影松弛术法【注释】〔为一种
快速摄影法。近来在

MRI 时, 特别强调摄影的快速化, 既要
缩短摄影时间, 又要获得优质的图像〕

RARS Refractory Anemia With Ring
Sideroblast 环 形铁粒幼红细胞性难治性
贫血

RAS Recurrent Aphthous Stomatitis 复
发性口疮性口炎

RAS Renal Artery Stenosis 肾动脉狭窄

RAS Renin- Angiotensin System 肾 素-血
管紧张素系统

RAS Reticular Activating System 网 状
激动系统

RAE 487 RAS
RAS Rheumatoid Arthritis Serum 类 风
湿性关节炎血清

RAST Radioallerogosorbent Test 过敏原
放免吸附试验; 放射过敏原吸附试验【注释】〔一
种测定抗某种过敏原特异抗
体 Ige 的放免分析法。将过敏原吸附到
纸板上, 被检血清中的抗体与之结合
后, 再结合标记 I125 的抗 Ige 抗体。根
据放射量对特异 Ige 进行定性定量〕

RA-Test Rheumatoid Arthritis Test 类风湿性关节炎试验【注释】〔为一种风湿因子的检测方法。

将人变性 Γ 球蛋白吸附到乳胶颗粒上,在载玻片上与患者血清进行凝集反应。即使是健康人也有 5 % 呈阳性〕

RATG Rabbit Anti-Human Thymocyte Globulin 兔抗人胸腺细胞球蛋白

RAVC Royal Army Veterinary Corps 皇家陆军兽医队〔英国〕

R/ AW/ Airway Resistance 气道阻力

RAW(Raw) Airway Resistance 气道阻力; 呼吸道阻力【注释】〔气道阻力=(气道开口部压

力- 肺胞内压力)/ 气流速度, 单位为

Cmh2o/ L/ 秒〕

RB Reflex Bradycardia 反射性心搏徐缓

RB Respiratory Burst 突发性呼吸

RB Retinoblastoma 成视网膜细胞瘤;视网膜母细胞瘤

R&B Rhytidectomy & Blepharoplasty 皱纹切除术与眼睑整容术

R-Band R 带

RBBB Right Bundle Branch Block 右束支传导阻滞【注释】〔心电图上显示的右束支兴奋性

刺激传导阻滞〕

RBC Red Blood Count 红细胞计数

RBC Relative Bone Conduction 相对骨导

RBC-CA Erythrocyte Carbonic Anhydrase

红 细胞碳酸酐酶

Rbce Red Blood Cell 红血球

RBC, Rbc Red Blood Cell(S) 红 细胞; 红 血球

RBD Recurrent Brief Depression 反复发 作的短暂性抑郁

RBD REM Sleep Behavior Disorder REM 睡眠行为障碍

RBE Relative Biological Effectiveness 相对生物学效果; 相对生物学效应【注释】 〔放射 生物学中, 即使是同一吸

收线量, 却也因为线质的不同, 引起不 同的生物学效应, RBE 能反应这种差 异〕

RBF Renal Blood Flow 肾血流量【注释】 〔流过肾 脏的血液量。 健康成年

人的肾血流量为 1 .1 ～ 1 .3L/ 分, 相当 于心输出量的 20% ～25 %〕

RBL Reid□s Base Line 雷 德基线【注释】 〔眼眶 下缘与外耳孔上缘之间的

连线, 用于头盖骨摄影时决定水平面的 角度〕

RBN Ret Robulbar Neuritis 球 后视神经 炎

RBP Renin-Binding Protein 肾素结合蛋 白

RBP Retinol-Binding Protein 视 黄醛结 合蛋白【注释】 〔结合并输送视黄醛(维生素 A1) 的蛋白质。 通常与前白蛋白形成复合 体。 其电泳条带位于 A2 球蛋白的位置〕

RBS Ribosome Binding Sequence 核 糖
体结合部位

RC Raymond-Céstan（Syndrome）雷
蒙德塞斯坦综合征

RC Red Cell 红细胞

RC Red Cross 红十字会; 红十字

RC Regional Colitis 局 限性结肠炎

RC Renal Carcinoma 肾癌

RC Respiratory Center 呼吸中枢

RC Routine Cholecystectomy 常 规胆囊
切除术

RAS 488 RC

RCA Radionuclide Cineangiography 放
射性核素血管电影造影术

RCA Regulators Of Complement Activa -
Tion 补体活性化调节剂〔人类细胞内的
一组蛋白〕

RCA Renal Cell Carcinoma 肾细胞癌

RCA Right Coronary Artery 右 冠状动脉

RCAG Radionuclide Cerebral Angiogra -
Phy 放射核素脑血管造影

Rcbf Regional Cerebral Blood Flow 局
部脑血流量【注释】〔从体外计测得到的局部脑
组织
的灌流血量〕

Rcbv Regional Cerebral Blood Volume
局部大脑血容量

RCC Rapid Cooling Contracture 快 速降
温性挛缩

RCC Read Clinical Classification 阅 读临
床分类

RCC Red Cell Count 红 细胞计数

RCC Relative Cytotoxic Capacity 相 对
细胞毒力

RCC Right Coronary Cusp 右 冠状尖

RCC, Rcc Renal Cell Carcinoma 肾 细胞
癌

RCC(Rcc) Radiochemical 放 射化学的

RCCT Randomized Controlled Clinical
Trial 随 机对照临床试验

RCCT Results Of Clinical Controlled Trial
临床对照试验结果

RCD Relative Cardiac Dullness 心 相对
浊音界

RCG Radiocardiogram 心 放射图; 放射
心电图

RCG Rheocardiography 心 电阻图描记
法

RC Gene RNA Control Gene 核 糖核酸
控制基因

RCH Rectocolic Hemorrhage 结 肠直肠
出血

RCIR Red Cell Iron Renewal 红 细胞铁
更新

RCIT Red Cell Iron Turnover 红 细胞铁
周转率

RCM Rate Chorionic Mamomt Ropin 促
绒(毛) 膜催乳激素

RCM Rheumatoid Cervical Myelopathy
类风湿颈脊髓病

Rcm Right Costal Margin 右肋缘

RCO Red Cell Ovecrriding 相 对心排血
量

RCP Regist Ry Of Comparative Pathology
比较病理学登记

RCS Red Cell Suspension 红细胞悬液

RCS Regimen Comprehension Scale 服
药理解能力评价标准【注释】〔为评价患者能否
正确理解 5 种
不同服药方法的药物和药袋上记载的
文字说明而设定的标准, 满分 10 分〕

Rcs Repeat Cesarean Section 重复剖腹产

RCT Recirculation Time 再循环时间【注释】〔静
脉注射指示剂, 以一定时间
间隔连续采集动脉血样检测其中的指
示剂, 从注入指示剂开始到其出现在动
脉血样中的时间即为 RCT。用来推算
血流速度和心输出量〕

RCT Registered Care Technologist 注 册
护理员【注释】〔为弥补护士人数的不足, 美国
医师协会在 1988 年建议设立的在病床
边照料病人的新职业, 帮助病人移动和
洗澡是其主要工作〕

RCT Retinal Circulation Time 视 网膜循
环时间

RCT Root Canal Therapy 根 管治疗术

RCU Respiratory Care Unit 呼吸监护病
房; 重症呼吸功能衰竭抢救室【注释】〔从 ICU 分
离出来的以重症呼吸
功能衰竭患者为对象的治疗部门, 与
CCU 相对应〕

RCV Red Cell Volume 红 细胞容量; 红
细胞体积

RCA 489 RCV

【注释】〔以 82 ～ 92μm3 为标准大小, 大
于此者称为大红细胞, 小于此者称为小
红细胞〕

RCVS Royal College Of Veterinary Surgeons
皇 家兽医外科学学会(英国)

Rcxr Repeat Chest X-Ray 重 复胸部 X 线
摄影

RD Rectal Distention 直肠扩张

R .D . Registered Dietician 注 册营养学
家

RD Renal Disease 肾脏病

RD Respiratory Disease 呼 吸道疾病

RD Respiratory Distress 呼吸性窘迫

RD Retinal Detachment 视网膜剥离

RD Revised Diagnosis 修改的诊断

RD Rheumatic Disease 风 湿病

RD Reaction Of Degeneration 变性反应

RDA Recommended Daily Allowance (S)
建议每日津贴; 推荐的每日供给量; 日最
佳定额量

RDA Right Displacement Of The Aboma -
Sum 皱胃右移

RDA Right-Sided Dispiacement Of Abomasum
皱胃右侧移位

RDC Research Diagnostic Criterion 研 究
用诊断标准

RDE Receptor Dest Roying Enzyme 受 体
破坏酶

RDEB Recessive Dyst Rophic Epidermolysis
Bullosa 隐性营养不良性大疱性表皮
松解

RDI Respiratory Disturbance Index 呼
吸障碍指数

Rdpase RNA-Dependent DNA Polymerase
R NA 依赖性 DNA 聚合酶

RDS Retinal Degeneration Slow 视网膜
缓慢退化蛋白【注释】〔定位于视网膜受体细胞
外片段
盘状膜的膜蛋白, 具 4 个跨膜区, 小鼠视
网膜缓慢退化蛋白的截短型突变体, 可
使外片段盘状膜发育异常、光受体再生
缓慢和失明〕

RDS Research Defense Society 科研防
御委员会

RDS Respiratory Difficult Syndrome 呼
吸困难综合征

RDS Respiratory Disease Syndrome 呼
吸系统疾病综合征

RDS Respiratory Distress Syndrome 呼
吸窘迫综合征【注释】〔肺泡腔内形成玻璃样体
而导致
呼吸困难。在生后数小时至数天期间,
表现出呼吸困难, 发绀。它是新生儿死
亡的一个原因〕

RDS(Rds) Downst Ream Resistance 下
游气道阻力

Rdss Respiratory Distress Syndrome 呼
吸窘迫综合征

RDW Red Cell Dist Ribution Width (Determination)

红细胞分布宽度(测定)

RDZ Radiation Danger Zone 辐射危险
区; 放射危险区

REA Rest Riction Enzyme Analysis 限制
酶分析

Reabd Rectus Abdominis 腹直肌〔解〕

Musculus R Ectus Abdominis〔拉〕
Readm Readmit 重新接纳

REAE Relapsing Experimental Allergic
Encephalomyelitis 复发性实验性过敏
性脑脊髓炎

Reanmos Reanastomosis 重新吻合

Rearr Respiratory Arrest 呼吸停止

Reatm Reattachment ① 复置术② 再附
着

REB Relative Biological Effectiveness
相对生物学效应; 相对生物学效果【注释】〔放射
学科用语, 指引起某种反
应所需的标准放射线吸收剂量与引起
同样反应所需的实际放射线吸收剂量
之比〕

R-EBA-L Recessive Epidermolysis Bul-
RCV 490 REB
Losa At Rophicans Local-Isata 隐性局部
性萎缩性大疱表皮松解 REB

R-EBA-Mitis Recessive Epidermolysis
Bullosa At Rophicans Generalisata Mitis
轻型隐性全身萎缩性大疱表皮松解

R-EBD-HS Recessive Epidermolysis Bullosa
Dyst Rophica-Hollopeau Siemens
隐性营养不良性大疱表皮松解

R-EBD-I Recessive Epidermolysi Bullosa Dystrophica Inversa 隐性反向营养不良性表皮松解

R-EBP Recessive Epidermolysis Bullosa Progressiva 隐性进行性大疱性表皮松解

Rebu Retrobulbar 脑桥后的; 眼球后的

REC Regional Enterocolitis 局限性小肠结肠炎

Recar Ret Rograde Cardioplegia 退行性心瘫痪

Recel Rectocele 直肠膨出

Rect Rectus ① 直的② 直肌

Recupd Recuperated 回流换热的; 回收的

RED Rapid Erythrocyte Degeneration 快速红细胞变性

RED Devil Seconal Capsule 速可眠胶囊; 速可巴比妥胶囊

Rede Retinal Detachment 视网膜剥离

Redi Respiratory Distress 呼吸窘迫

Redox . Reduction-Oxidation Reaction 还原- 氧化反应

Redrs Recreational Drugs 娱乐药

REE Resting Energy Expenditure 静息时能量消耗(量)

REF Renal Erythropoietic Factor 肾促红细胞生成因子

Refa Rectus Fascia 直肌筋膜; 直肠肌筋膜

Refai Respiratory Failure 呼吸衰竭

Reflx Ret Roflexed 后屈的

Refr Refract 使 折射

Refracg Refracting 折射望远镜

Refrd Refracted 骤 折的

REG Radioencephalography 放 射脑电
描记法

REG Rheoencephalography 脑 电阻描记
术; 脑血流描记术

Regr Retrograde ① 退行性的; 逆行的
②退化的; 衰退的; 异化的

Regra Retinography 视网膜照相术

REH Renin Essential Hypertension 原发
性肾素性高血压

Rehab Rehabilitation 康复; 恢复; 复原

Rehy Rehydrate 再 水化; 补充水分

Rehyd Rehydrated 再水合

REI Renal Excretory Index 肾 排泄指数【注释】
〔80 以下为正常〕

Reint Reintubate 重新插管

Reintd Reintubated 重新插管

Relg Releasing ① 释放; 释出② 分离
(的) ; 断开(的)

Relxn Relaxant 松弛剂; 弛缓的

Relxns Relaxants 松弛剂

REM Rapid Eye Movement (Sleep) 快
速眼动(睡眠) 【注释】 〔睡眠中多次或成群地出
现持续
2～ 3 秒的急速眼球运动, 此时脑波虽
是清醒型, 但人却处于深睡状态, 将受
试者唤醒, 有 80% 的人自述在做梦。

一个高质量的睡眠需要快波相与慢波相的适宜组合。全身麻醉状态下看不到 REM 期, 是其与深睡状态的一大不同点〕

Remed Rehabilitation Medicine 康复医学

REMS Rapid Eye Movement Sleep 快速眼动睡眠; 眼速动睡眠

Remu(S) Rectus Muscle (S) 直肌

Reno Retinopathy 视网膜病

Renot Retinotomy 视网膜造孔术

Ren Tran Renal Transplantation 肾脏移

REB 491 Ren

植

REO Virus Respiratory And Enteric Orphan Virus 呼吸道肠孤儿病毒

REP Retrograde Pyelogram 逆行性肾盂造影照片

REP Rifampin 利福平

REPE Re-Expansion Pulmonary Edema 再膨胀性肺水肿

Reper Retroperitoneum 腹膜后腔

Repe(R) L Ret Roperitoneal 腹膜后的

Reperly Ret Roperitoneally 腹膜后

Reph Referring Physician 咨询医生

Repha Relaxation Phase 舒张期

Repi Retinitis Pigmentosa 视网膜色素瘤

RER Resting Energy Requirement 储备能量需求

RER Rough (Surfaced) Endoplasmic Reticulum 粗面内质网

Rera Respiratory Rate 呼吸速率

Rero Recovery Room 恢复室〔手术后特
别病房〕

RES Reticuloendothelial System 网状内
皮系统【注释】〔包括淋巴结、脾、骨髓、肝
Kupffer
细胞、肾上腺皮质和结缔组织。它们
在功能上具有同一性, 能够吞噬清除异
物, 在发生学上均来自于间叶〕

Resco Resectoscope (经尿道) 前列腺切
除器

Rese Resect ①切掉; 切除② 外科切除手
术

Resed Resected 切除

Reseg Resecting 切除

Resen Resection ①切除术②后方交会法
③反切法; 截点法④ 交叉; 截断

RESEP Reent Ry Systems Environmental
Protection 再入(大气层) 系统环境保护

Reshe Rectus Sheath 直肌鞘

Resig Rectosigmoid 直肠乙状结肠

Resp Respiratory 呼吸(作用) 的; 呼吸器
官的; 呼吸系统的

RESPA Reticuloendothelial System
Phagocytic Activity 网状内皮系统吞噬
活性

Resp(I) Respiration 呼吸; 呼吸作用

Resq Rescue Squad 抢救队

Reste Ret Rosternal 胸骨后的

Restov Restorative 恢复药

Resun Resultant ① 生成物; (反应) 产物
②结果的; 结局的

Resut Resuture 再 缝术; 二期缝术

Resys Recurrent Symptoms 复 发症状

RET Rational Emotive Therapy 合 理情
绪疗法

Ret Reticulocyte 网织红细胞

RET Right Esot Ropia 右 内斜视

Retcol Ret Rocolic 结肠后的

Retcor Retrocorneal 角膜后的

Reth Recreational Therapy 娱 疗 〔精神医
学康复治疗法之一〕

Rethr Rethrombose 再次血栓形成

Rethrd Rethrombosed 再次血栓形成

Reti Retinaculum 支持带; 韧带

Retic Reticulocyte (S) 网 状细胞

Reticc Reticulocyte Count 网 织红细胞计
数

Retics Reticulocytes 网 织红细胞; 网状
细胞

Retir Retinacular 支持带的; 韧带的

Retra Recent T Rauma 近期创伤

Retrb Ret Ractable 可伸缩; 可收缩

Retro . Ret Rograde 退 行性的; 恶化的;
逆行的

RETRO Reverse Transcriptase Containing
Oncogenic 致 癌病毒反转录酶【注释】 〔具有反转
录酶活性的致癌病
毒, 又叫做 RNA 型致肿瘤病毒〕

Retrr Retractor 拉钩

Retrrs Ret Ractors 牵开器; 拉钩

Retsut Retention Suture 保持缝术

REO 492 Ret

RETT Radionuclide Esophageal T Ransit
Time 放射性核素食管通过时间

Ret(U)S Returns 回 炉料; 回炉物; 回用
料; 返回料

REV Reticuloendotheliosis Virus 网状内
皮组织增生病病毒

Reva Revascularize 再 血管化; 换…… 血
管以增加心脏的血液供应

Revad Revascularized 再血管化的

Revag Rectovaginal 直肠阴道的

Revaj Revascularization 血 管形成术; 血
管再通

Revej Reversion 回 复突变 〔突变后的基
因又回复为原有状态〕

Reverd Ret Rover Ted 后 倾的

Revir Retrovirus 逆 病毒 〔带有逆转录酶
的一组 RNA 病毒〕

Revis Return Visit 复诊

RF Radio Frequency 无线电频率

Rf Rate Of Flow 流 动速度; 流率; 移动
率; 通量强度

RF Renal Failure 肾 (功能) 衰竭

RF Respiratory Failure 呼 吸衰竭

RF Respiratory Frequency 呼 吸频率

RF Reticular Formation 网状结构

RF Rheumatic Fever 风湿热 【注释】 〔在关节和心
脏部位看到病变的

急性炎症性疾病, 由 A 型溶血性链球菌
感染引起。用最早记载此病之人的名
字命名, 又叫布优氏病〕

RFB Rheumatoid Factor Binding 结 合
的类风湿因子

RFC Roset Te Forming Cell 玫 瑰花结形
成细胞【注释】〔在用绵羊红细胞免疫的小鼠或
家兔的脾和淋巴结中发现的抗体产生
细胞。70 ％以上为大中小淋巴细胞〕

RFFIT Rabies Fluorescent Focus Inhibition
Test 狂犬病荧光抑制试验

RFI Renal Failure Index 肾衰指数

RFID Radio Frequency Identification Device
(Microchip) 无线电频率鉴定设备
(微芯片)

RFL Reiter-Feissinger-Leroy (Syndrome
) 赖 特尔菲新格勒鲁格〔综合
征〕

RFL Right Fronto-Lateral 右 额侧位〔胎
位〕

RFLP Restriction Fragment Length Polymorphisms
(Analysis) 限 制性内切酶
片段长度多态性(分析) 【注释】〔癌的基因水平
研究成果已被用
于癌的病理诊断。其中的一个方法就
是用限制酶将 DNA 切断, 特定区域片
段的长短因癌变而与正常的不同, 由此
可以作为癌症诊断的参考〕

RFM Rifampin 利 福平

Rfm Risk-Factor Modification 危 险因子

修正

RFNA Red Fuming Nit Ric Acid 红色发烟硝酸

RFP Rapid Filling Period 快速充盈期

RFP Rifampicin 利福平

RFP Right Frontoposterior 右额后

Rft Right Fallopian Tube 右输卵管

RFT Right Frontotransverse 右额横

Rfxs Reflexes 反射

Rg Regimen ①摄生法; 食物疗法②制度

RGBMT Renal Glomerular Basement Membrane Thickness 肾小球基底膜厚度

RGC Radio Gas Chromatography 放射气相色谱(法)

RGC Remnant Gastric Cancer 残胃癌

RGC Reticularis Gigantocellularis 网状巨细胞

Rgdi Regular Diet 常规饮食

Rgex Regular Exercise 定期训练; 按时训练

Rgs Regimens 摄生法; 食物疗法

RH Radial Hemolysis 辐射状溶血

RET 493 RH

RH Radiant Heat 辐射热

RH Reactive Histiocytosis 反应性组织细胞增生

RH Recurrent Herpes 复发性疱疹

RH Regional Heparinization 局部肝素化; 区域性肝素化

RH Relative Humidity 相对湿度【注释】〔通常用%表示的湿度。RH = 某
温度下空气中水蒸气压力/ 在该温度下
达到饱和状态时的水蒸气压力× 100〕

RH Renal Hypertension 肾性高血压

RH Retinal Hemorrhage 视 网膜出血

RH Retroperitoneal Hematoma 腹 膜后
血肿

Rh - Rh Negative Rh 阴性

Rh + Rh Positive Rh 阳性

RH Rhesus Blood Group 猕 猴血型; Rh
血型

Rh Rhesus Factor Rh 因子【注释】〔是一种血型抗
原, 也叫做恒河
猴因子。有 D , C, E, D , C , E 6 种 Rh 因
子。Rh 血型是根据用恒河猴红细胞免
疫的兔血清能与人红细胞发生凝集反
应来确定的。反复多次输血者的红细
胞如果与自体血清发生了同恒河猴免
疫的兔血清一样的凝集反应, 则应想到
此人有复杂的 Rh 血型〕

Rhpl Rhinoplasty 鼻成形术

Rhsv Rheumatology Service 风湿病学辅

RM Radical Mastectomy 根 治性乳房切
除术

RM Red Marrow 红 (骨) 髓

RM Respiratory Metabolism 呼吸代谢

RN Reactive Nitrogen 活 性氮

RN Reflux Nephropathy 反 流性肾病【注释】〔膀
胱中的尿液经输尿管逆流向

肾脏导致的肾萎缩等病态〕

Rnca Renal Calculus 肾结石

Rnci Renal Calculi 肾结石

Rnfa Renal Failure 肾 (功能) 衰竭

Rnin Renal Insufficiency 肾机能不全

RO Routine Observation 常 规观测

RS Raynaud□s Syndrome 雷 诺氏综合
征; 肢端动脉痉挛综合征; 继发性肢端动
脉痉挛现象【注释】〔指一组由多种病因所致的
伴有
肢端血管痉挛性皮肤颜色变化、感觉钝
麻、疼痛与灼热的综合病征〕

RS Rectal Suppository 直 肠坐药; 肛门
栓

RT Radiation Therapy 辐 射治疗; 放射
治疗

RV Rectovaginal 直 肠阴道的

RV Rhinovirus 鼻病毒

RV Rotavirus 轮状病毒

RV Rubella Vaccine 风 疹疫苗

RV Rubella Virus 风 疹病毒

Rvla Rhinovirus Type Ⅰ A 鼻 病毒Ⅰ

Japanese

R R 波 R-Wave

   ガス交換率 Respiratory Exchange Ratio

   呼吸 Respiration

   薬剤耐性 Resistance

右の　Right

レントゲン　Roentgen

RA　安静時狭心症　　Rest Angina

右心房　　Right Atrium

不応性貧血　Refractory Anemia

慢性関節リウマチ　Rheumatoid Arthritis

Ra　上部直腸　　Rectum Above The Peritoneal Reflection

ラジウム　　Radium

RAA　右心耳　　Right Atrial Appendage

右大動脈弓　Right Aortic Arch

RAD　右軸偏位　　Right Axis Deviation

Rad, Rad Ther　　放射線治療　Radiotherapy

Rad Op　　根治手術　　Radical Operation

RAG　腎動脈造影（法）　Renal Arteriography

RAHA リウマチ血球凝集試験　　Rheumatoid Arthritis Hemagglutination Test

RAMC Flap　腹直筋皮弁　Rectus Abdominis Musculocutaneous Flap

RAO　右前斜位　　Right Anterior Oblique

RAP　右房圧　　Right Atrial Pressure

反復性腹痛　Recurrent Abdominal Pain

網膜動脈血圧　　Retinal Arterial Pressure

RARS 鉄芽球性不応性貧血　　Refractory Anemia With Ringed Sideroblasts

RAS　腎動脈狭窄　Renal Artery Stenosis

Raw　気道抵抗　Airway Resistance

RB　腎生検　　Renal Biopsy

網膜芽細胞腫　　Retinoblastoma

網様体　　Reticular Body

リーメンビューゲル（先天性股関節脱臼治療用の装具）　Riemenbugel

Rb　下部直腸　Rectum Below The Peritoneal Reflection

RBBB 右脚ブロック　Right Bundle Branch Block

RBC, Rbc　赤血球（数）　Red Blood Cell(Count)

RBF　腎血流量　Renal Blood Flow

RC　呼吸中枢　Respiratory Center

　　呼吸停止　Respiration Cease

RCA　右冠状動脈　Right Coronary Artery

　　右結腸動脈　Right Colic Artery

Rca　直腸癌　Rectal Cancer

Rcbf　局所脳血流量　Regional Cerebral Blood Flow

RCC　腎細胞癌　Renal Cell Carcinoma

　　右冠尖　Right Coronary Cusp

RCG　心放射図　Radiocardiogram

RCIT 赤血球鉄代謝　Red Cell Iron Turnover

RCM　拘束型心筋症　Restrictive Cardiomyopathy

RCT　腱索断（破）裂　Ruptured Chordae Tendineae

　　無作為化臨床試験　Randomized Clinical Trial

　　無作為対象試験　Randomized Controlled Trial

RCU　呼吸集中治療室　Respiratory Care Unit

RCV　赤血球容積　Red Cell Volume

RD　呼吸窮迫　Respiretory Distress

網膜剝離　　Retinal Detachment

リウマチ性疾患　　Rheumatic Disease

RDS　呼吸窮迫症候群　　Respiretory Distress
Syndrome

Ref　反射　Reflex

Reg　規則的　　Regular

REGAP　　食道胃後上行枝　　Ramus
Esophagogastricus Ascendens Posterior

Reha, Rehabili　　リハビリテーション
Rehabilitation

REM　逆説睡眠、急速眼球運動睡眠、レム睡眠
Rapid Eye Movement(Sleep)

REP　逆行性腎盂造影(法) Retrograde Pyelography

REPE 再拡張性肺水腫　　Re-Expansion
Pulmonary Edema

Resp　呼吸　Respiration

Ret　網状赤血球　Reticulocyte

RF　呼吸不全　　Respiratory Failure

腎不全　　Renal Failure

リウマチ熱　Rheumatic Fever

RFA　右後前頭位(胎位)　Right
Frontoanterior(Position)

RFP　リファンピシン　　Rifampicin

RFT　右横前頭位(胎位)　Right
Frontotransverse(Position)

RGA　右胃動脈　Right Gastric Artery

RGE　右胃大網動脈　　Right Gastroepiploic
Artery

Rh　Rh 因子　Rhesus Factor

リウマチ　　Rheumatism

Rh　ラ音　Rhonchus

RHA　右肝動脈　　Right Hepatic Artery
RHC　右心カテーテル　　Right Heart
Catheterization
RHD　リウマチ性心疾患　Rheumatic Heart
Disease
RHV　右肝静脈　　Right Hepatic Vein
RI　　核医学検査　Radioisotope(Examination)
　　　レギュラーインスリン　　Regular Insulin

RICU 呼吸器疾患集中治療室　　Respiratory
Intensive Care Unit
RIF　右腸骨窩　　Right Iliac Fossa
RK　　直腸癌
RKM　ロキシタマイシン　Rokitamycin
R-L　右-左シャント　　Right-To-Left(Cardiac
Shunt)
RLE　右下肢　　Right Lower Extremity
RLL　右下肢　　Right Lower Limb
　　　右肺下葉　　Right Lower Lobe Of Lung
RLND 後腹膜リンパ節摘除(術)　Retroperitoneal
Lymph Node Dissection
RLQ　右下腹部　　Right Lower Quadrant
RMA　右頤前方位（胎位）　　Right
Mentoanterior(Position)
Rmbf　局所心筋血流量　　Regional Myocardial
Blood Flow
RMI　亜急性心筋梗塞　　Recent Mypcardial
Infarction
RML　右中外側　　Right Mediolateral
　　　右肺中葉　　Right Middle Lobe Of Lung
RMP　右頤後方位(胎位)　Right
Mentoposterior(Position)

RMT 右頤横位(胎位) Right Mentotransverse(Position)
RMV 分時呼吸量 Respiratory Minute Volume
RN 逆流性腎症 Reflex Nephropathy
ROA 右前方後頭位(胎位) Right Boccipitoanterior(Position)
ROM 関節可動域 Range Of Motion
破水 Rupture Of The Membranes
ROME 関節可動域訓練 Range Of Motion Exercise
ROMT 関節可動域テスト Range Of Motion Test

ROP 右後方後頭位(胎位) Right Occipitoposterior(Position)
未熟(児)網膜症 Retinopathy Of Prematurity
ROT 右後頭横位(胎位) Right Occipitotransverse(Position)
RP 逆行性腎盂造影(法) Retrograde Pyelography

Rp 処方せよ
RPA 右肺動脈 Right Pulmonary Artery
RQ 呼吸商 Respiratory Quotient
RR 回復室 Recovery Room
呼吸数 Respiratory Rate
RRP 相対不応期 Relative Refractory Period
RRPM 心拍応答型ペースメーカー Rate Responsive Pacemaker
RS 呼吸音 Respiratory Sound
レイノー症候群 Raynaud Syndrome
RSA 右仙骨前位（胎位） Right Sacroanterior(Position)

RSP　右仙骨後位(胎位）　Right Sacroposterior(Position)

RST　右仙骨横位(胎位）　Right Sacrotransverse(Position)

RSTI　右室収縮時間比　Right Systlic Time Interval

RT　呼吸療法　Respiratory Therapy

　　放射線療法　Radiotherapy, Radiation Therapy

R/T, R/T　～に関連した　Related To

Rt　右側臥位　Right Lateral Position

　　右の　Right

RTBD 逆行性経肝胆道ドレナージ

　　Retrograde Transhepatic Biliary Drainage

RUE　右上肢　Right Upper Extremity

RUL　右上肢　Right Upper Limb

　　右肺上葉　Right Upper Lobe Of Lung

RUM　残尿測定　Residual Urine Measurement

RUQ　右上腹部　Right Upper Quadrant

RV　右心室(枝)　Tight Ventricle(Branch)

　　残気量　Residual Volume

　　腎静脈　Renal Vein

RVAD右心補助人工心臓　Right Ventricular Assist Device

RVCD右室伝導遅延　Right Ventricular Conduction Delay

RVEDP　右室拡張終(末)期圧 Right Ventricular End-Diastolic Pressure

RVEF 右室駆出分画　Right Ventricular Ejection Fraction

RVET 右室駆出時間　Right Ventricular Ejection Time

RVG　右室造影(法) Right Ventriculography

RVH　右室肥大　　Right Ventricular Hypertrophy

　　　　腎血管性高血圧症　Renovascular
Hypertension

RVI　右室梗塞　　Right Ventricular Infarction

　　　残気率　　　Residual Volume Index

RVMDP　　右室平均拡張期圧　Right Ventricular
Mean Diastoric Pressure

RVP　右室圧　　　Right Ventricular Pressure

　　　腎静脈圧　　Renal Venous Pressure

RVR　腎血管抵抗　Renal Vascular Resistance

Rx　　処方、処方箋　　　　Prescription Or Take
Recipe Or Formula

RXM　ロキシスロマイシン　　　Roxithromycin

R-Y　ルー Y 型腸吻合(術)　　　Roux-En Y-
Anastomosis

S

French

SC Surface Corporelle, Sous-Cutané
Se Sensibilité
SEES Sonde D'entraînement Électrosystolique
SEP Sclérose En Plaque
SFA Souffrance Foetale Aiguë
SIDA Syndrome D'immunodéficience Acquise
SLA Sclérose Latérale Amyotrophique
SM Splénomégalie
SMP Syndrome Myélo-Prolifératif
SNA Système Nerveux Autonome
SNC Système Nerveux Central
SNP Système Nerveux Périphérique
SNV Système Nerveux Végétatif
SOS Système Orthosympathique
Sp Spécificité
SPS Système Parasympathique
Sttsyndrome Transfuseur Transfusé

English

S-A Sinoatrial; Sinoauricular
S&A Sickness And Accident; Sugar And Acetone
S/A Stent/Artery Ratio
Sa Most Anterior Point Of The Anterior Contour Of Sella Turcica; Saline; Staphylococcus Aureus
Sa Statampere
SAA Serum Amyloid A; Serum Amyloid–Associated [Protein]; Severe Aplastic Anemia; Starch Ampicillin Agar; Synthetic Amino Acid
SAAG Serum-Ascites Albumin Gradient
SAAP Selective Aortic Arch Perfusion
SAAQ Signal-Averaged Acoustic Quantification
SAARD Slow-Acting Antirheumatic Drug
SAAS Substance Abuse Attitude Survey
SAAST Self-Administered Alcohol Screening Test
SAB Scientific Advisory Board; Serum Albumin; Signal Above Baseline; Significant Asymptomatic Bacteriuria; Sinoatrial Block; Society Of American Bacteriologists; Spontaneous Abortion; Subarachnoid Block
Sab Spontaneous Abortion
SABER Stent-Assisted Balloon Angioplasty And Its Effects On Restenosis [Study]
SABOV Sabo Virus
SABP Spontaneous Acute Bacterial Peritonitis; Systolic Arterial Blood Pressure
SABV Saboya Virus
SAC Saccharin; Sacrum; Screening And Acute Care; Seasonal Acute Conjunctivitis; Self-Assessment Of Communication; Serum

Aminoglycoside Concentration; Short-Arm
Cast; Sideline Assessment Of Concussion
SAEM Society For Academic Emergency
Medicine
SAEP Salmonella Abortus Equi Pyrogen
SAF Scrapie-Associated Fibrils; Self-Articulating
Femoral; Serum Accelerator Factor; Simultaneous
Auditory Feedback; Standard Analytic
File
SAFA Soluble Antigen Fluorescent Antibody
SAFE Safety After Fifty Evaluation [Study];
Surgery, Antibiotics, Face Washing, Environmental
Change
SAFE-PACE Syncope And Falls In The
Elderly-Role Of Pacemaker [Study]
SAFHS Sonic-Accelerated Fracture-Healing
System
SAFIRE-D Symptomatic Atrial Fibrillation
Investigation And Randomized Evaluation Of
Dofetilide [Study]
SAFTEE Systematic Assessment For Treatment
Of Emergent Events
SAFTEE-GI Systematic Assessment For
Treatment Of Emergent Events-General Inquiry
SAFTEE-SI Systematic Assessment For Treatment
Of Emergent Events-Systematic Inquiry
SAFV Saint-Floris Virus
SAG Salicyl Acyl Glucuronide; Sodium
Antimony Gluconate; Sonoangiography;
Streptavidin-Gold; Superantigen; Swiss
Agammaglobulinemia
Sag Sagittal
SAGE Serial Analysis Of Gene Expression;
Systematic Assessment Of Geriatric Drug
Use Via Epidemiology [Study]

SAGES Signal-Averaged Electrocardiographic
Study
SAGM Sodium Chloride, Adenine, Glucose,
Mannitol
SAH S-Adenosyl-L-Homocysteine; Subarachnoid
Hemorrhage
SAHA Seborrhea, Hypertrichosis/Hirsutism,
Alopecia [Syndrome]; Suberoylanilide Hydroxamic
Acid
SAHCS Streptokinase-Aspirin-Heparin
Collaborative Study
SAHH S-Adenosylhomocysteine Hydrolase
SAHIGES Staphylococcus Aureus
Hyperimmunoglobulinemia
E Syndrome
SA-HRP Streptavidin-Conjugated Horseradish
Peroxidase
SAHS San Antonio Heart Study; Sleep
Apnea-Hypersomnolence [Syndrome]
SAHV St. Abb's Head Virus
SAI Self-Analysis Inventory; Sexual Arousability
Inventory; Social Adequacy Index;
Suppressor Of Anchorage Independence; Systemic
Active Immunotherapy
SAIC Science Applications International
Corporation
Saccat Stretch-Activated Channel Cations
Sacch Saccharin
SACD Subacute Combined Degeneration
SACE Serum Angiotensin-Converting Enzyme
SACH Small Animal Care Hospital; Solid
Ankle Cushioned Heel
SACK Suppression Of Asymmetric Cell Kinetics
SACNAS Society For The Advancement Of
Chicanos And Native Americans In Science

Saco2 Alveolar Carbon Dioxide Saturation
SACS Secondary Anticoagulation System
SACSF Subarachnoid Cerebrospinal Fluid
SACT Sinoatrial Conduction Time
SAD Scale Of Anxiety And Depression; Seasonal
Affective Disorder; Self-Assessment Depression
[Scale]; Separation Anxiety Disorder;
Serially Agitated Solution; Sinoaortic Denervation;
Small Airway Disease; Source-To-Axis Distance;
Standard American Diet; Sugar, Acetone,
And Diacetic Acid; Suppressor-Activating
Determinant
SADD Short-Alcohol Dependence Data
[Questionnaire]; Standardized Assessment
Of Depressive Disorders; Students Against
Drunk Driving
SADDAN Severe Achondroplasia With
Developmental
Delay And Acanthosis Nigricans
SADIA Small-Angle Double-Incidence Angiography
SADL Simulated Activities Of Daily Living
SADR Suspected Adverse Drug Reaction
SADS Schedule For Affective Disorders And
Schizophrenia; Self-Accelerating Decomposition
Temperature; Sudden Adult Death Survey;
Sudden Arrhythmic Death Syndrome
SADS-C Schedule For Affective Disorders
And Schizophrenia-Change
SADS-L Schedule For Affective Disorders
And Schizophrenia-Lifetime
SADT Stetson Auditory Discrimination
Test
Sadv Simian Adenovirus
SAE Serious Adverse Event; Sexual Assault
Evaluation; Short Above-Elbow [Cast]; Specific

Action Exercise; Subcortical Arteriosclerotic
Encephalopathy; Supported Arm Exercise
SAEB Sinoatrial Entrance Block
SAECG, Saecg Signal-Averaged Electrocardiogram
SAED Semiautomatic External Defibrillator
SAEFVSS Serious Adverse Events Following
Vaccination Surveillance Scheme
SAMIT Streptokinase And Angioplasty
Myocardial Infarction Trial
SAMMEC Smoking-Attributable Mortality,
Morbidity, And Economic Costs [Study]
SAMO Senior Administrative Medical Officer
SAMPLE Study On Ambulatory Monitoring
Of Pressure And Lisinopril Evaluation
SAMS Society For Advanced Medical Systems;
Substrate Adhesion Molecule
S-AMY Salivary Amylase; Serum Amylase
SAN Sinoatrial Node; Sinoauricular Node;
Slept All Night; Solitary Autonomous Nodule;
Storage Area Network
SANA Sinoatrial Node Artery
Sanat Sanatorium
SANDR Sinoatrial Nodal Reentry
SANE Sexual Assault Nurse Examiner; Single
Assessment Numerical Evaluation
SANE-A Sexual Assault Nurse Examineradult/
Adolescent
SANE-P Sexual Assault Nurse Examinerpediatric
Sang Sanguineous
SANGUIS Safe And Good Use Of Blood In
Surgery [Study]
Sanit Sanitary, Sanitation
SANS Scale For The Assessment Of Negative
Symptoms
SANV Sango Virus

SANWS Sinoatrial Node Weakness Syndrome
SAO Small Airway Obstruction; Splanchnic
Artery Occlusion; Subvalvular Aortic Obstruction
SAO2 Oxygen Saturation In Alveolar Gas
Sao2 Oxygen Saturation
Sao2 Oxygen Saturation In Arterial Blood
SAP Sensory Action Potential; Serum Acid
Phosphatase; Serum Alkaline Phosphatase;
Serum Amyloid P; Shrimp Alkaline Phosphatase;
Situs Ambiguus With Polysplenia; Sphingolipid
Activator Protein; Stable Angina
Pectoris; Staphylococcus Aureus Protease;
Subjective And Physical; Surfactant-Associated
Protein; Systemic Arterial Pressure; Systolic
Arterial Pressure
SAPA Scan Along Polygonal Approximation;
Spatial Average, Pulse Average
SAPALDIA Swiss Study Of Air Pollution
And Lung Diseases In Adults
SAPAT Swedish Angina Pectoris Aspirin
Trial
SAPD Short Action Potential Duration;
Signal-Averaged P-Wave Duration; Sphingolipid
Activator Protein Deficiency
SAPF Simultaneous Anterior And Posterior
Fusion
Saph Saphenous
SAICAR Sylaminoimidazole Carboxylase
SAID Specific Adaptation To Imposed Demand
SAIDS Sexually Acquired Immunodeficiency
Syndrome; Simian Acquired Immune Deficiency
Syndrome
SAIF Shigella Boulardii Antiinflammatory
Factor
SAIMS Student Applicant Information Management

System
SAKV Sakhalin Virus
SAL Sensorineural Activity Level; Sterility Assurance
Level; Suction-Assisted Lipectomy;
Suction-Assisted Lipoplasty
Sal Salicylate, Salicylic; Salmonella
Sal Serum Aluminum [Level]
Sal Salicylate, Salicylic; Saline; Saliva
SALAD Surgery Vs. Angioplasty For Proximal
Left Anterior Descending Coronary Artery
Stenosis [Trial]
Salm Salmonella
SALP Salpingectomy; Salpingography; Serum
Alkaline Phosphatase
Salpx Salpingectomy
SALT Skin-Associated Lymphoid Tissue;
Swedish Aspirin In Low Dose Trial
SALTS Strategic Alternatives With Ticlopidine
In Stenting [Study]
SALV Salehebad Virus
SAM S-Adenosyl-L-Methionine; Scanning
Acoustic Microscope; Self-Assembled Monolayer;
Senescence-Accelerated Mouse; Sex
Arousal Mechanism; Short-Arc Motion;
Smoking-Attributable Mortality; Staphylococcal
Absorption Method; Stepwatch Activity
Monitor; Subject Area Model; Substrate Adhesion
Molecule; Sulfated Acid Mucopolysaccharide;
Surface Active Material; System For
Assembling Markers; Systolic Anterior Motion
SAMA Schizoaffective Mania, Mainly Affective;
South African Medical Association;
Student American Medical Association
SAMBA Society Of Ambulatory Anesthesiologists;
Staffordshire Arthritis, Musculoskeletal,

And Back Assessment
SAMD S-Adenosyl-L-Methionine Decarboxylase
SAM-DC S-Adenosyl-L-Methionine Decarboxylase
Same S-Adenosyl-L-Methionine
SAMHSA Substance Abuse And Mental
Health Services Administration
SAMI Streptokinase And Angioplasty In
Myocardial Infarction [Trial]; Streptokinase
In Acute Myocardial Infarction [Study]; Students
For Advancement Of Medical Instrumentation
SAMII Survey Of Acute Myocardial Ischemia
And Infarction [Study]
SAST Selective Arterial Secretin Injection
Test; Self-Administered Alcoholism Screening
Test; Serum Aspartate Aminotransferase
SAT Saliva Alcohol Test; Saruplase Alteplase
Study; Satellite; Satisfactibility; Saturated,
Saturation; Serum Antitrypsin; Shifting Attention;
Single-Agent Chemotherapy; Slide Agglutination
Test; Sodium Ammonium Thiosulfate;
Solitary Arterial Trunk; Spermatogenic Activity
Test; Spontaneous Activity Test; Subacute
Thrombosis; Subacute Thyroiditis; Subcutaneous
Adipose Tissue; Sulfate Adenyltransferase;
Symptomless Autoimmune Thyroiditis; Systematic
Assertive Therapy; Systematic Axis
Transform; Systolic Acceleration Time
Sat, Sat Saturated, Saturation
SATA Spatial Average, Temporal Average
SATB Special Aptitude Test Battery
Satd Saturated
SATE Safety Antiarrhythmic Trial Evaluation
SATL Surgical Achilles Tendon Lengthening
SATP Spatial Average, Temporal Peak
SATS Substance, Amount Ingested, Time Ingested,

Symptoms
SATSA Swedish Adoption-Twin Study Of
Aging
SATT Scottish Adjuvant Tamoxifen Trial
SATV Sathuperi Virus
SAU Statistical Analysis Unit
SAUDIS Sudden And Unexpected Death In
Sports [Study]
SAV San Angelo Virus; Sequential Atrioventricular;
Sikhote-Alyn Virus
SAVD Spontaneous Assisted Vaginal Delivery
SAVE Saved-Young-Life Equivalent; Sudden
A Ventilatory Event; Survival And Ventricular
Enlargement [Trial]
SAVED Saphenous Vein De Novo
SAW Surface Acoustic Wave
SAX Short Axis; Surface Antigen, X-Linked
Sax Short Axis
SAX-APEX Short-Axis Plane, Apical
SAX-MV Short-Axis Plane, Mitral Valve
SAX-PM Short-Axis Plane, Papillary Muscle
SB Bachelor Of Science; Schwartz-Bartter
[Syndrome]; Serum Bilirubin; Shortness Of
Breath; Sick Bay; Sideroblast; Single Blind;
Single Breath; Sinus Bradycardia; Small
Bowel; Sodium Balance; Sodium Bisulfite;
Southern Blotting; Soybean; Spike Burst;
Spina Bifida; Spontaneous Blastogenesis;
Spontaneous Breathing; Standard Bed; Stanford-
Binet [Intelligence Scale]; Stereotyped
Behavior; Sternal Border; Stillbirth; Sudan
Black [Stain]; Surface Binding
S-B Sengstaken-Blakemore [Tube]; Suppression
Burst
SAPHO Synovitis, Acne, Pustulosis Hyperostosis,

Osteomyelitis [Syndrome]
SAPK Stress-Activated Protein Kinase
SA-PMP Streptavidin-Paramagnetic Particle
SAPPHIRE Stanford Asian Pacific Program
In Hypertension And Insulin Resistance
SAPS Simplified Acute Physiology Score;
Staphylococcus Aureus Protease Sensitivity
SAPV Sapphire Virus
SAPX Salivary Peroxidase
SAQ Saquinavir; Self-Applied Questionnaire;
Short Arc Quadriceps
SAQC Statistical Analysis Of Quality Control
SAR Scaffold Attachment Region; Scatter/
Air Ratio; Seasonal Allergic Rhinitis; Sexual
Attitude Reassessment; Slowly Adapting
Receptor; Specific Absorption Rate; Structureactivity
Relationship; Supplied Air Respirator;
Supraaortic Ridge; Supraaortic Ring; Synthetic
Aperture Radar
SARA Sexually Acquired Reactive Arthritis;
Superfund Amendments And Reauthorization
SARB Statistical Application And Research
Branch
SARI Serotonin-2 Antagonist Reuptake Inhibitor
SARS San Antonio Rotablator Study; Severe
Acute Respiratory Syndrome
SARS-Cov Severe Acute Respiratory Syndrome–
Associated Coronavirus
SART Simultaneous Algebraic Reconstruction
Technique; Society For Assisted Reproductive
Technology
SARV Santa Rosa Virus
SAS Sarcoma Amplified Sequence; Scandinavian
Angiopeptin Study; Scottish Ambulance
Service; Sedation-Agitation Scale; Self-Rating

Anxiety Scale; Severe Aortic Stenosis; Short
Arm Splint; Sklar Aphasia Scale; Sleep Apnea
Syndrome; Small Animal Surgery; Small Aorta
Syndrome; Social Adjustment Scale; Sodium
Amylosulfate; Space Adaptation Syndrome;
Specific Activity Scale; Statistical Analysis System;
Sterile Aqueous Solution; Sterile Aqueous
Suspension; Subaortic Stenosis; Subarachnoid
Space; Sulfasalazine; Supravalvular Aortic Stenosis;
Surface-Active Substance; Synchronous
Atrial Stimulation
SASA Solvent-Accessible Surface Area
SASD State Ambulatory Surgery Database
SASMAS Skin-Adipose Superficial
Musculoaponeurotic
System
SASP Salicylazosulfapyridine
SASPP Syndrome Of Absence Of Septum Pellucidum
With Preencephaly
SASS Syngen Acute Stroke Study
SAS-SR Social Adjustment Scale, Self-Report
SASSY Seniors Active Spirits Staying
Young [Program]
SAPHO Synovitis, Acne, Pustulosis Hyperostosis,
Osteomyelitis [Syndrome]
SAPK Stress-Activated Protein Kinase
SA-PMP Streptavidin-Paramagnetic Particle
SAPPHIRE Stanford Asian Pacific Program
In Hypertension And Insulin Resistance
SAPS Simplified Acute Physiology Score;
Staphylococcus Aureus Protease Sensitivity
SAPV Sapphire Virus
SAPX Salivary Peroxidase
SAQ Saquinavir; Self-Applied Questionnaire;
Short Arc Quadriceps

SAQC Statistical Analysis Of Quality Control
SAR Scaffold Attachment Region; Scatter/
Air Ratio; Seasonal Allergic Rhinitis; Sexual
Attitude Reassessment; Slowly Adapting
Receptor; Specific Absorption Rate; Structureactivity
Relationship; Supplied Air Respirator;
Supraaortic Ridge; Supraaortic Ring; Synthetic
Aperture Radar
SARA Sexually Acquired Reactive Arthritis;
Superfund Amendments And Reauthorization
SARB Statistical Application And Research
Branch
SARI Serotonin-2 Antagonist Reuptake Inhibitor
SARS San Antonio Rotablator Study; Severe
Acute Respiratory Syndrome
SARS-Cov Severe Acute Respiratory Syndrome–
Associated Coronavirus
SART Simultaneous Algebraic Reconstruction
Technique; Society For Assisted Reproductive
Technology
SARV Santa Rosa Virus
SAS Sarcoma Amplified Sequence; Scandinavian
Angiopeptin Study; Scottish Ambulance
Service; Sedation-Agitation Scale; Self-Rating
Anxiety Scale; Severe Aortic Stenosis; Short
Arm Splint; Sklar Aphasia Scale; Sleep Apnea
Syndrome; Small Animal Surgery; Small Aorta
Syndrome; Social Adjustment Scale; Sodium
Amylosulfate; Space Adaptation Syndrome;
Specific Activity Scale; Statistical Analysis System;
Sterile Aqueous Solution; Sterile Aqueous
Suspension; Subaortic Stenosis; Subarachnoid
Space; Sulfasalazine; Supravalvular Aortic Stenosis;
Surface-Active Substance; Synchronous
Atrial Stimulation

SASA Solvent-Accessible Surface Area
SASD State Ambulatory Surgery Database
SASMAS Skin-Adipose Superficial
Musculoaponeurotic
System
SASP Salicylazosulfapyridine
SASPP Syndrome Of Absence Of Septum Pellucidum
With Preencephaly
SASS Syngen Acute Stroke Study
SAS-SR Social Adjustment Scale, Self-Report
SASSY Seniors Active Spirits Staying
Young [Program]
SBO Small Bowel Obstruction; Spina Bifida
Occulta
SBOM Soybean Oil Meal
SBP Schizobipolar; Serotonin-Binding Protein;
Spontaneous Bacterial Peritonitis;
Steroid-Binding Plasma; Sulfobromophthalein;
Symmetric Biphasic; Systemic Blood
Pressure; Systolic Blood Pressure
SBQ Smoking Behavior Questionnaire
SBQC Small-Base Quad Cane
SBR Small Bowel Resection; Small Box Respirator;
Spleen/Body [Weight] Ratio; Strict Bed
Rest; Styrene-Butadiene Rubber
SB-RDC Sleep Bruxism Research Diagnostic
Criteria
SBRN Sensory Branch Of Radial Nerve
SBRS Senior Biomedical Research Service
SBRT Split-Beam Rotation Therapy
SBS Secondary Bilateral Synchrony; Shaken
Baby Syndrome; Short Bowel Syndrome; Sick
Building Syndrome; Sinobronchial Syndrome;
Skull Base Surgery; Small Bowel Series; Social
Breakdown Syndrome; Straight Back Syndrome;

Substrate-Binding Strand
SBSL-Ltx Sequential Bilateral Single-Lung–
Liver Transplantation
SBSP Simultaneous Bilateral Spontaneous
Pneumothorax
SBSS Seligmann's Buffered Salt Solution
SBT Sequence-Based Typing; Serum Bactericidal
Titer; Single-Breath Test; Sulbactam
SBTI Soybean Trypsin Inhibitor
SBTPE State Boards Test Pool Examination
SBTT Small Bowel Transit Time
Sbtx Small Bowel Transplantation
SBV Singular Binocular Vision; Soilborne
Virus
SBV Pentavalent Antimonial
SBW Standard Body Weight
SC Conditioned Stimulus; Sacrococcygeal;
Sanitary Corps; Sarcomatous Component;
Scalenus; Scan Computer; Scapula; Schüller-
Christian [Disease]; Schwann Cell; Schwarz
Criterion; Sciatica; Science; Sclerosing Cholangitis;
Secondary Cleavage; Secretory Component;
Self-Care; Semicircular; Semilunar
Valve Closure; Serum Complement; Serum Creatinine;
Service Connected; Sex Chromatin;
Sézary Cell; Short Circuit; Sick Call; Sickle
Cell; Sieving Coefficient; Sigmoid Colon; Silicone
Coated; Single Chemical; Skin Conduction;
Slice Collimation; Slow Component;
Snellen Chart; Sodium Citrate; Soluble Complex;
Special Care; Specialty Clinic; Spinal
Canal; Spinal Cord; Squamous Carcinoma; Start
Conversion; Statistical Control; Stepped Care;
Sternoclavicular; Stratum Corneum; Subcellular;
Subclavian; Subcorneal; Subcortical;

Subcostal; Subcutaneous; Subtotal Colectomy;

S/B Sickle Cell Beta-Thalassemia

S/B Sickle Cell Beta-Thalassemia

Sb Strabismus

SBA Serum Bactericidal Activity; Serum Bile Acid; Soybean Agglutinin; Spina Bifida Aperta; Stand-By Assist

SBAHC School-Based Adolescent Health Care

SBB Stimulation-Bound Behavior

SBBT Specialist In Blood Bank Technology

SBC School-Based Clinic; Schwarz Bayesian Criterion; Serum Bactericidal Concentration; Strict Bed Confinement

SBCS Stockholm Breast Cancer Study

SBD Selective Bowel Decontamination; Senile Brain Disease

S-BD Seizure–Brain Damage

Sbdh Sorbitol Dehydrogenase

SBDX Scanning Beam Digital X-Ray

SBE Breast Self-Examination; Short Belowelbow [Cast]; Shortness Of Breath On Exertion; Small Bowel Enema; Small Bowel Enteroscopy; Subacute Bacterial Endocarditis

SBEH Social Behavior

SBEPI Sinusoidal Blipped Echo-Planar Imaging

SBET Society For Biomedical Engineering Technicians; Standby Emergency Treatment

SBF Serologic Blocking Factor; Simulated Body Fluid; Skin Blood Flow; Specific Blocking Factor; Splanchnic Blood Flow; Systemic Blood Flow

SBFT Small Bowel Follow-Through

SBG Selenite Brilliant Green

SBH Sabra Hypertensive [Rat]; Sea-Blue Histiocyte; Small Basophilic Hemocyte

SBHC School-Based Health Center
SBI Shape-Based Interpolation
SBIAB Secondary Bacterial Infection Acute
Bronchitis
SBIS Stanford-Binet Intelligence Scale
SBL Soybean Lecithin
Sbl Sporadic Burkitt Lymphoma
SBLA Sarcoma, Breast And Brain Tumors, Leukemia,
Laryngeal And Lung Cancer, And Adrenal
Cortical Carcinoma
SB-LM Stanford-Binet Intelligence Test-
Form L-M
SBM Scientific Basis Of Medicine; Sexual
Intercourse Between Men; Solomon-Bloembergen-
Morgan [Equation]
SBMA Spinal Bulbar Muscular Atrophy
Sbmd Standardized Bone Mass Density
SBMLC Synchronous Bilateral Multiple Lung
Cancers
SBN State Board Of Nursing
SBN2 Single-Breath Nitrogen [Test]
SBNS Society Of British Neurological Surgeons
SBNT Single-Breath Nitrogen Test
SBNW Single-Breath Nitrogen Washout
SCAT Sheep Cell Agglutination Test; Sickle
Cell Anemia Test; Simvastatin And Enalapril
Coronary Atherosclerosis Trial; Sports Competition
Anxiety Test
SCAV Sunday Canyon Virus
SCAVF Spinal Cord Arteriovenous Fistula
SCAVM Spinal Cord Arteriovenous Malformation
SCB Strictly Confined To Bed
SCBA Self-Contained Breathing Apparatus
SCBE Single-Contrast Barium Enema
SCBF Spinal Cord Blood Flow

SCBG Symmetric Calcification Of The Basal
Cerebral Ganglia
SCBH Systemic Cutaneous Basophil Hypersensitivity
SCBP Stratum Corneum Basic Protein
SCC Self-Care Center; Sequential Combination
Chemotherapy; Services For Crippled Children;
Short-Course Chemotherapy; Sickle Cell
Disease; Side-Chain Cleavage; Small Cell
Carcinoma; Small Cleaved Cell; Spinal Cord
Compression; Squamous Cell Carcinoma;
Standardized
Coding And Classification; Symptom
Cluster Constraint
SC4C Subcostal Four-Chamber [View]
SCCA Single-Cell Cytotoxicity Assay; Small
Cell Carcinoma
SCCB Small Cell Carcinoma Of The Bronchus
SCCC Squamous Cell Cervical Carcinoma
SCCH Sternocostoclavicular Hyperostosis
SCCHN Squamous Cell Carcinoma Of The
Head And Neck
SCCHO Sternocostoclavicular Hyperostosis
SCCL Small Cell Carcinoma Of The Lung
SCCM Sertoli Cell Culture Medium; Society
Of Critical Care Medicine
SCCOR Specialized Centers Of Clinically
Oriented Research
SCCT Severe Cerebrocranial Trauma
SCD Scleroderma; Sequential Compression
Device; Service-Connected Disability; Sickle
Cell Disease; Spinocerebellar Degeneration;
Subacute Combined Degeneration; Subacute
Coronary Disease; Sudden Cardiac Death; Sudden
Coronary Death; Support Clinical Database;
Systemic Carnitine Deficiency

Scd Doctor Of Science

SCDA Situational Control Of Daily Activities
[Scale]; Special Care Dentistry Association

Scda Right Scapuloanterior [Lat. Scapulodextra
Anterior]

SCDAI Simplified Crohn Disease Activity
Index

SCDF Skin Condition Data Form

SCD-Heft Sudden Cardiac Death In Heart
Failure: Trial Of Prophylactic Amiodarone Vs.
Implantable Defibrillator Therapy

SCDNT Self-Care Deficit Nursing Theory
Containing;
Supercoil Cruciform; Supercomputing;
Superior Colliculus; Supportive Care;
Supraclavicular; Surface Colony; Surface
Cooling; Switching Circuit; Systemic Candidiasis;
Systolic Click

S/C Subcutaneous; Sugar Coated

S-C Sickle Cell

S&C Sclerae And Conjunctivae

Sc Scandium; Scapula; Science, Scientific;
Screening

Sc Statcoulomb

Sc Subcutaneous

SCA Self-Care Agency; Senescent Cell Antigen;
Severe Congenital Anomaly; Sickle Cell
Anemia; Single-Camera Autostereoscopy;
Single-Channel Analyzer; Sperm-Coating Antigen;
Spinocerebellar Ataxia; Starburst Calcification;
Steroidal-Cell Antibody; Subclavian
Artery; Superior Cerebellar Artery; Suppressor
Cell Activity; Survivor Of Cardiac Arrest

Sca-1 Stem Cell Antigen 1

SCAA Skin Care Association Of America;

Sporadic Cerebral Amyloid Angiopathy
SCABG Single Coronary Artery Bypass
Graft
SCAD Segmental Colitis Associated With
Diverticulosis
[Syndrome]; Short-Chain Acylcoenzyme
A Dehydrogenase; Spontaneous
Coronary Artery Dissection
SCAG Sandoz Clinical Assessment-
Geriatric [Rating]
SCAI Society For Cardiac Angiography And
Interventions
SCAM Statistical Classification Of Activities
Of Molecules
SCAMC Symposium On Computer Applications
In Medical Care
SCAMIA Symposium On Computer Applications
In Medical Care
SCAMIN Self-Concept And Motivation Inventory
SCAMP Stanford Coronary Artery Monitoring
Project
SCAN Schedules For Clinical Assessment Of
Neuropsychiatry; Suspected Child Abuse And
Neglect; Systolic Coronary Artery Narrowing
SCAP Scapula
SCAR Sequence Characterized Amplified Region;
Severe Cutaneous Adverse Reactions;
Society For Computer Application In Radiology
SCARF Skeletal Abnormalities, Cutis Laxa,
Craniostenosis, Psychomotor Retardation, Facial
Abnormalities [Syndrome]
SCARI Spinal Cord Injury Assessment Of
Risk Index
SCARMD Severe Childhood Autosomal Recessive
Muscular Dystrophy

Containing;
Supercoil Cruciform; Supercomputing;
Superior Colliculus; Supportive Care;
Supraclavicular; Surface Colony; Surface
Cooling; Switching Circuit; Systemic Candidiasis;
Systolic Click
S/C Subcutaneous; Sugar Coated
S-C Sickle Cell
S&C Sclerae And Conjunctivae
Sc Scandium; Scapula; Science, Scientific;
Screening
Sc Statcoulomb
Sc Subcutaneous
SCA Self-Care Agency; Senescent Cell Antigen;
Severe Congenital Anomaly; Sickle Cell
Anemia; Single-Camera Autostereoscopy;
Single-Channel Analyzer; Sperm-Coating Antigen;
Spinocerebellar Ataxia; Starburst Calcification;
Steroidal-Cell Antibody; Subclavian
Artery; Superior Cerebellar Artery; Suppressor
Cell Activity; Survivor Of Cardiac Arrest
Sca-1 Stem Cell Antigen 1
SCAA Skin Care Association Of America;
Sporadic Cerebral Amyloid Angiopathy
SCABG Single Coronary Artery Bypass
Graft
SCAD Segmental Colitis Associated With
Diverticulosis
[Syndrome]; Short-Chain Acylcoenzyme
A Dehydrogenase; Spontaneous
Coronary Artery Dissection
SCAG Sandoz Clinical Assessment-
Geriatric [Rating]
SCAI Society For Cardiac Angiography And
Interventions

SCAM Statistical Classification Of Activities
Of Molecules
SCAMC Symposium On Computer Applications
In Medical Care
SCAMIA Symposium On Computer Applications
In Medical Care
SCAMIN Self-Concept And Motivation Inventory
SCAMP Stanford Coronary Artery Monitoring
Project
SCAN Schedules For Clinical Assessment Of
Neuropsychiatry; Suspected Child Abuse And
Neglect; Systolic Coronary Artery Narrowing
SCAP Scapula
SCAR Sequence Characterized Amplified Region;
Severe Cutaneous Adverse Reactions;
Society For Computer Application In Radiology
SCARF Skeletal Abnormalities, Cutis Laxa,
Craniostenosis, Psychomotor Retardation, Facial
Abnormalities [Syndrome]
SCARI Spinal Cord Injury Assessment Of
Risk Index
SCARMD Severe Childhood Autosomal Recessive
Muscular Dystrophy
Sternoclavicular
Joint; Sternocostal Joint
Scjd Sporadic Creutzfeldt-Jakob Disease
SCK Serum Creatine Kinase
SCL Scleroderma; Serum Copper Level; Sinus
Cycle Length; Skin Conductance Level; Soft Contact
Lens; Stromal Cell Line; Subcostal Lateral
[View]; Symptom Checklist; Syndrome Checklist
SCL-90 Symptom Checklist 90
Scl Sclerosed, Sclerosis, Sclerotic
Scla Left Scapuloanterior [Lat. Scapulolaeva
Anterior]

SCLBCL Secondary Cutaneous Large B-Cell
Lymphoma
SCLC Small Cell Lung Carcinoma
SCLD Sickle Cell Chronic Lung Disease
SCLE Subacute Cutaneous Lupus Erythematosus
Scler Scleroderma, Sclerosis
SCLH Subcortical Laminar Heterotopia
Sclp Left Scapuloposterior [Lat. Scapulolaeva
Posterior]
SCL-90-R Symptom Checklist 90, Revised
SCLS Systemic Capillary Leak Syndrome
SCM Scanning Capacitance Microscopy;
Schwann Cell Membrane; Sensation, Circulation,
And Motion; Society Of Computer
Medicine; Soluble Cytotoxic Medium; Spleen
Cell–Conditioned Medium; Split Cord Malformation;
Spondylitic Caudal Myelopathy;
State Certified Midwife; Sternocleidomastoid;
Streptococcal Cell Membrane; Subclavius
Muscle; Subcutaneous Mastectomy;
Supernumerary Marker Chromosome;
Surfaceconnecting
Membrane
SCMC Spontaneous Cell-Mediated Cytotoxicity
SCMHR Society For Clinical And Medical
Hair Removal
SCMO Senior Clerical Medical Officer
SCMPT Sperm–Cervical Mucus Penetration
Test
SCN Coagulase-Negative Staphylococcus;
Severe Chronic Neutropenia; Severe Congenital
Neutropenia; Special Care Nursing; Suprachiasmatic
Nucleus
SCN1A Sodium Channel, Neuronal Alphasubunit
Type 1

SCN5A Sodium Channel Gene

SCNS Subcutaneous Nerve Stimulation

SCNT Somatic Cell Nuclear Transfer

Scnv-20S Saccharomyces Cerevisiae Narnavirus 20S

Scnv-23S Saccharomyces Cerevisiae Narnavirus 23S

SCO Sclerocystic Ovary; Somatic Crossingover; Subcommissural Organ

SCOFF Sick, Control, One Stone, Fat, Food [Questionnaire]

Scdp Right Scapuloposterior [Lat. Scapulodextra Posterior]

SCE Secretory Carcinoma Of The Endometrium; Serious Cardiac Event; Sister Chromatid Exchange; Split Hand, Cleft Lip/Palate, Ectodermal [Dysplasia]; Subcutaneous Emphysema

Sce Somatic Cell

SCED Single-Case Experimental Design

SCEP Sandwich Counterelectrophoresis; Spinal Cord Evoked Potential

SCER Sister Chromatid Exchange Rate

SCES Subjective Computer Experience Scale

SCETI Stanford Computer-Based Educator Training Intervention

Scety1v To 5V Saccharomyces Cerevisiae Ty1 Virus To Ty5 Virus

SCF Sinusoid Containing Blood Flow; Skin Cancer Foundation; Stem Cell Factor; Subcostal Frontal [View]

SCFA Short-Chain Fatty Acid

SCFE Slipped Capital Femoral Epiphysis

SCG Scaled Conjugate Gradient; Serum Chemistry Graft; Serum Chemogram; Sodium Cromoglycate; Superior Cervical Ganglion

SCGE Single-Cell Gel Electrophoresis
SCH Student Contact Hour; Succinylcholine
Sch Succinylchloride; Succinylcholine
Sche Serum Cholinesterase
SCHIP State Children's Health Insurance
Program
Schiz Schizophrenia
SCHL Subcapsular Hematoma Of The Liver
SCI Science Citation Index; Scottish Care
Information; Serial Communication Interface;
Sperm Capacitation Index; Spinal Cord Injury;
Structured Clinical Interview
Sci Science, Scientific
SCID Severe Combined Immunodeficiency;
Soft Copy Image Display; Structured Clinical
Interview For DSM IV
SCI/D Spinal Cord Injury/Disorder
SCIDS Severe Combined Immunodeficiency
Syndrome
SCIDX Severe Combined Immunodeficiency
Disease, X-Linked
SCIE Social Care Institute For Excellence
SCIEH Scottish Centre For Infection And
Environmental
Health
SCII Strong-Campbell Interest Inventory
SCIM Spinal Cord Injury Medicine
SCINT, Scint Scintigraphy
SCIS Spinal Cord Injury Service
SCIU Spinal Cord Injury Unit
SCIV Subcutaneous Intravenous; Subcutaneous
Vs. Intravenous Heparin In Deep Venous
Thrombosis [Study]
SCIWORA Spinal Cord Injury Without Radiographic
Abnormality

SCRIP Stanford Coronary Risk Intervention
Project
SCRIPPS Scripps Coronary Radiation To
Inhibit Proliferation Post Stenting [Trial]
SCRIPT Smoking Cessation-Reduction In
Pregnancy Trial
Scrna Small Cytoplasmic Ribonucleic Acid
SCRT Stereotactic Conformation Radiotherapy
SCS Saethre-Chotzen Syndrome; Seven
Country Study; Shared Computer System;
Silicon-Controlled Switch; Slow Channel Syndrome;
Society Of Clinical Surgery; Specialized
Chromatin Structure; Spinal Canal
Stenosis; Spinal Cord Stimulation; Splattercontrol
Shield; Splint Classification System;
Synovial Chondrosarcoma; Systolic Click Syndrome
SCSA Sperm Chromatin Structure Assay; Subcostal
Short Axis
SCSB Static Charge–Sensitive Bed
SCSI Small Computer System Interface
SCSIT Southern California Sensory Integration
Test
SCSR Standard Cervical Spine Radiography
SCT Salmon Calcitonin; Secretin; Sertoli Cell
Tumor; Sex Chromatin Test; Sexual Compatibility
Test; Sickle Cell Trait; Solid Cystic Tumor;
Sperm Cytotoxicity; Spinocervicothalamic;
Spiral Computed Tomography; Staphylococcal
Clumping Test; Star Cancellation Test; Stem Cell
Transplantation; Sugar-Coated Tablet
S-CT Spiral Computed Tomography
SCT Serum Creatinine
SCTA Spiral Computed Tomography Angiography
SCTAT Sex Cord Tumor With Annular Tubules
SCTBIFR South Carolina Traumatic Brain

Injury Follow-Up Registry
SCTN South Carolina Telemedicine Network
SCTR Secretin Receptor
Sctx Spinal Cervical Traction
SCU Self-Care Unit; Special Care Unit
SCUBA Self-Contained Underwater Breathing
Apparatus
SCUD Septicemic Cutaneous Ulcerative Disease
SCUF Slow Continuous Ultrafiltration
SCUP Skin Cancer Utrecht–Philadelphia
[Study]
SCU-PA Single-Chain Urokinase Plasminogen
Activator
SCUT Schizophrenia, Chronic Undifferentiated
Type
SCV Sensory Nerve Conduction Velocity;
Smooth, Capsulated, Virulent; Squamous Cell
Carcinoma Of The Vulva; Subclavian Vein
Scv Saccharomyces Cerevisiae Virus
SCOP Scopolamine; Structural Classification
Of Proteins; Systematic Classification Of Proteins
SCOPE Scientific Committee On Problems
Of The Environment; Specialist Certification
Of Obesity Professionals In Europe; Study Of
Cognition And Prognosis In The Elderly; Surveillance
And Control Of Pathogens Of Epidemiologic
Importance [Study]
SCOPEG Symmetric, Centrally Ordered,
Phase-Encoded Group [Imaging]
SCOPME Standing Committee On Postgraduate
Medical And Dental Education
SCOR Specialized Center For Research
SCORE Status, Connections, Occupation,
Resources, Events
SCORES Stent Comparative Restenosis

[Trial]; SCORES Saphenous Vein Graft Registry
SCOT Social Construction Of Technology;
Subcostal Outflow [View]
SCP Single-Celled Protein; Smoking Cessation
Program; Sodium Cellulose Phosphate;
Soluble Cytoplasmic Protein; Specialty Care
Physician; Standard Care Plan; Sterol Carrier
Protein; Submucous Cleft Palate; Superior Cerebral
Peduncle
Scp Spastic Cerebral Palsy
Scp Spherical Candle Power
SCPE Simplified Collective Protective Equipment
SCPK Serum Creatine Phosphokinase
SCPL Supracricoid Partial Laryngectomy
SCPM Somatic Crossover Point Mapping
SCPN Serum Carboxypeptidase N
SCPNT Southern California Postrotary Nystagmus
Test
SCPR Standard Cardiopulmonary Resuscitation
S-CPR Standard Postcompression Remodeling
SCPS Skin Cancer Prevention Study
SCPT Schizophrenic Chronic Paranoid Type
SCQ Social Communication Questionnaire
SCR Schick Conversion Rate; Short Consensus
Repeat; Silicon-Controlled Rectifier;
Skin Conductance Response; Slow-Cycling
Rhodopsin; Spondylitic Caudal Radiculopathy
Scr, Scr Serum Creatinine
Scr1 Soluble Complement Receptor Type 1
Scr Scruple
SCRAM Speech-Controlled Respirometer For
Ambulation Measurement
SCRAS Sheehan Clinician-Rated Anxiety
Scale
SCRF Surface Coil Rotating Frame; Systematized

Nomenclature In Medicine Cross-Reference Field

SDCL Symptom Distress Checklist

SDCN Neural Syndectan; N-Syndectan

SDD Selective Decontamination Of The Digestive Tract; Skeletal Dysplasia Diagnostician [Database]; Sporadic Depressive Disease; Sterile Dry Dressing

SDDS 2-Sulfamoyl-4,4'-Diaminodiphenylsulfone

SDE Simulation Development Environment; Specific Dynamic Effect; Standard-Dose Epinephrine; Structured Data Entry; Subdural Empyema

SDEEG Stereotactic Depth Electroencephalography

SDES Symptomatic Diffuse Esophageal Spasm

SDF Slow Death Factor; Standard Data Format; Stress Distribution Factor; Stromal-Derived Factor; Structured Data File

SDFV Syr-Daria Valley Virus

SDG Sucrose Density Gradient

SDGF Schwannoma-Derived Growth Factor

SDH Serine Dehydratase; Sorbitol Dehydrogenase; Spinal Dorsal Horn; Subdural Hematoma; Succinate Dehydrogenase

SDHD Sudden Death Heart Disease

SDI Selective Dissemination Of Information; Standard Deviation Interval; Survey Diagnostic Instrument

SDIF Standard Generalized Markup Language Document Interchange Format

SDIHD Sudden Death Ischemic Heart Disease

SDILINE Selective Dissemination Of Information Online [Databank]

SDIS Stockholm Diabetes Intervention Study

SDL Serum Digoxin Level; Speech Discrimination

Level

Sdl Sideline; Subline

SDM Semantic Data Model; Sensory Detection
Method; Sparse Distributed Memory;
Standard Deviation Of The Mean; System Of
Decision Making; System Development Method;
Systematized Nomenclature In Medicine
Digital Imaging And Communications In
Medicine Microglossary

SDMD Sulfadimethoxine

SDMS Society Of Diagnostic Medical Sonography

SDN Sexually Dimorphic Nucleus

SDNF Sliding Discrete Fourier Transform
Narrow Band Filter

SDNV Serra Do Navio Virus

SDO Standards Development Organization;
Sudden Dosage Onset

SDP Right Sacroposterior [Lat. Sacrodextra
Posterior]; Shared Decision-Making Program;
Signal Density Plot

SDR Shared Data Research; Skeletal Dysplasia
Registry; Spontaneously Diabetic Rat;

Scv-BC Saccharomyces Cerevisiae Virus
L-BC

SCV-CPR Simultaneous Compression Ventilation–
Cardiopulmonary Resuscitation

SCVIR Society Of Cardiovascular And Interventional
Radiology

Scv-L-A Saccharomyces Cerevisiae Virus
L-A

SCWM Subcortical White Matter

SCZ Schizophrenia

SD Sandhoff Disease; Selective Decontamination;
Semidry; Senile Dementia; Septal Defect;
Serologically Defined; Serologically

Detectable; Serologically Determined; Serum
Defect; Shine-Dalgarno [Sequence]; Short Dialysis;
Shoulder Disarticulation; Shy-Draper
[Syndrome]; Skin Destruction; Skin Dose;
Solvent/Detergent; Somatization Disorder;
Spatial Deconvolution; Spatial Embedding Dimension;
Speech Delay; Sphincter Dilation;
Spontaneous Delivery; Sporadic Depression;
Sprague-Dawley [Rat]; Spreading Depression;
Stable Disease; Standard Definition; Standard
Deviation; Statistical Documentation; Stensen
Duct; Still Disease; Stone Disintegration;
Straight Drainage; Strength Duration; Streptodornase;
Structural Deterioration; Sudden
Death; Superoxide Dismutase; Synchronous
Detector; Systolic Discharge
S-D Sickle Cell Hemoglobin D; Suicidedepression
S/D Sharp/Dull; Shine-Dalgarno [Region];
Systolic/Diastolic
Sd Standard; Standard Deviation Of Differences
Of Sample; Stimulus Drive
Sd Discriminative Stimulus
SDA Right Sacroanterior [Lat. Sacrodextra
Anterior]; Sabouraud Dextrose Agar; Serotonin-
Dopamine Antagonist; Sialodacryoadenitis;
Specific Dynamic Action; Strand
Displacement Amplification; Structural Displacement
Amplification; Succinic Dehydrogenase
Activity
SDAI Simplified Disease Activity Index
SDAT Senile Dementia Of Alzheimer Type;
Surface Digitalization Accuracy Test
SDAV Sialodacryoadenitis Virus
SDAVF Spinal Dural Arteriovenous Fistula
SDB Shared Database; Sleep-Disordered

Breathing

SDBP Seated (Or Standing, Or Supine) Diastolic
Blood Pressure

SDC Serum Digoxin Concentration; Singledispensing
Container; Smith Delay Compensator;
Sodium Deoxycholate; Sodium
Dichromate; Subacute Combined Degeneration;
Subclavian Hemodialysis Catheter; Succinyldicholine;
Symptomatic Developmental
Complex; Syndectan

SEADS-C Self-Efficacy And Dyspnea Strategies-
Confidence

SEAL Steric And Electrostatic Alignment

SEAP Secreted Alkaline Phosphatase

SEARCH Study Of The Effectiveness Of Additional
Reductions Of Cholesterol And Homocysteine

SEAT Sheep Erythrocyte Agglutination Test

SEB Seborrhea; Staphylococcal Enterotoxin B

SE(B) Standard Error Of Regression Coefficient

SEBA Staphylococcal Enterotoxin B Antiserum

SEBI Stereotactic External Beam Irradiation

SEBL Self-Emptying Blind Loop

SEBM Society For Experimental Biology
And Medicine

SEBOV Sudan Ebola Virus

SEBT Star Excursion Balance Test

SEC Screening End Code; Secretin; S-Ethylcysteine;
Singapore Epidemic Conjunctivitis;
Size-Exclusion Chromatography; Soft
Elastic Capsule; Spontaneous
Echo/Echocardiographic
Contrast Swollen Endothelial
Cell

Sec Seconal; Selenocysteine

Sec Second; Secondary; Section

Sec-Bu Sec-Butyl
Secd Service For The Care Of Drug Addicts
SECG Stress Electrocardiography
SECON Sequential Continuity
SECORDS South-Eastern Consortium On
Racial Differences In Stroke
SECRET Stiffness Of Joint, Elderly Individuals,
Constitutional Symptoms, Arthritis,
Elevated Erythrocyte Sedimentation Rate, Temporal
Arthritis [Mnemonic]
SECSY Spin-Echo Correlated Spectroscopy
Sect Section
SECURE Study To Evaluate Carotid Ultrasound
Changes With Ramipril And Vitamin E
SED Sedimentation Rate; Skin Erythema Dose;
Spondyloepiphyseal Dysplasia; Standard Error
Of Deviation; Standard Erythema Dose;
Staphylococcal
Enterotoxin D
Sed Sedimentation; Stool [Lat. Sedes]
SEDL Spondyloepiphyseal Dysplasia, Late
Sed Rt Sedimentation Rate
SEDT Spondyloepiphyseal Dysplasia Tarda
SEDT-PA Spondyloepiphyseal Dysplasia
Tarda–Progressive Arthropathy
SEE Standard Error Of Estimate; Staphylococcal
Enterotoxin E; Substernal Epicardial
Echocardiography
SEEG Stereotactic Electroencephalography
SEER Surveillance Epidemiology And End
Results [Program]
SEF Somatosensory Evoked Magnetic Field;
Spectral Edge Frequency; Staphylococcal
Anthropometry;
Stimulated Fibrinolytic Activity; Superficial

Femoral Artery
SFAP Single-Fiber Action Potential
SFB Sanfilippo Syndrome Type B; Saphenofemoral
Bypass; Surgical Foreign Body
SFBL Self-Filling Blind Loop
SFC Soluble Fibrin Complex; Soluble Fibrin–
Fibrinogen Complex; Spinal Fluid Count
SFCP Stanford Five City Project
SFD Silo Filler's Disease; Skin-Film Distance;
Small For Dates; Source-Film Distance; Spectral
Frequency Distribution
SFE Slipped Femoral Epiphysis
SFEMG Single-Fiber Electromyography
SFFA Serum Free Fatty Acid
SFFF Sedimentation Field Flow Fractionation
SFFV Spleen Focus-Forming Virus
SFG Spotted Fever Group; Subglottic Foreign
Body
SFH Schizophrenia Family History; Serumfree
Hemoglobin; Stroma-Free Hemoglobin
SF/HGF Scatter Factor/Hepatocyte Growth
Factor
SFI Sexual Function Index; Social Function
Index
SFIS Structural Family Interaction Scale
SFJ Saphenofemoral Junction
SFJT Saphenofemoral Junction Thrombophlebitis
SFL Scalar Fuzzy Logic; Synovial Fluid Lymphocyte
SFM Scanning Force Microscopy; Schimmelpenning-
Fuerstein-Mims [Syndrome];
Self-Fitting Face Mask; Serum-Free Medium;
Solution-Focused Management; Streptozocin,
5-Fluorouracil, And Mitomycin C
SFMC Soluble Fibrin Monomer Complex
SFMS Smith-Fineman-Myers Syndrome

SFN Society For Neuroeconomics
SFNM Standard Finite Normal Mixture
SFNV Sabin Virus; Sandfly Fever Naples
Virus
SFO Subfornical Organ
SFP Screen Filtration Pressure; Simultaneous
Foveal Perception; Spinal Fluid Pressure;
Stopped Flow Pressure
SFR Screen Filtration Resistance; Stenosis
Flow Reserve; Stroke With Full Recovery
SFS Serial Foveal Seizures; Skin And Fascia
Stapler; Social Functioning Schedule; Sodium
Formaldehyde Sulfoxylate; Spatial Frequency
Spectrum; Split Function Study
SFSV Sandfly Fever Sicilian Virus
SFT Sabin-Feldman Test; Second Field Tumor;
Sensory Feedback Therapy; Skinfold Thickness
SFTP Secure File Transfer Protocol [Telemedicine]
SERHOLD National Biomedical Serials
Holding Database
Holding Database
SERLINE Serials Online
SERM Selective Estrogen Receptor Modulator
Sero, Serol Serologic, Serology
SERP Somatosensory Event–Related Potential
SERPIN Serpine Protease Inhibitor
SERS Stimulus Evaluation/Response Selection
[Test]
SERT Sustained Ethanol Release Tube
Serv Keep, Preserve [Lat. Serva]; Service
SERVHEL Service And Health Records
SES Sirolimus-Eluting Stent; Society Of Eye
Surgeons; Socioeconomic Status; Spatial
Emotional Stimulus; Sphenoethmoidal Suture;
Subendothelial Space

SESAM Study In Europe Of Saruplase And
Alteplase In Myocardial Infarction
SESAP Surgical Educational And Self-
Assessment Program
SES-CD Simple Endoscopic Score–Crohn
Disease
SESE Somatosensory Evoked Spike Epilepsy
SESIP Safety Engineered Sharp Injury Protection
SET Scar Entry Technique; Secure Electronic
Transaction; Single Electron Transistor; Single
Embryo Transfer; Surrogate Embryo Transfer;
Systolic Ejection Time
SET-N Software Evaluation Tool For Nursing
SETTS Subjective Experience Of Therapeutic
Touch Survey
SEV 1 To 18, 125, 203 Simian Enteroviruses
1 To 18, 125, 203
Sev Sendai Virus
Sev Severe; Severed
SEW Slice Excitation Wave
SEWHO Shoulder-Elbow-Wrist-Hand Orthosis
SE(X) Standard Error Of The Mean
SF Sabin-Feldman [Test]; Safety Factor; Salt
Free; Scarlet Fever; Scatter Factor; Screen Film;
Seminal Fluid; Serosal Fluid; Serum Factor;
Serum Ferritin; Serum Fibrinogen; Sham Feeding;
Shell Fragment; Shunt Flow; Sickle Cell–
Hemoglobin F [Disease]; Simian Foam Virus;
Skin Fibroblast; Skinfold; Soft Feces; Spinal
Fluid; Spontaneous Fibrillation; Stable Factor;
Steel Factor; Sterile Female; Steroidogenic Factor;
Stress Formula; Sugar Free; Superior Facet;
Suppressor Factor; Suprasternal Fossa; Surviving
Fraction; Svedberg Flotation [Unit]; Swine
Fever; Symptom Free; Synovial Fluid

S1F Steel Factor
SF-1 Steroidogenic Factor 1
SF-36 Short-Form Health Survey
Sf Spinal Fluid; Streptococcus Faecalis
Sf Svedberg Flotation Unit

German

S - Sakralsegment

SA - Soziale Anamnese

S.C. - Subcutan

Serol - Serologisch, Serologie

Sin - Sinister

SM - Schrittmacher

ST - Steiltyp Im EKG

St.Pr. - Status Praesens

Sup - Superior

SVES - Supraventrikuläre Extrasystole

SW - Sakralwirbel

Sy(Ndr) - Syndrom

Italian

S

SCA Sindrome Coronarica Acuta
SCA Spinocerebellar Ataxia
SF Soluzione Fisiologica
SLA Sindrome Laterale Amiotrofica
SM Sclerosi
SNC Sistema Nervoso Centrale
SNG Sondino Naso-Gastrico
SNP Sistema Nervoso Periferico
Stemiinfarto Del Miocardio Con Sopraslivellamento
ST (ST Elevation Myocardial Infarction)
SV Stato Vegetativo

Russian

S/A
Sugar And Acetone
Сахар И Ацетон
SA
Sinoatrial
Синоатриальный [Узел]
SAH
Subarachnoid Hernorrhage
Субарахноидальное Кровоизлияние
Sat
Saturated
Насыщеный
SBE
Subacute Bacterial (Intfective) Endocarditis
Подострый Бактериальный (Инфекционный)
Эндокардит
SBP
Spontancous Bacterial Peritonitis
Спонтанный Бактериальный Перитонит
Sbp
Systolic Blood Pressure
Систолическое Артериальное Давление
SC, SQ, Subcu
Subcutaneous
Подкожный
SL
Sublingual
Сублингвальный
SLA
Soluble Liver Antigens

Растворимые Печеночные Антигены
SLE
Systemic Lupus Erythematosus
Системная Красная Волчанка (СКВ)
SMS
Somatostatin
Соматостатин
SO2
Oxvgen Saturation
Сатурация Кислорода
SOB
Short Of Breath, Shortness Of Breath
Одышка, Затруднение Дыхания
SOC
State Of Consciousness
Уровень (Состояние) Сознания
S/P, S/P
Status Post
Состояние После [Заболевания, Операции]
SQ, SC, Subcu
Subcutaneous
Подкожный
SR
Slow Release
Медленно Высвобождающийся [В Названии
Лекарственного Препарата]
SS
Sjogren's Syndrome
Синдром Шегрена
SSS
Sick Sinus Syndrome
Синдром Слабости Синусного Узла (СССУ)
STD
Sexually Transmitted Disease

Заболевания, Передающиеся Половым Путем
(Венерические Болезни)

STS

Serologic Test For Syphilis

Серологический Тест На Сифилис

Subcu, SC, SQ

Subcutaneous

Подкожный

Supp

Suppository

Суппозиторий

Surg

Surgery

Хирургия

Susp

Suspension

Суспензия

SVC

Superior Vena Cava

Верхняя Полая Вена

SVR

Systemic Vascular Resistance

Системное Сосудистое Сопротивление

SVT

Supraventricular Tachycardia

Суправентрикулярная Тахикардия

Sx

Symptoms

Симптомы

Syr

Syrup

Сироп

Chinese

S

S4 Four Th Heart Sound (An Abnormal
Hear T Sound) 第 四心音〔一种异常心
音〕

S Percentage Of Saturation 饱 和百分数
〔氧合血红蛋白或二氧化碳血红蛋白〕

S Saturation Of Hemoglobin 血红蛋白饱
和度

S Sella Turcica 蝶鞍点; 鞍〔土耳其鞍〕

S Sevoflurane 七 氟醚【注释】〔一种挥发性麻醉
剂〕

S Spine Sacral 骶脊柱

S Svedberg Unit 斯 韦德贝格单位〔沉降
系数单位〕

S- Symmet Ric Isomer 对 称性(同分) 异
构体

S3 Third Hear T Sound (An Abnormal Heart
Sound) 第 三心音〔一种异常心音〕

SA Sarcoma 肉瘤

SA Sensory Aphasia 感觉性失语(症)

SA Serum Albumin 血 清清蛋白; 血清白
蛋白

SA Siali Acid 唾液酸

SA Sideroblastic Anemia 铁 粒幼细胞贫
血

SA Sinoatrial 窦 房的

SA Sinoauricular 窦 房的

SA Small Animal 小 家畜

SA Storage Area 存 储区(数据)

S&A Sugar & Acetone 糖与丙酮

SAA Serum Amyloid A (Protein) 血 清 淀粉样蛋白 A

SAA Surface Active Agent 表面活性剂

SAARD Slow-Acting Antirheumatic Drug 缓用抗风湿药; 二线抗风湿药【注释】〔慢性风湿性关节炎病人经数年 使用阿斯匹林或其他非甾体类抗炎药 治疗后, 仍在 X 线片上发现关节病变 时, 才考虑使用的功效强大但副作用也 大的抗风湿药物(指甾体激素类)〕

SAB Selective Alveolobronchography 选择性肺泡支气管造影【注释】〔为了解末梢支气管和肺泡状态 而进行的有选择的小范围的造影。 也 就是将导管插入到所选部位, 用喷雾器 将造影剂喷到局部的造影方法〕

SAB Spontaneous Abor Tion 自 发流产; 自然流产

SAB Subarachnoid Block 蛛网膜下腔阻 滞【注释】 〔即通常所说的脊椎麻醉。在疼 痛临床领域, 针对癌症引起的疼痛, 有 时采用将微量的神经破坏药(苯酚甘 油) 以 45°体位注入到蛛网膜下腔中, 保 持体位 1 小时左右将脊髓后根局部破坏 的方法进行治疗〕

SA Block Sinoat Rial Block 窦 房传导阻 滞【注释】 〔窦房结和心房间的兴奋性刺激

传导障碍〕

SAC Scot Tish Agricultural Colleges 苏
格兰农业学院

SA(C) Staphylococcus Aureus 金 黄色
葡萄球菌; 金黄色酿脓葡萄球菌

Saca Short Arm Cast 短 臂管型

SACE Serum Angiotensin Converting Enzyme
血清血管紧张素转化酶

SACH Solid Ankle Cushion Heel SACH
足【注释】 〔无足关节、脚跟部有胶垫的一
种假肢的足部〕

Sacl Satinsky□s Clamp 萨 丁斯基(氏)
钳; 无损伤钳

Saclu Scapholunate 舟月骨

SACO Swedish Confederation Of Professional
Associations 瑞典职业协会联盟

Sacou Substance Abuse Counseling 药 物
滥用咨询服务

SACT Sinoatrial Conduction Time 窦 房
传导时间

SAD Seasonal Affective Disorder 季 节性
情感障碍

SADD Schedule For A Standardized Assessment
Of Patients With Depressive
Disorders 抑 郁症标准化评价计划表 【注释】
〔WHO 制定的由 37 项内容组成
的抑郁症标准化评价计划, 虽未普及,
但适用于国际间的合作研究〕

SAECG Signal Average Elect Rocardiography
信 号平均心电描记术

SAEM Society For Academic Emergency

Medicine 传统急诊医学会

SAF Small Abattoir Federation 小屠场
联合会

Sagec Salpingectomy 输卵管切除术

SAH Subarachnoid Hemorrhage 蛛网膜
下腔出血

SAIDS Simian Acquired Immunodeficiency
Syndrome 类 人猿获得性免疫缺
陷综合征

Sail Sacroiliac 骶髂的

Saju Saphenofemoral Junction 隐静脉股
静脉连接

Salaj Sacculation ① 小囊; 袋② 成囊

Salajs Sacculations 小 囊形成

Salar Saccular 囊 形的

SALINET Satellite Library Information
Network 卫星图书情报网络

Salm Salmonella 沙 门菌属

SAM Senile (Senescence) Activating
Mouse 促衰老模型小鼠【注释】 〔某种小鼠在传
代过程中, 会偶
然发生快速衰老的现象, 传代后其子代
仍保留这一特征。促衰老模型小鼠指
的就是以这种小鼠所作的动物模型〕

SAM Surface Active Material 表 面活性
材料

SAM Systolic Anterior Motion 收 缩期
前向活动

SAM Systolic Anterior Movement 收 缩

期前向活动【注释】〔肥大型心肌病所见, 三尖瓣的

尖部在收缩期向前方伸展而非后退关

闭瓣膜, 造成三尖瓣部分闭锁不全, 心

室血液逆流至心房。同时多伴有室中

隔非对称性肥厚和主动脉瓣闭锁不全〕

SAMCF Sheep-Associated Malignant
Catarrhal Fever (Virus) 羊 相关恶性卡
他热(病毒)

SAMS Sow Abortion And Mor Tality Syndrome
母 猪流产死亡综合征

SAMU Serviced□ Aide Medicale Urgente
地域医疗急救体系【注释】〔特指法国的由医师组成的地域

性医疗急救体系〕

Saoo Salpingo-Oophorectomy 卵 巢输卵
管切除术; 输卵管卵巢切除术

Sao2 Ar Terial Oxygen Saturation 动脉血
氧饱和度【注释】〔根据血中氧分压和 Ph 计算出
来的血氧饱和度(％) , 采血者用普通的
血液气体分析装置即可测定。动脉血
中的氧饱和度具有较大意义〕

Sap . Saponification 皂化(作用)

SAP Sensory Action Potential 感觉动作
电位

SAP Serum Alkaline Phosphatase 血 清
碱性磷酸酶

SAP Serum Amyloid P Component 血清
Sac 506 SAP
淀粉样物质 P 成分

SAP Systemic Arterial Pressure 体 循环
动脉压

SAP Systolic Ar Terial Pressure 动脉收缩
压

Sapro Sacral Prominence 骶 骨隆突

SAPS Simplified Acute Physiology Score
简化紧急生理计分法【注释】 〔用于评价急救重
症患者病情严

重程度的计分法〕

Sar Sarcoid 结节病的

SARA Subacute Ruminal Acidosis 亚 急
性瘤胃酸中毒

SARDA Search And Rescue Dog Association
犬类搜寻与营救协会

Sars Sarcoidosis 类 肉瘤病

SARS Severe Acute Respiratory Syndrome
严重急性呼吸系统综合征

SART Specific St Ress Caused By Alterna -
Tion Of Rhythm In Temperature 温度应
激动物【注释】 〔为研究自律神经调节功能而制
作的病态模型动物, 通过周期性改变饲
养环境的温度作成的副交感神经紧张
型的病态动物。 呈现呼吸心率增加、 心
室内刺激传导时间延长、 血压下降、 胆
碱反应性降低等〕

SAS Sleep Apnea Syndrome 睡 眠呼吸暂
停综合征【注释】 〔睡眠中频发呼吸暂停, 导致夜
间睡眠不良和白天困倦, 进一步引起低
氧血症、 高碳酸血症并进而出现呼吸循
环功能障碍〕

SAS Subarachnoid Space 蛛 网膜下腔
〔解〕

Sasa Sagittal Saw 矢 状锯

SASAS South African Society Of Animal
Science 南非动物科学学会

SASBLIA South African Stud Book And
Livestock Improvement Association
南非优良马中及牲畜改良协会

Saso Saline-Soaked 盐 水浸泡

Sasp Sacral Spine 骶 椎骨

SASP Sulfasalazine Salicylazosulfapyridine
柳 氮磺胺吡啶

Sast Skin And Subcutaneous Tissue 皮肤
与皮下组织

SAT Subacute Thyroiditis 亚 急性甲状
腺炎

SATS Short-Actin Thyroid Stimulator
短效甲状腺刺激素

Saud Saucerized 碟形手术

SAVA South African Veterinary Association
南 非兽医协会

SAVAB Small Animal Veterinary Association
Of Belgium 比 利时小动物兽医
协会

Savei Saphenous Vein 隐 静脉

SAVMA Student American Veterinary
Medical Association 美 国学生兽医医
药协会

SB Share Base 共 享库

SB Shower Bath 泼水疗法; 淋浴

SB Sinus Bradycardia 窦性心动过缓

SB Standard Bicarbonate 标准碳酸氢盐【注释】〔指在 37℃ , Pco2 40mmhg 下与 CO2 达到平衡时的血中 HCO - 3 浓度。

正常值为 24 (23 ～26)Meq/ L〕

SB Sternal Border 胸骨缘

SBD Senile Brain Disease 老年性脑病

Sbd Sharp And Blunt Dissection 锐器与钝器分解

SBE Sporadic Bovine Encephalomyelitis 牛散发性脑脊髓炎

SBE Standard Base Excess 标准碱过剩

SBE Subacute Bacterial Endocarditis 亚急性细菌性心内膜炎【注释】〔亚急性、慢性经过的败血症性

心内膜炎。来自于体内病灶的细菌附着在心内膜上繁殖发病, 难以医治〕

SBF Splanchnic Blood Flow 内脏血流量

SAP 507 SBF

SBFT(Sbft) Small-Bowel Follow- Through 小肠通畅

SBO Small Bowel Obst Ruction 小肠梗阻

Sbos Specific Behavioral Objectives 特殊行为目标【注释】〔医学教育用语〕

SBP Spontaneous Bacterial Peritonitis 自发性细菌性腹膜炎【注释】〔在肝硬化腹水的基础上发生的

感染性腹膜炎, 感染源尚不清楚。也叫 Conn 综合征〕

SBP Systolic Blood Pressure 收缩期血

压

Sbpr Scleral Buckle Procedure 巩膜扣操
作

SBS Sinobronchial Syndrome 鼻窦支气
管综合征

SBTPC Sultamicillin 舒它西林

SC Society For Cryobiology 低温生物学
会

SC Spinal Cord 脊髓〔解〕

SC St Reptococcus 链球菌

SC Subcutaneous(Ly) 皮下

SC Synaptonemal Complex 联会复合体

Sca Scar 瘢痕

SCA Sickle Cell Anemia 镰状细胞性贫
血

SCA Subclavian Ar Tery 锁骨下动脉〔解〕

Scaf Schizoaffective 分裂情感性

Scag Scarring ①伤痕; 瘢痕②瘢痕形成

SCAHAW Scientific Committee For Animal
Health And Welfare (Of The European
Commission) (欧盟) 动物健康福
利科学委员会

SCAIMVS South Central Australia Institute
Of Medical And Veterinary Science
澳大利亚南中部医学和兽医学协
会

Scani Sclera Are Anicteric 巩膜无黄疸

Scap Scapula 肩胛骨〔解〕

Scaph Scaphoid 舟状骨

Scapr Scapular 肩胛(骨) 的

Scaps Scapulas 肩胛骨

Scard Scarred 瘢痕性的

Scas Scars 瘢痕

SCAS Society For Companion Animal
Studies 伴侣动物研究协会

Scatg Scattering 散射

SCAW Scientists□ Center For Animal
Welfare 动物福利科学中心

Scbl Scalpel Blade 解剖刀片

Scbu Scleral Buckle 巩膜卡子; 巩膜扣

Scc Small-Cell Carcinoma 小细胞癌

SCC Squamous Cell Carcinoma 鳞 状细
胞癌【注释】〔扁平上皮的恶性肿瘤, 由皮肤、
黏膜、气管等的鳞状上皮细胞癌变形
成〕

SCC Succinylcholine Chloride 氯 琥珀胆
碱【注释】〔肌肉松弛剂〕

Scc Squamous Cell Carcinoma 鳞状细胞
癌

Scca Scarification ①划痕; 划破② 切刺
疗法③松土

Scch Sclerosing Cholangitis 硬 化性胆管
炎

Sccl Sclera Are Clear 巩 膜清晰

Sccos Scrotal Contents 阴 囊内容物

Sccys Schistocytes 裂 细胞

SCD Sterile Connection Device 无 菌连
接装置【注释】〔小儿自我输血时, 为减少穿刺
次数, 用带有 Y 型管的采血袋将采血与
回输连续进行, 一次穿刺即可〕

SCD Sudden Cardiac Death 心 脏猝死

SCDC Subacute Combined Degeneration
Of Spinal Cord 亚 急性脊髓联合变性【注释】〔先
是脊髓后束、侧束受损, 进而
引起末梢神经和大脑白质的变性, 伴有

SBF 508 SCD
恶性贫血是其特点。由维生素 B12 缺乏
导致〕

Scde Scleroderma 硬皮病

Scdep Scleral Depression 巩 膜凹陷

Scdi Scattered Diverticula 散在憩室

Scdrg Scrubbing And Draping 擦洗覆盖

SCE Sister Chromatid Exchanges 姐 妹
染色单体交换【注释】〔在培养淋巴细胞过程中
经常见
到的染色体异常, 同源的染色体之间发
生交换〕

SCE Subcutaneous Emphysema 皮 下气
肿

SCF Stem Cell Factor 干 细胞因子

Scfa Scarpa□s Fascia 史 卡巴筋膜; 斯卡
帕氏筋膜

Scfe Scarlet Fever 猩红热

Scfl Scalp Flap 头 皮瓣

SCG Sodium Cromoglycate 色 甘酸钠
〔抗过敏药〕

Scgr Scleral Groove 巩 膜沟

SCH Subconjunctival Hemorrhage 结 膜
下出血

SCH(D)F Slow Continuous Hemodiafilt

Ration 徐缓连续血液透析滤过【注释】〔血液环
路中加入小型过滤器,
将从这里滤出的体液弃去, 根据需要静
脉点滴药厂生产的补充液。这一方法
可有效地除去尿素、肌酐等〕

Sche Serum Cholinesterase 血清胆碱酯
酶

SCH(Seh) Succinylcholine 琥 珀胆碱

SCHUD Slow Continuous Hemo-Ultrafilt
Ration Dialysis 徐缓连续血液透析滤过

SCI Science Citation Index 科 学引文
索引【注释】〔作为评价科学研究水平的指
标, 覆盖了全世界可利用文献的 80%。
医学杂志发表的部分文献也在其收录
范围〕

SCI Spinal Cord Injury 脊髓损伤

Scia Sciatica 坐骨神经痛

Scic Scleral Icterus 巩膜黄疸

SCID Severe Complex (Combined)
Immunodeficiency
重症复合型免疫缺陷【注释】〔以体液免疫功能
和细胞免疫功
能的双重缺陷为特征, 是 X 染色体劣性
遗传病〕

SCID Structured Clinical Interview For
DSMIII-R 为 了 DSMⅢ -R 的临床交谈
机制【注释】〔事先拟好提问项目, 通过 Yes
或 No 的回答达到可以正确诊断的做法,
作为研修医生的诊断训练或客观诊断
的手段都是有用的, 在美国被广泛推

行〕

SCIWORA Spinal Cord Injury Without
Radiological Abnormality 无 放射性异常
的脊髓损伤

SCJ Squamocolumnar Junction 扁 平圆
柱状上皮交界处【注释】〔指子宫阴道部的黏膜,
是宫颈
癌的多发部位〕

Scl Sclera 巩膜〔解〕

SCL Sof T Contact Lens 软 接触镜

Sclae Scapulae 肩胛骨

Scll Scleral 巩 膜的

Sclot Sclerotomy 巩膜切开术

Sclots Sclerotomies 巩 膜切开术

Scls Scleras 巩膜

Scm Sternocleidomastoid Muscle 胸 锁
乳突肌〔解〕

Scmi Scopolamine 东 莨菪碱

Scmu Sclera Are Muddy 巩膜混浊

Scne Sciatic Nerve 坐骨神经〔解〕

SCO2 Computed Ar Terial Oxygen Saturation
计 算机显示的动脉血氧饱和度【注释】〔计算机
与质量分析仪联机, 根
据质量分析仪测得的终末呼气氧分压
和二氧化碳分压, 经计算机计算后自动
显示出的动脉血氧饱和度〕

SCP Single Cell Protein 单细胞蛋白

Scd 509 SCP

SCP Sodium Cellulose Phosphate 磷 酸
钠纤维素

SCP Sterol Carrier Protein 固 醇载体
蛋白

Scph Schizophrenia 精神分裂症

Scphc Schizophrenic 精神分裂症的

Scphf Schizophreniform 精神分裂症样

Scpks Serial Cpks 肌酸磷酸激酶序列

Scpl Scalpel 解剖刀; 手术刀

Scrg Screening ① 筛选(检查) ② 遮蔽
③荧光屏检查

Scri Schatzki□s Ring Schiazki 环

Scrog Sclerosing 致硬化的; 发生硬化的

SCS Spinal Cord Stimulation 脊髓刺激 【注释】
〔利用电刺激脊髓治疗难治性疼
痛的方法。现多用一种埋入型电刺激
疼痛控制仪进行操作〕

SCT Sentence Completion Test 造 句测
验【注释】 〔给出多个单词或词组, 让受试
者造句, 从中了解受试者性格的方法〕

Scth Sclerotherapy 硬 化疗法

Scti Scar Tissue 瘢 痕组织

Sctu Scleral Tunnel 巩 膜管

Scty Schizotypical 分裂型

SCU Scottish Crofters Union 苏格兰小
农场主联合会

SCU Self Care Unit 轻症病室【注释】 〔P PC 的最
轻病情患者入住的病
室〕

SCU Shock Care Unit 休 克监护病房

SCU Single Chain Urokinase 单 链尿激
酶

SCU Special Care Unit 特护病室

SCUD Septicemic Cutaneous Ulcerative
Disease 败血性皮肤溃疡病

SCUI Surgically Curable Urinary Incontinence
外科可治性尿失禁

SCV Sensory Nerve Conduction Velocity
感觉神经传导速度

Scv Subclavian Vein 锁骨下静脉〔解〕

Ve Na Subclavia〔拉〕

SCVMPH Scientific Committee For Veterinary
Measures Relating To Public
Health (Of The European Commission)
公共卫生兽医科学委员会

Scwu Scalp Wound 头 皮损伤

Scwzs Scattered Wheezes 散在喘鸣音

SD Scleroderma 硬皮病【注释】〔一种胶原性疾病〕

SD Senile Dementia 老 年痴呆

SD Septal Defect 中 隔缺损

S/ D Sharp/ Dull 高音低音之比

SD Standard Deviation 标 准差【注释】〔统计学用
语, 表示来自一个总
体的各个测定值的离散程度〕

SD Streptodornase 链道酶

SD Sudden Death 猝死【注释】 〔看上去很健康的
人完全出乎意
料的突然死亡。原因多为患者自身潜
伏了致死性病灶而没有注意到〕

SD Superoxide Dismutase 超 氧化物歧
化酶

SD Suspected Diagnosis 可 疑诊断

SDA Scottish Dairy Association 苏格兰乳制品协会

SDA Sialodacryoadenitis 唾液腺类腺炎

SDA Single Domain Antibody 单域抗体

SDA Specific Dynamic Action 特殊动力作用【注释】〔进食时能量代谢亢进的现象。食入蛋白质可使能量代谢速率加快30%, 食入脂肪加快 4%, 食入糖加快 6 %〕

SDB Society For Developmental Biology 发育生物学会

SDB Superficial Dermal Burn 浅层皮肤烫(烧)伤【注释】〔指比真皮乳头层浅的 II 度烫(烧)伤〕

SDCM Serum Drug Concent Ration Moni-SCP 510 SDC Toring 血清药物浓度监测

SDD Selective Decontamination Of The Digestive Tract (Selective Digestive Decontamination) 选择性消化道内杀菌【注释】〔为预防重症患者的住院感染特别是肺部感染, 对口腔、鼻咽部、消化道分别有选择地局部给予抗菌素, 通过这种净化措施, 防止感染物向下呼吸道的污染〕

SDF Synchronous Diaphragmatic Flutter 同步膈扑动; 重击声

SDH Sorbitol Dehydrogenase 山梨醇脱氢酶

SDHD Sudden Death Hear T Disease 心脏病猝死

SDI Selective Dissemination Of Informa - Tion 定题情报服务

SDI On-Line Selective Dissemination Of Information On-Line 联机定题情报服务

SDLC Synchronous Data Link Cont Rol 同步数据链路控制

Sdms Sharp Disc Margins SHARP 光盘的空白区

SDR Simple Diabetic Retinopathy 单纯性糖尿病性视网膜病

SDS Self-Rating Depression Scale 抑郁症自我评价尺度【注释】〔由 Zung WWK 建议的自我评价抑郁症的尺度。包括 20 项内容, 满分为 100 分。受试者按项对照自己有无相应表现, 自我打分。正常人 33 分(25 ～ 43 分) , 人格障碍 53 分(42 ～ 68 分) , 应门诊治疗 64 分(50 ～ 78 分) , 应住院治疗 74 分(63 ～90 分)〕

SDS Shy-Drager Syndrome 夏- 德综合征【注释】〔原因不明的一种自律神经功能失调(站立性低血压、尿失禁、少汗、性器萎缩、缩瞳、睡眠呼吸暂停) , 伴有运动障碍, 几乎都伴有小脑功能失调症状〕

Sdt Saline Drop Test 盐水点滴试验

SDT Speech Detection Threshold 言语检察阈

Sdu(S) Sacral Decubitus Ulcer (S) 骶骨褥疮溃疡

SDV Specific Desensitizing Vaccine 特
异性脱敏疫苗

SE Saline Enema 盐水灌肠

SE Status Epilepticus 癫痫持续状态【注释】〔癫痫
大发作在短时间内反复出
现, 呈几乎不间断地、连续地发作的危
重状态〕

SEAC Spongiform Encephalopathy Advisory
Committee 海 绵状脑病咨询委
员会

Sea(R) T(H) Septic Arthritis 脓毒性关节
炎

SEAT Sheep Erythrocyte Agglutination
Test 绵 羊红细胞凝集试验

SEB Society For Experimental Biology
实验生物学会

Seba Sebaceous ① 脂肪的; 皮脂的② 分
泌脂质的

Seca Senile Cataract 年龄相关性白内障

Secgs Serial Electrocardiograms 连 续心
电图监测

Seclj Seclusion 隔 离; 闭塞过程

Seco Second Course 二 道锉纹

Secre Serum Creatinine 血清肌酐

Sectd Sectioned 切片的

Sectg Sectioning 切 片

Secy Sebaceous Cyst 皮脂囊肿

SED Skin Erythema Dose 皮肤红斑剂量【注释】
〔所谓 1 个皮肤红斑剂量, 指的
是 1 次照射 1 ～ 3 周后, 能使皮肤产生

一过性红斑的放射线剂量〕

SED Spondyloepiphyseal Dysplasia 脊椎骨骺发育不良

Sedad Sedated 镇静

Sedag Sedating 镇静

SDD 511 Sed

Sedaj Sedation 镇静(作用);镇静状态

Sedav Sedative ① 镇静的 ② 镇静剂

Sedavs Sedatives 镇静药

Sede Septal Deviation 鼻中隔偏离

Sedef Sensory Deficit 感觉缺陷

Sedefs Sensory Deficits 感觉缺乏

Sedem Senile Dementia 老年性痴呆

Seder Seborrheic Dermatitis 脂溢性皮炎

Sedg Secondary Diagnosis 辅助诊断

Sed Rate Sedimentation Rate 沉降率

Seemb Septic Embolism 脓毒性栓子

Seens Serial Enzymes 连续酶学检查

Seex Self- Examination 自我检查

Seexa Sensory Examination 感觉检查

Sefl Serous Fluid 浆液

Sehcs Serial Hematocrits 系列红细胞压积

Sehn Severe Hypertension 严重高血压

SEI Stockholm Environment Institute 斯德哥尔摩环境研究所

Seis Serial Isoenzymes 系列同工酶

Sekes Seborrheic Keratoses 脂溢性角化病

Seloc Serologic 血清学的

Selocl Serological 血清学的
Selocly Serologically 血清学的
Seloy Serology 血清学
SEM Scanning Elect Ron Microscope 扫
描电子显微镜
SEM Scanning Electron Microscopy 扫
描电子显微镜术; 扫描电子显微镜法
SEM Secondary Enrichment Medium
二次增菌培养基; 二次强化培养基
SEM Systolic Ejection Murmur 收 缩期
射血杂音
Sema Serratia Marcescens 黏 质沙雷菌;
黏质沙雷(氏) 杆菌
SEMI Subendocardial Myocardial Infarction
心内膜下心肌梗死
Semods Sensory Modalities 感 觉形式
Semu Seromuscular 浆 膜肌膜的
Sene Sensorineural 感 觉神经的
Sento Sensitive To 对…… 敏感
Senu Sensory Neuropathy 感 觉神经病
Seos Serum Osmolality 血 清渗透压
SEP Serum Electrophoresis 血清电泳
SEP Somatosensory Evoked Potential
躯体感觉诱导电位 【注释】 〔人对于感觉刺激的
脑诱发电位
之一。通过其可以获得在各种感觉传
导路的不同部位障碍的诊断等脑波中
所不能获得的情报。也就是说, 由于将
构成背景的自发电活动(脑波) 进行平
均后去除, 加算诱发电位, 使数量变

大, 因此易于观察]

SEP Spinal Evoked Potential 脊髓诱发电位

SEP Systolic Ejection Period 收缩射血期

SEPA Scottish Environmental Protection Agency 苏格兰环境保护局

Sepjs Separations 分色片

Sepl Septoplasty 鼻中隔成形术

Sepols Sessile Polyps 无柄息肉

Sepos Sensory Evoked Potentials 感觉激发电位

Sepr Semi-Pressure 半压力

Seps Sepsis 脓毒症

Septo . Septoplasty 鼻中隔成形术

Sepv Separative 分离的(分离性的)

Sepy Separately 分别地; 个别地; 独立地; 借助外力地

Seq Sequence 序列分析

Seql Sequential 顺序的; 顺序取样

Seqla Sequela 后遗症

Seqle Sequelae 后发病; 结局

SER Serine (Aminoacid) 丝氨酸

SER Smooth Endoplasmic Reticulum 滑面内质网

SERAD Scottish Executive Rural Afsed 512 SER Fairs Depar Tment 苏格兰乡村事务管理局

Serat Sedimentation Rate 沉降速率; 沉

降率

SERM Selective Estrogen Receptor Modulator
选 择性雌激素受体修饰因子【注释】〔虽然对于
生殖器官上具有抗雌
激素作用或没有任何作用, 但对于骨组
织具有与雌激素相同的作用。 目前, 作
为维持改善骨组织和脂肪代谢及克服
雌激素副作用的药物而受关注〕

Sero Serosa 浆 膜; 绒(毛) 膜

Serol Serosal 浆膜的

SES Staphylococcal Enterotoxin 葡 萄球
菌产生的毒素

Sesa Sesamoid ① 籽骨的②籽骨

Sesan Serosanguineous 血清血液的

Seso Sensorium 感 觉机制

SETAC Society Of Environmental Toxicology
And Chemistry 环 境毒理学与化
学会

Sete Seldinger Technique 塞尔丁格(氏)
技术 〔下腔静脉造影时, 病人捏鼻屏气,
使显影良好〕

Setiy Sensitivity 感光性; 灵敏性

Setiys Sensitivities 敏感; 灵敏性

Setox Serum Toxicology 血清毒理学

Setu Sella Turcica 蝶鞍

Sevd Severanced 切断

Seve Seminal Vesicle 精 囊 〔某些无脊椎
动物和低等脊椎动物贮存精子的器官〕

Seves Seminal Vesicles 精 囊

Sevg Severancing 切 断

SF Shipping Fever 航运热

SF Spayed Female 切除卵巢的雌体

SF Spinal Fluid 脊 髓液

SF Spontaneous Fracture 自发性骨折

SFA Saturated Fatty Acid 饱和脂肪酸

SFA Superficial Femoral Artery 股 浅动
脉

SFA Suppressive Factor Of Allergy 变态
反应抑制因子

SFACET Scot Tish Farm And Countryside
Educational Trust 苏 格兰农场乡
村教育信托公司

SFBR Southwest Foundation For
Biomedical Research 生物医学研究西
南基金会

SFC Society For Cryobiology 低 温生物
学会

SFC Supercritical Fluid Chromatography
超临界温度液相色谱法; 超临界温度液相
层析法

SFD Small For Dates (Infant) 出生时未
成熟婴儿【注释】 〔与相同周数婴儿的平均体重
相
比显著轻的婴儿。另外, 其程度进一步
加重者, 称为 IUGR〕

SFE Supercritical Fluid Extraction 超临
界流体抽提

SFEC Specialization & Further Education
Committee (Of The RCVS) 专 业
进修委员会(皇家外科兽医协会)

SFF Société Francaise De Félinotechnie

(France) 法国猫技术学会

SFM Simple Face Mask 简易面罩

SFM Stimulation-Facilitation-Motivation 刺激-促进-诱导〔失语症治疗三概念〕

SFP Spinal Fluid Pressure 脊髓液压力

SFTA Société Francaise De Toxicologie Analytique 法国毒理分析学会

Sfv Superficial Femoral Vein 股浅静脉

SG Secondary Glaucoma 继发性青光眼

SG Specific Gravity 比重

SG Substantial Gelatinosa 胶状质

SGA Small For Gestational Age 小于孕龄儿

SGB Satellite Ganglion Block 星状神经节阻断【注释】〔颈下交感神经节和 T1 合并的神经节, 位于第 7 颈椎横突的前面, 如

Ser 513 SGB
果将其用 1% 局部麻醉药封闭时, 出现霍纳氏综合征状而发挥效果。应用于其所支配区域的血流障碍性疾病和疼痛性疾病等〕

Sgbs Satellite Ganglion Blocks 星状神经节阻滞

SGC Swan-Ganz Catheter Swa N-Ganz 导管【注释】〔带有 3 个小孔, 且其顶端带有小气球的探管。它可以从前腔静脉入右心房, 再通过血流经右心室至肺动脉。通过其测定肺动脉压、中心静脉压及测定左心室扩张末期压和心输出量〕

SGD Sodium Gradient Dialysis 钠梯度透析

SGE Second Gas Effect 第 二气体效果【注释】
〔导入两种混合的麻醉气体时,
其中一种气体为高浓度(第一气体) , 在
血中的移行速度很快。在这种情况下,
另一低浓度(第二气体) 的导入气体的
移行速度也变快。在实际上, 第一气体
为笑气, 第二气体为氟烷、安氟醚等〕
SGG Sirognathograph 下颌运动描记仪
Sgl Surgical 外科的; 外科手术的
SGM Society For General Microbiology
普 通微生物学会
SGML Standard Generalized Markup
Language 标准通用标注语言
SGOT Serum Glutamic-Oxaloacetic
Transaminase 血 清谷氨酸草酰乙酸转
氨酶; 血清谷草转氨酶
Sgpt Serum Glutamate-Pyruvate (Glutamic-
Pyruvic) Transaminase / Alanine
Aminot Ransferase 血 清谷丙转氨酶; 血
清谷氨酸丙酮酸转氨酶
SGR Sachs-Georgi Reaction 萨 - 乔二氏
反应; 缓慢胆固醇反应
SG(Sg) Specific Gravity 比 重
SGTT Standard Glucose Tolerance Test
标准葡萄糖耐量试验
SGV Schweizerische Gesellschaft Für
Versuchstierkunde
(Swiss Laboratory Animal
Science Association) 瑞 士实验动
物科学协会
SGV Society Of Greyhound Veterinarians

灰狗兽医社团

SH Serum Hepatitis 血 清性肝炎【注释】〔由输血
等导致的 B 型肝炎〕

SH Sex Hormone 性 激素

SH Stimulating Hormone 兴奋性激素

SHA Stockholm Herpetological Association
(Sweden) 斯德哥尔摩两栖爬行类
学会〔瑞典〕

SHAA-Ab Serum Hepatitis- Associated
Antigen Antibody 血 清肝炎相关抗原抗
体

SHA-Ab Serum Hepatitis-Associating Antibody
血 清肝炎相关抗体

SHB Shoe Horn Brace 塑 料制小腿假肢【注释】
〔与 SLB 一样的小腿假肢〕

SHBG Sex Hormone Binding Globulin
性激素结合球蛋白

Shbl Sharp And Blunt 锐器与钝器

Shbly Sharply And Bluntly 锐 利的与钝
性的

Shca Shiley Catheter 导管

Shchs Shaking Chills 寒 战

Shcu Sharp Curettage 锐 器刮除术

SHD Syphilitic Hear T Disease 梅 毒性心
脏病

Shdid Sharply Dissected 锐器分解

Shdij Sharp Dissection 锐器解剖法

Shdu Shifting Dullness 移动性浊音

She Sheep Erythrocytes 绵 羊红细胞

Sheas Sheaths 鞘

Shedg Shelving Edge 支 架边缘

SHEFC Scottish Higher Education
Funding Council 苏格兰高等教育基金
会

Shfi Shellfish 贝 (壳) 类; 甲壳类

SHG Sonohysterography 声 谱子宫收缩
Sgb 514 SHG
描计法

Shh She Has Had 她 已经患有

SHH Syndrome Of Hyporeninemic
Hypoaldosteronism
低 肾素性低醛固酮综
合征

SHIS Shared Hospital Information System
共 享型医院信息系统; 共享医院信
息系统

SHO Syndrome Hyperstimulation Ovarienne
卵巢过度刺激综合征

Shous Shoulders 割 面肩; 侧翼

Shpa Sharp Pain 锐 痛

Shpai Shoulder Pain 肩痛

SHR Spontaneous Hyper Tensive Rat 自
发性高血压大鼠【注释】 〔实验性高血压动物模
型, 被认
为是脑干部位的交感神经抑制机制的
遗传缺陷所致〕

Shs Second Heart Sound 第二心音

SHS Shoulder-Hand Syndrome 肩 -手综
合征【注释】 〔肩部疼痛性活动受限, 与病肩
同侧的手软组织肿胀、 潮红、 发热和烧
灼性疼痛〕

SHS Supine Hypotensive Syndrome 仰

卧低血压综合征

SHS Swollen Head Syndrome 头部肿胀
综合征

SHT Speech And Hearing Therapy 语听
疗法

Shu Shunt 分流器; 逃避

Shus Shunts 分流

SI Safety Index 安全指数

SI Saturation Index 饱和指数

SI Serum Iron 血清铁

SI Severity Of Illness Scale 疾病严重程
度量表

SI Small Intestine 小肠

SI Smear Index 涂片指数

SI Soluble Insulin 可溶性胰岛素

SI Stroke Index 心搏指数

SIADH Syndrome Of Inappropriate Secretion
Of ADH (Antidiuretic Hormone)
ADH(抗利尿激素) 不当分泌综合征【注释】 〔尽
管体内已处于血浆渗透压低
下状态, 抗利尿激素还继续分泌, 结果
导致低渗透压血症, 严重者会出现意识
障碍〕

Siar Sinus Arrhythmia 窦性心律不齐

SIAS St Roke Impairment Assessment Set
脑卒中后功能障碍评价【注释】 〔综合掌握脑卒
中患者的功能障
碍为目的, 用 22 项测验进行评价的方
法。 开始康复后, 重点观察患者坐位时
的功能障碍〕

Sibal Sitting Balance 坐姿平衡

Sibi Side-Biting 侧 痛的

SIBO Small Intestinal Bacterial Overgrowth
小肠细菌生长过度

Sibr Sinus Bradycardia 窦性心动过缓

Sibrs Side Branches 侧 枝

Sibs Siblings 同科

SICB Society For Integrative And Comparative
Biology 综合与比较生物学会

Sice Sickle Cell 镰状细胞〔红细胞〕

Sich Single-Channel 单通路; 单信道的

Sico Sigmoid Colon 乙状结肠〔解〕

Sicon Sinus Congestion 鼻 窦充血

SIDS Sudden Infant Death Syndrome
婴儿猝死综合征【注释】〔由呼吸中枢的呼吸自
动调控机
制异常所致。也有许多病例是与脑炎、
脑肿瘤有关〕

Sief Side Effect 副作用

Siefs Side Effects 副作用

Sifa Similar Fashion 类似式样

Sig Sigmoidoscopy 乙 状结肠镜检查(术)

Sigm Sigmoid ①S 形的② 乙状结肠(的)

Sigmsc Sigmoidoscope 乙 状结肠镜

SIHF Systolic Insufficiency Heart Failure
Shh 515 SIH
收缩功能不全性心力衰竭

Siin Sinus Infection 鼻 窦感染

Sij Sacroiliac Joint 骶骨关节

SIL Speech Interference Level 言语干扰
级

SIL Squamous Int Raepithelial Lesion(S)
鳞状表皮内病损

Silu Single Lumen 单管腔

SIMV Synchronized Intermittent
Mandatory Ventilation 同 步间歇性强
迫换气

Sinsi Sinusitis 窦炎

Sioi Silicone Oil 硅 油

SIP Sympathetically Independent Pain
交感神经不依赖性疼痛【注释】 〔与神经损伤有
关的疼痛有两种
情况, 一种是对交感神经阻滞起反应
的, 另一种则是对交感神经阻滞不起反
应的, SI P 指后者〕

Sipl Side Plate 边板

Sipo Sit Ting Position 坐位; 坐姿

Sipor Side Por T 侧孔; 侧喷火口

Sipr Similar Procedure 类似操作

Sipy Sigmoid Polyp 乙状结肠息肉

SIRF Severely Impaired Renal Function
重度肾功能损害

Sirh Sinus Rhythm 窦性心律

SIRS Systemic Inflammatory Response
Syndrome 全 身性炎症反应综合征【注释】 〔新近
提出的败血症系统化概
念。 与败血症相伴随的一系列脏器损
害, 引起 TEF、IL、PAF 一类炎症介质
的活化, 这些因子的活化在肺炎等局部
感染时作为一种机体的防御反应是有
意义的, 但对败血症这样的全身性感

染, 则会对患者产生种种不良影响。系
统地观察这类全身性的脏器损害, 命名
为 SIRS 似乎比败血症更恰当。实质是
一种败血症综合征〕

SISI Super-Large -Scale Integration 超
大规模集成电路

Sisys Signs And Symptoms 症 状与体征

SIT Serum Inhibitory Titer 血清抑制滴
度

Sita Sinus Tachycardia 窦 性心动过速

Siten Sinus Tenderness 鼻窦压痛

Sitn Sinus Tenderness 鼻窦压痛

Sitr Sinus T Ract 窦道

SIV Simian Immunodeficiency Virus 猴
免疫缺陷病毒【注释】〔与人免疫缺陷病毒(HIV-I ,
爱
滋病毒) 类似的感染猴的病毒, 作为爱
滋病研究的模型被用于抗爱滋病药物
的开发研究〕

SIV Swine Influenza Virus 猪流感病毒

Sive Single-Vessel 单血管

SJS Stevens-Johnson Syndrome
Stevens-Johnson 综合征; 口腔黏膜皮
肤眼综合征

SK Sarcome De Kaposi 卡波济肉瘤

SK St Reptokinase 链激酶

Skba Skull Base 颅 底

Skbr Skin Breakdown 表面裂纹

Skca Skin Cancer 皮肤癌

Skcar Skin Care 皮 肤护理

Skchs Skin Changes 皮肤改变

Skcls Skin Clips 皮 肤夹

Skcr Skin Crease 皮 肤皱褶

Skeds Skin Edges 皮 肤边缘

Skeld Skeletonized 骨 骼化

Skelg Skeletonizing 绘制草图

Skelj Skeletonization 成骨架; 骨骼化

Skelz Skeletonize 极 度消瘦

Skex Skin Examination 皮肤检查

Skfl Skin Flap 皮瓣

Skfls Skin Flaps 皮瓣

Skfo Skin Fold 皮褶

Skfx Skull Fracture 颅骨折

Skgr Skin Graft 皮肤移植片; 植皮

Skgrg Skin Graf Ting 皮 移植术; 植皮术

Skgrs Skin Grafts 皮肤移植

Sii 516 Skg

Skhos Skin Hooks 皮 肤牵引钩

Skinc Skin Incision 皮肤切口

Sklz Skin Lesion 皮 肤损害

Sklzs Skin Lesions 皮 肤病变

Skpo Skin Popping 肌注麻醉药品

Skra Skin Rash 皮 疹

Sksava Slovakian Small Animal Vet -
Erinary Association 斯洛伐克小动物兽
医协会

SKSD St Reptokinase St Reptodornase 双
链酶; 链激酶- 链道酶

Sksts Skin Staples 皮肤 U 型钉

Skta Skin Tag 皮赘

Sktas Skin Tags 皮赘

Sku Skull 颅骨

Skul Skin Ulcer 皮 肤溃疡

Skza Skeletonization 成骨架; 骨骼化

SL Sensation Level 感觉级

SL Sigmoid Lophophore S 形触手冠 〔动〕

SL Sublingual 舌 下的

Sla Sleep Apnea 睡 眠窒息

SLAC Scapholunate Advanced Collapse
舟月区进行性萎缩

Slc Shor T Leg Cast 短 腿管型

Sldi Sleep Disturbance 睡 眠障碍

SLE Slit Lamp Examination 裂隙灯检查

SLE(Slex) Systemic Lupus Erythematosus
系 统性红斑狼疮

SLIA Subst Rate-Labeled Immunoassay
基质标记免疫测定 〔免〕

SLIL Scapholunate Interosseous Liga -
Ment 舟月区骨间韧带

SLIP Serial Line Internet Protocol 串 行
线路互联网协议

Slkn Slit Knife 裂 隙刀

Slln Sleeplessness 失眠

SLM Sound Level Meter 声 音等级计;
噪声等级计

Slng Sublingual Nit Roglycerin 舌 下含服
硝酸甘油

SLO Streptolysin O 链球菌溶血素

SLO Scanning Laser Ophthalmoscope 激
光扫描检眼镜

Slp Speech-Language Pathology 言 语病

理学

Slpis Sleeping Pills 安 眠药

SLR Straight-Leg Raising (Test) 直 伸抬
腿试验

SLS Streptococcal Lymphadenitis 链 球
菌性淋巴结炎

SLS Streptococcal Lymphadenitis Of
Swine 猪链球菌淋巴腺

Slsc Sliding Scale 滑尺; 比例增减制

Slsp Slurred Speech 急促不清的言语

Slta Slow Taper 缓慢变细

SLUD Salivation , Lacrimation , Urination
, Defecation 流涎, 流泪, 排尿, 排
便

SM Simple Mastectomy 单 纯乳房切除
术

SM Sinusitis Maxillas 上颌窦炎

SM Skim Milk 脱脂乳

SM Smooth Muscle 平滑肌

SM Somatomedin 促软骨素; 生长调节
素

SM Sphingomyelin (神经) 鞘髓磷脂

SM St Reptomycin 链 霉素

SM Synaptic Membrane 突 触膜

SM Systolic Murmur 收缩期杂音

SMA Smooth Muscle Antibody 平 滑肌
抗体【注释】 〔以大鼠胃壁平滑肌作为抗原,
在患者血清中检出的一种与肝脏病变
有关的自身抗体。类狼疮肝炎或慢性
活动性肝炎时呈阳性〕

SMA Spinal Muscular Atrophy 脊髓性
肌萎缩

SMA Superior Mesenteric Artery 肠系
膜上动脉

SMAF Specific Macrophage Activating
Skh 517 SMA

Factor 特异巨噬细胞活化因子【注释】〔由巨噬细
胞提供的抗原信息和
白细胞介素 I 所激活的致敏 T 细胞中产
生的抗原特异性 SMAF，它激活巨噬细
胞，使其发挥吞噬功能〕

Smag Smith Antigen 史密斯抗原

SMAS Subcutaneous And Musculoaponeurotic
System 皮下和肌腱膜系
统

Smax Superior Mesenteric Artery 肠系
膜上动脉〔解〕

Smbo Small Bowel 小肠

Smbw- Small-Bowel 小肠

Smce- Small-Cell 小细胞

SMD Slow Migration Dimmer Of Actin
肌动蛋白慢迁移二体【注释】〔以亚苯基二顺丁
烯二酰亚胺为
交联剂时所形成的肌动蛋白交联的二
体，在变性凝胶上电泳迁移率慢〕

SMD Senile Macular Degeneration 老年
性黄斑变性

SMD Sulfamethoxydiazin 磺胺-5-甲氧
二嘧啶

SMD Sulfametoxydiazine 磺胺对甲氧
嘧啶

SMD Sulfameter 消炎磺; 磺胺-5-甲氧
嘧啶

SMEDI Stillborn-Mummification Embryonic
Death-Infertility (Syndrome)
斯梅迪猪流产、木乃伊胎、胚胎死亡、不孕
(综合征)

SMI Silent Myocardial Ischemia 无症状
心肌缺血【注释】〔表示无症状的一过性心肌缺
血
的新的临床概念, 由于随身携带型心电
图等检查方法的进步, 这一疾病最近引
起人们关注。Cohn 将其分为三种类型〕

SMI Simplified Menopausal Index 简 略
更年期指数【注释】〔反映更年期症状严重程度
的库
茨帕曼指数已在临床上使用了 40 多年,
但有些医院为方便门诊而将其进行了
简化处理, SMI 即指这种简化后的指
数〕

Smin Small Incision 小 切口

SMM Society Of Marine Mammalogists
海洋哺乳动物学家协会

SMM Sulfamonomethoxine 磺 胺间甲
氧嘧啶

SMON Subacute Myelo-Optico (Optical)
Neuropathy 亚急性脊髓视神经病【注释】〔由止
泻药喹典方引起的伴有腹
泻症状的脑脊髓炎, 出现视力障碍、感
觉异常和运动障碍〕

SMP Sulfamethoxypyridazine 磺 胺甲

氧嗪

SMP Sympathetically Maintained Pain
交感神经依赖性疼痛【注释】〔与交感神经有关
的疼痛中, 有
的对交感神经阻滞起反应, 而有的则不
起反应, SMP 指前者〕

SMR Standardized Mor Tality Ratio 标准
化死亡比

SMR Submucous Resection Of Nasal Septum
鼻中隔黏膜下切除术

SMSV San Miguel Sea Lion Virus 圣 米
格尔海狮病毒

Smve(S) Small Vessel(S) 小 血管

SMVT Sustained Monomorphic Ventri
Cular Tachycardia 持 续单一型室心动过
速

SMX Sulfamethoxazole 磺胺甲异□唑

SMZ Sulfamethazine 磺 胺二甲嘧啶

SN Sensory Neuron 感 觉神经元

SN Serum Neut Ralization (Test) 血 清中
和(试验)

S/ N Signal- To-Noise Ratio 信噪比

SN Sinus Node 窦结

SN Spinal Needle 脊 椎穿刺针; 腰椎穿
刺针

SN Spontaneous Nystagmus 自 发性眼
震

Sma 518 SN

SN Substantia Nigra 黑 质

Sncs Sponge And Needle Counts 棉 球与
针计数

SNCV Sensory Nerve Conduction Velocity
感觉神经传导速度

SND Normal Spontaneous Delivery 正 常
自然分娩

SND Single Needle Dialysis 单针透析

SND Striatonigral Degeneration 纹 状体
黑质变性【注释】 〔大脑基底核内有尾状核和豆
状
核, 其邻接部位有黑质存在, 它们的病
变导致异常运动(舞蹈病) 和肌张力障
碍(帕金森氏病)〕

SNF Skilled Nursin Facility 高 级保健
所

SNGPF Single Nephron Glomerular Plasma
Flow 单个肾单位肾小球血浆流量

SNHL Sensorineural Hearing Loss 神 经
性听力损失

Snob Shortness Of Breath 呼 吸急促; 气
促

SNOP Systematized Nomenclature Of
Pathology 病理学统一用语【注释】 〔1965 年美国
病理学会编集, 由
4 章组成〕

SNP Single Nucleotide Polymorphism
单核酸多态性【注释】 〔个体间的差异是由于
DNA 的
不同所导致的。 DNA 序列上只要有一
个碱基不同, 就会改变某种遗传性状,
这就是所谓的单核酸多态性〕

SNP Sodium Nit Roprusside 硝 普钠(硝

基氢氰酸钠)【注释】〔一种直接作用于血管平滑肌使
血管扩张的药物, 用于低血压麻醉〕

SNS Somatic Nervous System 躯体神经系统

SNS Sympathetic Nervous System 交感神经系统

SNVI Swedish National Veterinary Institute 瑞典国家兽医研究所

SNVQ Scottish National Vocational Qualification 苏格兰国家职业资格认证委员会

S&O Salpingectomy & Oophorectomy 输卵管与卵巢切除术

SOAD Sleep , Orientation , Activity , Demand 护士为了观察记录重症患者的精神症状所采用的一种简易打分评价法【注释】〔评价 4 个项目:" 睡眠觉醒节律","方位辨别", " 身体活动、语言活动","需求、诉说"〕

SOAP Subjective And Objective Data , Assessment Of Patient Response , Plan Of Action 主观信息、客观信息、病人反应评价、活动计划

SOB Shortness Of Breath 呼吸急促; 气促

SOC Sense Of Coherence (Psychology) 相干感〔心理学〕

Soca South Carolina 南卡罗莱纳州

Soch Sodium Chloride 氯化钠

Sod Sodium 钠

SOD Superoxide Dismutase 过 氧化物歧化酶【注释】〔氧在体内也以活性氧的形式存在, 它在体内大量生成时, 就会攻击细胞, 使细胞膜脂质过氧化, 引起种种伤害。在消除这种活性氧的一个重要成员" 过氧化物"的反应中起作用的酶就是 SOD(1968 年发现) 。近年利用基因重组技术已能生产, 作为许多疾病的治疗药而引人注目〕

SOD1 Superoxide Dismutase , Soluble 可溶性超氧化物歧化酶

SOG Standard Operating Guidelines 标准操作指南

Sogr Sonogram 语图; 声波图

SOLVD Studies Of Left Vent Ricular Dysfunction 左 心室障碍研究【注释】 〔关于药物对心功能不全特别是

SN 519 SOL
左心功能不全的治疗以及预防的调查性研究〕

SOM Serous Otitis Media 浆液性中耳炎

SOM Solitary Osseous Myeloma 独 立性骨的骨髓瘤

SOM Somatostatin 生长抑素【注释】 〔位于肠壁神经丛的多肽神经元所含有的一种多肽, 与肠内反射、蠕动反射有关〕

SOM Somatotrophin 生 长激素

Somnt Somnolent 嗜 眠的; 嗜睡的

SOP Society Of Protozoologists 原 生动

物学家协会

SOP Standard Operating Procedure 标准操作程序; 标准手术程序

SOS Secure Operating System 安全操作系统

SOT Society Of Toxicology 毒理学会

Soth Sore Throat 咽喉痛

Soti Soft Tissue 软组织; 松软组织

Sotis Soft Tissues 软组织

Soug Sounding 探通术

Sowor Social Worker 社会(服务) 工作者 (管理医疗福利事业的人)

SP Serum Protein 血清蛋白质

Sp . Speech Function Test 言语功能测试

Sp . Splint 夹板

SP Standardized Patient Or Simulated Pa - Tient 标准或模拟患者【注释】 〔为医学临床教育及其成果评价
而设置的一种教育资源。选用没有医学背景的普通人充当, 对他们进行模拟各种疾病症状的训练, 使他们能像演员那样可以逼真而且随时地重现各种疾病的症状。由美国的 St Illma N 等人创立〕

S/ P Status Post 病后状态

SP St Rip Package 铝铂包装; 孔膜包装【注释】 〔药物的一种包装方式〕

SP Substance P P 物质【注释】 〔由 11 个氨基酸组成的小肽, 具
有强烈降压作用和消化道收缩作用。

而且, 作为一级感觉神经元的兴奋性神
经递质存在于后根神经节发出的 Aδ 或
C 纤维中, 将来自皮肤的痛觉信息传递
给脊髓后角〕

SP Systolic Pressure 收 缩压

SPA Single Photon Absorptiometry 单
光子吸收法【注释】〔一种骨扫描测量法。用于
评价
治疗退行性骨质疏松症等的药物的疗
效〕

SPA Spinal Progressive Amyot Rophy 脊
髓性进行性肌萎缩症【注释】〔因脊髓前角运动
神经元退行性
变化和末梢运动神经的变性, 引起进行
性肌肉萎缩的疾病, 被看作是肌萎缩性
侧索硬化症的下位神经元型。有 Ar An-
Duch Enn E 型和 Vulpian-Bernhard 型〕

SPA Staphylococcal Protein A 葡 萄球
菌 A 蛋白

SPA Stimulation Produced Analgesia 刺
激镇痛机制【注释】〔从镇痛机制角度分析, 有从
高
位水平抑制疼痛的机制, 也有作用在网
状体(来自末梢的痛觉刺激上行到脑的
一个重要通道结构) 的下行性抑制机
制, 将它们笼统称为 SPA〕

SPANA Society For The Protection Of
Animals Abroad 防 止动物迁移境外协
会

Spasc Spastic 痉 挛的; 强直的

Spasy Spasticity 痉挛状态; 强直状态

Spat Spatula 压舌板

Spatd Spatulated 调拌的

SPC Synthesizing Protein Complex 合成蛋白复合物

SPCA Serum Prothrombin Conversion Accelerator 血清凝血酶原转化促进因子【注释】〔第Ⅶ因子, 是位于外因性凝血系统起始点的因子, 在 Ca2 + 存在下, 与组织凝血激酶结合, 活化第 X 因子〕

SOM 520 SPC

SPCA Serum Prothrombin Conversion Accelerator , Coagulation Factor Ⅶ 血清凝血酶原转变加速因子, 凝固因子Ⅶ

SPCA Short Posterior Ciliary Artery 睫后短动脉

Spcan Spinal Canal 脊椎管

Spcas Spica Cast 人字形管型

Spce Spermatocele 精子囊肿

SPCM Spectinomycin 壮观霉素

Spcol Spastic Colon 结肠痉挛

Spcus Sputum Cultures 痰培养

Spcy Spherocyte 球形红细胞

Spcyos Spherocytosis 球形红细胞贫血症

Spcys Spherocytes 球形红细胞

SPD Salmon Poisoning Disease 鲑鱼中毒病

SPD Storage Pool Disease (Deficiency) 贮存缺乏病【注释】〔通常情况下血小板受刺激后会

释放出所贮存的颗粒。SPD 则指因先
天或后天原因导致的血小板内无颗粒
释放的病态〕

SPECT Single Photon Emission Computed(
Computerized) Tomtgraphy 单 光子
放射型计算机断层摄影【注释】〔ECT 中有 2 种,
与使用正电子
放射性核素的 PET 不同, 它们是使用
能够放射光子或 Γ 线的各种示踪剂, 待
其在特定组织或脏器中聚集后, 进行计
算机断层扫描的技术。它不仅能显示
形态, 而且能反映血液量和代射功能等
方面的信息。S PECT 与 PE T 接近〕

Spet Sphenoethmoid 蝶 筛(骨) 的

SPF Specific Pathogen Free 无 特定病原
体的

SPFA Specific Pathogen Free Animals
无特定病原动物

Spfi Spine Film 脊 柱 X 光片

Spfis Spine Films 脊 柱 X 光片

Spflu Spinal Fluid 脊髓液

Spfu Spinal Fusion 脊柱融合术

Sp .Gr . Specific Gravity 比重

Sph Spherical Lens 球镜片

Sph Sphincter 括 约肌

Sphc Sphincteric 括约肌的

Sphe Sphenoid ① 楔形的②蝶骨③ 蝶骨
的

Sphei Sphenoiditis 蝶 窦炎

Sphel Sphenoidal 蝶骨的

Spheots Sphenoidostomies 蝶窦切开术

Sphot Sphincterotomy 括约肌切开术

Sphots Sphincterotomies 括约肌切开术

Sphpl Sphincteroplasty 括约肌成形术

Sphs Sphincters 括约肌

Sphto Sphincterotome 括约肌切开器

Spi Spine ①棘; 突; 刺②脊柱③ 马蹄嵴

SPK Serum Pyruvate Kinase 血清丙酮
酸激酶

SPK Superficial Punctuate Keratitis 浅
层点状角膜炎

Spkd Speckled 有斑点的

SPL Sound Pressure Level 声压强度

Spl Spleen 脾

Splac Spironolactone 螺甾内酯; 螺旋内
酯固醇; 安体舒通

Splc Splenic 脾的

Splec Splenectomy 脾切除术

Splig Split Ting 分裂; 分解; 分离; (牲
畜) 剥皮; 裂缝; 劈开

SPM Suppressor-Promoter-Mutator System
玉米的一种转座子系统

Spma Sphenomaxillary 蝶上颌骨的

SPMA Spinal Progressive Muscular At Rophy
脊髓性进行性肌萎缩症【注释】〔脊髓下位神经
元变性的疾病,
是肌萎缩侧索硬化症的一个亚型〕

Spme Splenomegaly 脾 (肿) 大

Spmet Spirometry 肺量测定法; 呼吸量
测定法

SPMI Severely & Persistently Mentally
SPC 521 SPM
Ill 严重与持续性精神疾病

Spn Spinal ① 脊髓的; 脊柱的② 脊髓麻
醉

SPO Stimulated Pepsin Output 刺 激时
胃蛋白酶分泌量

SPO2 Peripheral Oxygen Saturation 外
周氧饱和度

Spo2 Pulse Oximeter Saturation 脉 搏氧
饱和度仪所显示的氧饱和度【注释】〔通过在指
端或耳朵处装上探针
就能不抽血连续显示动脉血氧饱和度
的脉搏氧饱和度仪所测得的饱和度
（％）。Spo2 这一缩写词从 1987 年前后
开始使用〕

SPP Suprapubic Prostatectomy 耻 骨上
前列腺切除术

Sppa Speech Pathology 言 语病理学

Sppat Speckled Pat Tern 斑点型

Sppr Spinous Process 棘突 〔解〕

Spprs Spinous Processes 棘 突

Spr Superior Prosthion 上 颌中切牙牙
槽嵴顶点

SPRIA Solid Phase Radioimmunoassay
固相放射免疫测定

Sproy Spirometry 肺 量测定法; 呼吸量
测定法

SPS Simple Par Tial Seizure 简 单部分发
作

SPS Sleep Promoting Substance 促进睡眠物质

Spsm Spasm 痉挛

Spsti Sponge Stick 棉球棒

Sptap Spinal Tap 腰椎穿刺

Sptaps Spinal Taps 腰椎穿刺

Sptc Septic 腐败性的; 脓毒性的; 败血病的; 腐败剂; 腐烂物

SPTI Systolic Pressure-Time Index 收缩期压时间指数【注释】〔心肌的外部工作量指标〕

Sptl Septal 中隔的; 间隔的

Sptm Septum 隔膜〔软体动物〕

SPVS Society Of Practising Veterinary Surgeons 兽医开业外科医师学会

SQA Scottish Qualifications Authority 苏格兰资格认证机构

Sqcc Squamous Cell Carcinoma 鳞状细胞癌

SQL Structured Query Language 结构式查询语言

SR Seizure Resistant 抗癫痫发作

SR Sinus Rhythm 窦性节律

SR Slow Release 慢释; 缓慢释放

SR Spontaneous Respiration 自发呼吸

SR Stomach Rumble 胃鸣音; 胃部隆隆声

SR Superior Rectus 上直肌〔解〕

SR Sustained Release 持久释放

SR Systems Review 系统复习〔病历记录

内容之一〕

SRBC Sheep Red Blood Cells 绵 羊红细胞【注释】〔绵羊红细胞在兔抗绵羊红细胞抗体及豚鼠血清或人补体存在下发生敏感的溶血反应, 所以是免疫学领域研究或开发中传统使用的血细胞。近年用于人淋巴细胞的分离和作为免疫化学反应的载体〕

SRDA Search And Rescue Dog Association 犬 类搜寻与营救协会

SRE Serum Responsive Element 血 清应答元素

SRF Serum Response Factor 血 清刺激应答因子【注释】〔肿瘤增殖过程中, 该因子与肿瘤结合, 刺激肿瘤基因的表达〕

SRF Somatotropin Releasing Factor 生长激素释放因子

SRF Subretinal Fluid 视网膜下积液

SRFOA(SRF-A) Slow-Reacting Factor Of Anaphylaxis 过 敏反应迟缓反应因子

SRFS Split Renal Function Study 分肾功能检查

Spn 522 SRF
【注释】〔为确定是否为肾血管性高血压的手术适应症, 通过左右输尿管插管分别采取左右肾的尿液进行检查的方法〕

SRID Single Radial Immunodiffusion 单向放射免疫扩散

SRIF Somatotropin Release Inhibiting Factor 生长激素释放抑制因子

SRM Search-Rescue-Medical 搜寻-救护-
医疗【注释】〔救灾时作为医疗队的活动原则
提出的其操作顺序容易记住的口号〕

SRM Specified Risk Materials 特 定危险
材料

Srma Seroma 血 清肿〔组织内有肿瘤样
的血清积液〕

Srmu Superior Rectus Muscle 上 直肌
〔动〕

SRN State Registered Nurse 洲 注册护士

SRN Subretinal Neovascularization 视
网膜下新血管形成

SRNV Subretinal Neovascularization 视
网膜下新血管形成

SRO Single Room Occupancy 单间居住

SROM Spontaneous Rupture Of Membrane
自发性膜破裂

SRP Signal Recognition Par Ticle 信 号识
别颗粒

SRS Slow-Reacting Substance 慢 反应物
质【注释】〔使支气管平滑肌缓慢收缩的一
种物质〕

SRS Slow Reacting Substance 慢 反应物
质

SRS-A Slow Reactin Substance-A 慢 反
应物质-A

SRS-A Slow-Reacting Substance Of Ana -
Phylaxis 过敏反应慢性反应物质【注释】〔过敏反
应时被分离出来的一种
物质, 其作用不能用抗组胺剂抑制, 比

组织胺作用慢, 具有使某种平滑肌特别
是支气管平滑肌收缩、血管通透性增大
的作用〕

SR (S/ R) Schizophrenic Reaction 精神
分裂症反应

SR (S .R .) Sedimentation Rate 沉 降速
率; 沉降率

SRT Speech Reception Threshold 言 语
接受阈【注释】〔使用第 57～ 67 项语音听力检查
用语表的数字语表测定, 回答正确率达
到 50% 时的水平〕

SS Saline Solution 盐 溶液

SS Saturated Solution 饱 和溶液

SS Sclera Spur 巩 膜距

SS Single Strength 一 倍浓度(单一浓度)

综 合征; 口眼干

燥关节炎综合征

生长抑素【注释】〔存在于中枢神经系统和胰腺、

消化道等部位, 作为神经递质起作用。
能抑制胰岛素和胰高血糖素等消化道
激素的分泌以及肠管的蠕动〕

系 统性硬化病

放 射线源

表面距离

【注释】〔放射线照射时放射线源与皮肤
表面间的距离。亦即沿射线束中心轴
测到的从放射线源表面到被照射物体
表面的距离〕

类固醇硫酸酯酶缺乏病

休 克疗法【注释】〔精神科中的休克疗法, 指的是
胰岛素休克疗法和痉挛疗法。但在其

他多个领域也被用于指冲击性强的疗

法〕

胺甲异□唑甲氧苄氨嘧啶

颞浅动

脉〔解〕

萄球菌性的

① 厩舍② 马厩值勤③ 稳定

的; 固定的; 安定的④坚固的; 牢固的

斜 视

间控制【注释】〔心脏超声检查用语〕

肿瘤间距离【注释】〔放疗时, 从放射线射出孔到
肿

瘤表面间的距离。用于决定放射量〕

性传染病【注释】〔通过男女性交或同性恋者的
性

行为导致的传染病, 包括外阴疱疹、病

毒性肝炎、细胞巨病毒感染症、阴道滴

虫病、爱滋病等〕

甾 体; 甾类; 甾类化合物

甾体; 激素; 激素类

促 生长激

素; 生长激素【注释】〔脑垂体前叶激素, 由前叶
的嗜

酸性细胞分泌, 受下丘脑生长激素释放

激素的促进, 而受生长激素释放抑制激

素抑制〕

子 宫亚全

切除术

促生长素释放因子

滚压; 压合; 缝缀

刺 激的; 有刺激性的

① 刺激器② 刺激物;

刺激剂

刺激物; 刺激

穿刺伤

应激性失禁

穿刺伤

缝线

(脑) 卒中

中风

缝合线状的

周 围红斑

应激性尿失禁

外科手术

上外侧的

槽 ; (大脑) 回间沟; 沟

舌 下的

耻骨上地

上直肌〔解〕

基因敏感突变型【注释】〔通过抑制剂使表型恢复的突变体〕

缝 合; 颅缝

手 术疤痕

手 术部位

悬浮液

缝 合

自发通气

动脉瓣上狭窄

慢 肺活量

腔静脉综合征【注释】〔由于上腔静脉受压、变窄、堵塞

等产生的一系列症状。包括① 上半身

浮肿, 发红; ② 呼吸困难, 咳嗽; ③ 颅

压增高; ④上肢静脉压上升等。多由肺

癌引起〕

自 动

阴道分娩

体循 环血管阻力【注释】〔体循环血管阻力= (平均动脉

压- 中心静脉压)/ 心输出量×79 .9〕

室上性心动过速

可 感蒸发

蜡 下(汗油)

外 科(学) ; 外科手术

性 滥交

性 活跃

性功能

性交

性 倾向

滑膜液

滑膜

昏厥

梅毒

注射器

发作; 癫痫发作

癫 痫预防

癫痫发作

Japanese

略語	日本語の意味	スペル	読み方
S	S 波	S-Wave	
	血清	Serum	
	主観的情報	Subjective Date	
	精神分裂病	Schizophrenia	
	仙骨、仙骨の、仙髄の	Sacrum, Sacral	
	左の	Sinister(ラ)	
	飽和脂肪酸	Saturated Fat	
	老人（性）の、老年の	Senile	
S Ⅱ	第 2 心音	Second Heart Sound	
S Ⅲ	第 3 心音	Third Heart Sound	
S Ⅳ	第 4 心音	Fourth Heart Sound	
S	秒	Second	
SA	安静型狭心症	Stable Angina	
	感覚失語	Sensory Aphasia	
	自殺未遂、自殺企図	Suicide Attempt	
	自然流産	Spontaneous (Natural) Abortion	
	スルファニルアミド、サルファ剤	Sulfanilamide	
	体表面積	Surface Area	
	単心房	Single Artium	
	洞房の	Sinoatrial	
	脾動脈	Splenic Artery	
SAB	選択的肺胞気管支造影（法）	Selective Alveolar Bronchography	

洞房ブロック　　　　Sinoatrial Block

SACT 洞房伝導時間　　　Sinoatrial Conduction Time

SAH　クモ膜下出血　　　Subarachnoid Hemorrhage

SAN　洞房結節　　Sinoatrial Node

Sao2　動脈血酸素飽和度　Saturation Of Arterial Blood Oxygen

Sar　サルコイドーシス　Sarcoidosis

SAS　睡眠時無呼吸症候群　　　Sleep Apnea Syndrome

SAS(S)　　大動脈弁上狭窄（症候群）
　　　　Supravalvular Aortic Stenosis(Syndrome)

SB　自発呼吸　Spontaneous Breathing
　　石鹸清拭　Soap Bath

S-B　セングステークン・ブレークモア食道静脈瘤止血用チューブ、SB チューブ Sengstaken-Blakemore Tube

SBD　老人性脳疾患　　　Senile Brain Disease

SBE　亜急性細菌性心内膜炎　　Subacute Bacterial Endocarditis
　　　乳房自己検査法　Self-Breast Examination

SBP　最大（収縮期）血圧　　　Systolic Blood Pressure
　　　特（自）発性細菌性腹膜炎
　　　Spontaneous Bacterial Peritonitis

SBPC スルホベンジルペニシリン（スルベニシリン）　Sulfobenzylpenicillin(Sulbenicillin)

SBR　小腸大量切除（術）　　　Small Bowel Massive Resection

SBS　脊髄延髄脊髄反射　Spino-Bulbo-Spinal(Reflex)

SC　皮下（注射）　Subcutaneous(Injection)

Sc　肩甲骨　Scapula
　　精神分裂病　Schizophrenia

Sc　胸鎖関節の　Sternoclavicular
　　鎖骨上窩リンパ節郭清（乳癌）
　　Supraclavicular
　　皮下の　Subcutaneous

SCA　鎌状赤血球貧血　Sickle Cell Anemia
　　鎖骨下動脈　Subclavian Artery
　　上小脳動脈　Superior Cerebellar Artery
　　選択的腹腔動脈造影(法)　Selective Caeliac Angiography

SCC　小細胞癌　Small Cell Carcinoma
　　扁平上皮癌　Squamous Cell Carcinoma

SCD　脊髄小脳変性（症）　Spinocerebellar Degeneration

SCFE　大腿骨頭すべり症　Slipped Capital Femoral Epiphysis

Schiz　精神分裂病　Schizophrenia

SCI　脊髄損傷　Spinal Cord Injury

Sci　硬性型（胃癌）　Scirrhous Type

SCIA　浅腸骨回旋動脈　Superficial Circumflex Iliac Artery

SCID　重症複合免疫不全症　Severe Combined Immunodeficiency

Scicti　シンチレーション、シンチグラム　Scintillation, Scintigram

SCIS　重症複合免疫不全症候群　Severe Combined Immunodeficiency Syndrome

SCLC 小細胞肺癌　Small Cell Lung Cancer

SCM　胸鎖乳突筋　Sternocleidomastoid Muscle

SCR, Scr　　血清クレアチニン　Serum Creatinine

SCT　スパイナル（脊髄）CT　　Spinal Computed
Tomography

SD　変形性脊椎症　　　Spondylosis Deformans

老年期痴呆　Senile Dementia

SDAT アルツハイマー型老年痴呆　　　Senil
Dementia Of Alzheimer Type

SDB　真皮浅層熱傷　　　Superficial Dermal Burn

SDH　硬膜下血腫　Subdural Hematoma

硬膜下出血　Subdural Hemosshage

SDR　単純型糖尿病性網膜症　　　Simple Diabetic
Retinopathy

SEP　（冠状動脈）中隔穿通枝　Septal Coronary
Perforating Artery(Branch)

SEV　セボフルレン　　　Sevofluren

SFD　妊娠期間に比して小さい　Small-For-
Dates(Infant)

SG　比重　Specific Gravity

SGA　短胃動脈　Short Gastric Artery

妊娠期間に比して小さい　Small For
Gestational Age

SGC　スワン・ガンツカテーテル　　　Swan-
Ganz Catherer

SGN　上殿神経　Superior Bluteal Nerve

SGO　外科・産婦人科　Surgery, Gynecology
And Obstetrics

SGOT 血清グルタミン酸オキサロ酢酸トランスアミナーゼ　Serum Glutamic-Oxaloacetic Transaminase

SGPT 血清グルタミン酸ピルビン酸トランスアミナーゼ　Serum Glitamic-Pyruvic Transaminase

Sgt　妊娠

SH　血清肝炎　Serum Hepatitis

SHP　二次性副甲状腺機能亢進症　Secondary Hyperparethyroidism

SHS　仰臥位低血圧症候群　Supine Hypotensive Syndrome

SI　1回拍出係数　Stroke Index
　　ショック指数　Shock Index
　　仙腸の　Sacroiliac

SIDS　乳幼児突然死症候群　Sudden Infant Death Syndrome

SIMV 周期的間歇的強制換気法　Synchronized Intermittent Mandatory Ventilation

Sin　左の

SIRS　全身性炎症反応症候群　Systemic Inflammatory Response Syndrome

SISO　シソマイシン　Sisomicin

SIT　スタンフォード知能テスト　Stanford Intelligence Test

SK　ストレプトキナーゼ　Streptokinase

SKA(O)　長下肢装具　Supra Knee Ankle(Orthosis)

SKI　皮膚　Skin

SK-SD ストレプトキナーゼ・ストレプトドルナーゼ　Streptokinase-Streptodornase

SL　ストレプトリジン　Streptolysin

SLB　短下肢装具　Short-Leg Brace
SLC　短下肢ギプス　　　Short-Leg Cast
SLE　全身性エリテマトーデス、全身性紅斑性狼瘡　Systemic Lupus Erythematosus
SLV　左室性単心室　　　Single Left Ventricle
SM　収縮期雑音　Systolic Murmur
　　　ストレプトマイシン　　　Streptomycin
SMA　上腸間膜動脈　　　Superior Mesenteric Artery
SMBG血糖自己測定　　　Self Monitoring Of Blood Glucose
SMC　自己乳房管理　　　Self Mamma Control
SMDS 青壮年急死症候群　Sudden Manhood Death Syndrome
SMI　無症候性心筋虚血　Silent Myocardial Ischemia
SMON亜急性脊髄視神経障害、スモン病　Subecute Myelo-Optico-Neuropthy
SMV　上腸間膜動脈　　　Superior Mesenteric Vein
SN　洞房結節　Sinus Node
SNRT 洞結節回復時間　　Sinus Node Recovery Time
SNS　交感神経系　Sympathetic Nervous System

S/O　～の疑い　Suspect Of
SO2　酸素飽和度　Oxygen Saturation
SOB　息切れ　Shortness Of Breath
Sol, Sol, Soln　溶液　Solution
SP　脊椎　Spinal
　　　痰　　Sputum
S/P　～の後の状態　　　Status Post

Sp　　棘波　Spike
　　　脊椎麻酔　　Spinal Anesthesia
SPCA 短後毛様体動脈　　Shoet Posterior Ciliary Artery
SPCM スペクチノマイシン　　　Spectinomycin

SPFX スパルフロキサシン　　　Sparfloxacin
Spgr　比重　Specific Gravity
SPMA 脊髄性進行性筋萎縮症　　Spinal Progressive Muscular Atrophy
SPO2，Spo2 （パルスオキシメーターによる）動脈血酸素飽和度　　Oxygen Saturation Of Arterial Blood Measured By Pulse Oximeter
Sppc　慢性化膿性副鼻腔炎
Sp&W 棘徐波複合　Spike And Wave Complex
SQ　　皮下の　　　Subcutaneous
Sq　　扁平上皮癌　Squamous Cell Carcinoma
SR　　正常調律　　Sinus Rhythm
　　　赤血球沈降速度　　Sedimentation Rate
　　　抜糸　Sutures Removed
　　　伴性劣性遺伝　　　Sex-Linked Recessive Inheritance
SRA　上直腸動脈　Superior Rectal Artery
SRRD 睡眠関連呼吸障害　Sleep Related Respiratory Disturbance
SRT　洞結節回復時間　　Sinus Node Recovery Time
SRV　右室性単心室　　Single Right Ventricle

SS　　鎌状赤血球　Sickle Cell
　　　妊娠

SSM　丸山ワクチン　　　　Specific Substance
Maruyama
SSS　洞不全症候群　　　　Sick Sinus Syndrome
ST　　ST 部分（心電図）　ST-Segment
　　　言語療法（士）　　　Speech
Therapy(Therapist)
　　　硬化療法　　　Sclerotherapy
　　　皮膚試験　　　Skin Test
St I 〜Ⅳ　　　胃癌の肉眼的進行度を示す記号

St I 〜Ⅳ　　　胃癌の組織学的進行度を示す記号

STA-MCA　　浅側頭動脈・中大脳動脈吻合術
　　　　　Superficial Temporal Artery-Middle Cerebral
Artery(Anastomosis)
Staph　ブドウ球菌
Stat　直ちに、至急
STD　性（行為）感染症　Sexually Transmitted
Disease
STH　ステロイドホルモン　　　Steroid Hormone

STI　　（心）収縮時間　Systolic Time Interval

Strept 連鎖球菌
STZ　ストレプトゾトシン　　　Streptozotocin
SU　スルホニル尿素　Sulfonyl Urea
Subcu，Subcut　　皮下の　　　Subcutaneous
Subdura　　硬膜下血腫　Subdural Hematoma
SUD　内因性急死　Sudden Unexpected Natural
Death
SUED 原因の明らかな突然死　　　Sudden
Unexpected But Explained Death

Supp　坐剤　Suppository

Sut　縫合（単数）

Sutt　縫合（複数）

SUUD 原因不明の突然死　Sudden Unexpected And
Unexplained Death

SV　　１回拍出量　Stroke Volume
　　　静脈洞
　　　単心室　　　　Single Ventricle
　　　脾静脈　　　Splenic Vein

SVASS　　　大動脈弁上狭窄症候群
　　　　Supravalvular Aortic Stenosis Sydrome

SVC　上大静脈　　Superior Vena Cava

SVCG 上大静脈（造影）　Superior Vena
Cavography

SVCS 上大静脈症候群　　Surerior Vena Cava
Syndrome

SVD　一枝病変　Single Vessel Dosease

SVG　伏在静脈移植片　　Saphenous Vein Graft

Svo2，Svo2　混合静脈血酸素飽和度　　Mixed
Venous Oxygen Saturation

SVPC 上室期外収縮　　　Supraventricular
Premature Contraction

SVR　体血管抵抗　Systemic Vascular Resistance

SVT　上室頻拍　　　Supraventricular Tachycardia

SW　１回仕事量　Stroke Work
　　　ソーシャルワーカー　　Social Worker

S&W，SWC 棘徐波複合　Spike And Wave
Complex

SWI　１回仕事量係数　　Stroke Work Index

SWR 血清ワッセルマン反応 Serum
Wasserman Reaction

Russian

S/A   Sugar And Acetone   Сахар И Ацетон
        Синоатриальный [Узел]
        Субарахноидальное Кровоизлияние
Насыщеный
        Подострый Бактериальный (Инфекционный)
Эндокардит
        Спонтанный Бактериальный Перитонит
        Систолическое Артериальное Давление
Подкожный
        Сублингвальный
        Растворимые Печеночные Антигены
        Системная Красная Волчанка (СКВ)
        Соматостатин
        Сатурация Кислорода
        Одышка, Затруднение Дыхания
Уровень (Состояние) Сознания
        Состояние После [Заболевания, Операции]
        Подкожный
Медленно Высвобождающийся [В Названии
Лекарственного Препарата]
Синдром Шегрена
Синдром Слабости Синусного Узла (СССУ)
        Заболевания, Передающиеся Половым
Путем (Венерические Болезни)
        Подкожный
Суппозиторий
Surgery   Хирургия
        Суспензия
        Верхняя Полая Вена
        Системное Сосудистое Сопротивление

Суправентрикулярная Тахикардия
Симптомы

T
French

T3 Triiodotyronine
T4 Tétraiodotyronine
TA Tentative D'autolyse
TAC Traitement Anticoagulant
Tartraitement Antireflux
TCA Temps De Céphaline Activé
TCK Temps De Céphaline Kaolin
TDM Tomodensitométrie
TG Triglycérides
THS Traitement Hormonal Substitutif
TJ Turgescence Jugulaire
TP Taux De Prothrombine
TQ Temps De Quick
TR Toucher Rectal
TRT Traitement
TS Temps De Saignement, Tentative De Suicide
TSH Thyroïd Stimulating Hormone
TV Toucher Vaginal, Tachycardie Ventriculaire
TVP Thrombose Veineuse Profonde

English

TAB Tape-Automated Bonding; Total Autonomic
Blockage; Typhoid, Paratyphoid A, And
Paratyphoid B [Vaccine]

Tab Therapeutic Abortion

Tab Tablet

TABC Total Aerobic Bacteria Count; Typhoid,
Paratyphoid A, Paratyphoid B, And Paratyphoid
C [Vaccine]

TABP Type A Behavior Pattern

Tabs Tablets

Tabs Absorption Time

TABT Typhoid, Paratyphoid A, Paratyphoid
B, And Tetanus Toxoid [Vaccine]

TABTD Typhoid, Paratyphoid A, Paratyphoid
B, Tetanus Toxoid, And Diphtheria Toxoid [Vaccine]

TABV Tamana Bat Virus

TAC Tachykinin; Temporary Abdominal Closure;
Terminal Antrum Contraction; Tetracaine,
Adrenalin, And Cocaine; Time-Activity Curve;
Total Abdominal Colectomy; Total Aganglionosis
Coli; Total Allergen Content; Total Antioxidant
Capacity; Transient Aplastic Crisis;
Triamcinolone Cream; Truncus Arteriosus Communis

TAC-1 Tachykinin-1

TAC-2 Tachykinin-2

TACC Thoracic Aorta Cross Clamping

TACE Chlorotrianisene; Teichoic Acid Crude
Extract; Transarterial Chemoembolization;
Tumor-Necrosis Factor Alpha–Converting Enzyme

Tachy Tachycardia

TACI Total Anterior Circulation Infarct

TACIP Triflusal Vs Aspirin In Cerebral Infarction
Prevention [Study]

TACR Tachykinin Receptor

TACS Thrombolysis And Angioplasty In
Cardiogenic Shock [Study]

TACT Thermoacoustic Computed Tomography;
Ticlopidine Angioplasty Coronary Trial;
Ticlopidine Vs. Placebo For Prevention Of
Acute Closure After Angioplasty Trial; Tuned
Aperture Computed Tomography

TACTICS Thrombolysis And Counterpulsation
To Improve Cardiogenic Shock Survival
[Trial]

TACTICS-TIMI 18 Treat Angina With Aggrastat
And Determine Cost Of Therapy With
An Invasive Or Conservative Strategy-
Thrombolysis In Myocardial Infarction
[Trial]

TAD Test Of Auditory Discrimination; Thoracic
Asphyxiant Dystrophy; Tobacco, Alcohol,
And Drugs; Traffic Accident Deformity
[Scale]; Transactivation Domain; Transient
Acantholytic

Dermatosis T4 Thyroxine

T-7 Free Thyroxine Factor

T90 Time Required For 90% Mortality In A
Population Of Microorganisms Exposed To A
Toxic Agent

T Duration; Small T [Antigen]; Student T Test;
Teaspoonful; Temperature; Temporal; Terminal;
Tertiary; Test Of Significance; Three Times
[Lat. Ter]; Time; Tissue; Tonne; Transformer;
Translocation

T T Value From T Distribution

T Lowercase Greek Letter Tau; Life [Of
Radioisotope];
Relaxation Time; Shear Stress; Spectral
Transmittance; Transmission Coefficient
Θ Lowercase Greek Letter Theta; An Angular
Coordinate Variable; Customary Temperature;
Temperature Interval
T? Time After Infusion
T1/2 Half-Life
T2 Time At The End Of Inspiration
TA Alkaline Tuberculin; Arterial Tension; Axillary
Temperature; Tactile Afferent; Takayasu
Arteritis; Technology Assessment; Teichoic
Acid; Temporal Abstraction; Temporal Arteritis;
Terminal Antrum; Therapeutic Abortion;
Thermophilic
Actinomyces; Thymidine Analogue;
Thymocytotoxic Autoantibody; Thyroarytenoid;
Thyroglobulin Autoprecipitation; Thyroid
Antibody; Thyroid Autoimmunity; Tibialis
Anterior; Tissue Adhesive; Titratable Acid; Total
Alkaloids; Total Antibody; Toxic Adenoma;
Toxin-Antitoxin; Traffic Accident; Transactional
Analysis; Transaldolase; Transaminase; Transantral;
Transplantation Antigen; Transposition
Of Aorta; Trapped Air; Triamcinolone Acetonide;
Tricuspid Atresia; Trophoblast Antigen;
True Anomaly; Truncus Arteriosus; Tryptamine;
Tryptose Agar; Tube Agglutination; Tubular Atrophy;
Tumor Associated; Typical Absences
T-A Toxin-Antitoxin; Transfusion Associated
T&A Tonsillectomy And Adenoidectomy;
Tonsils And Adenoids
T/A Time And Amount
TA-4 Tumor-Associated Antigen 4

Ta Tantalum; Tarsal
T1a Breast Tumor 0.1 To 0.5 Cm
T4a Breast Tumor With Extension To Chest
Wall
Tα T Value Corresponding To Specified Tail Area
Alpha
TAA Thioacetamide; Thoracic Aortic Aneurysm;
Total Ankle Arthroplasty; Transverse
Aortic Arch; Tumor-Associated Antigen
TAAA Thoracoabdominal Aortic Aneurysm
TAAD Type A Aortic Dissection
TAAF Thromboplastic Activity Of The Amniotic
Fluid
TA-AIDS Transfusion-Associated Acquired
Immunodeficiency Syndrome

German

Tbc - Tuberkulose
Tbk - Tuberkulose
Tbl - Tablette
Tct - Tinktur
TEE - Transoesophageale Echocardiographie
Th - Thorakalwirbel
TIPS - Transhepatischer Intravenöser
Portosystemischer (Stent)Shunt
TPO - Thyreoperoxidase (TPO-Ak =
Thyreoperoxidase-Antikörper)
Tr. - Tractus, Truncus
TSR - Trizepssehnenreflex
Tx - Transplantation

Italian

T
Taterapia Antalgica
Tabterapia Antibiotica
Tactomografia Assiale Computerizzata
Taoterapia Anticoagulante Orale
Tctomografia Computerizzata
Tccorporea
Teatromboendoarteriectomia
Teptromboembolia Polmonare
Titerapia Infusiva
TIPO Terapia Intensiva Post Operatoria

Russian

T4
Thyroxine
Тироксин
T&A
Tonsillectomy And Adenoidectomy
Тонзиллэктомия И Аденоидэктомия
Tab
Tablet
Таблетка
TB
Tuberculosis
Туберкулез
TBG
Thyroxine Binding Globulin
Тироксинсвязывающий Глобулин
TBIL
Total Bilirubin
Общий Билирубин
Tbsp
Tablespoon
Столовая Ложка
Temp
Temperature
Температура
TENS
Transcutaneous Electrical Nerve Stimulation
Чрезкожная Электрическая Стимуляция Нерва
Tg
Thyroglobulin

Тироглобулин
TIA
Transient Ischemic Attack
Транзиторная Ишемическая Атака (ТИА),
Динамическое Нарушение Моз- Гового
Кровообращения
Tid
Three Times Daily
Три Раза В День
Tinc
Tincture
Настойка
TMP-SMX
Trimethoprim/Sulfamethoxazole
Триметоприм+Сульфаметаксозол (Бактрим,
Бисептол)
TNF
Tumor Necrosis Factor
Фактор Некроза Опухолей
Tpa
Tissue Plasminogen Activator
Тканевой Активатор Плазминогена
TP
Total Protein
Общий Белок
TPI
Treponema Pallidum Immobilization
Иммобилизация Бледных Трепонем (РИБТ)
TPR
Temperature, Pulse, And Respiration
Температура, Пульс И Частота Дыхания
TR
Tricuspid Regurgitation
Недостаточность Трикуспидального
(Трехстворчатого) Клапана

TRIG
Triglycerides
Триглицериды
TS
Tricuspid Stenosis
Стеноз Трикуспидального (Трехстворчатого)
Клапана
Tsp
Teaspoon
Чайная Ложка
TT
Thrombin Time
Тромбиновое Время
TUR
Transurethral Resection
Трансуретральная Резекция (ТУР)
Tx
Therapy
Терапия

Chinese

T Absolute Temperature 绝对温度

T Spine Thoracic 胸 脊柱

T + 1 . . Stages Of Increased Intraocular
Tension 表示眼压升高程度的符号

T Temperature 温 度; 体温

T Testosterone 睾 酮

T Tetracycline 四环素

T Thoracic Ver Tebrae 胸 椎 〔解〕

T Thorax 胸 廓

T Thymine 胸腺嘧啶; 胸腺碱

3T Triage- T Retment- Transpor Tation 判
断- 应急处置- 后方运送【注释】 〔在灾害现场所
要三项重要措
施, 3T 就是其三个单词的组合略语〕

T3 T Riiodothyronine 三碘甲状腺原氨酸【注释】
〔表示甲状腺功能的一个指标。

$122 \pm 41mg/ Dl$〕

T4 Tetraiodothyronine , Thyroxin 甲 状
腺素; 四碘甲腺原氨酸【注释】 〔表示甲状腺功能
的一个指标。

$117 \pm 7pg/ Ml$〕

TA Temporal Ar Teritis 颞动脉炎

TA Tension Artérielle 动 脉压

Ta Tension By Applanation 扁 平张力

T&A Tonsils And Adenoids 扁桃体与增
殖腺

TA Tricuspid At Resia 三尖瓣闭锁

TAA Tumor Associated Antigen 肿 瘤相

关抗原【注释】〔来自近交系动物的植入性肿瘤
引起近交系宿主出现免疫应答和肿瘤
移植排斥反应的抗原〕

Taar Tachyarrhythmia 快速型心律失常

TAB Salmonella Typhia And S . Paratyphoid
A And B (Vaccine) 伤寒杆菌与甲
型和乙型副伤寒杆菌疫苗

Tabr Tachycardia-Bradycardia 心动过
速-心动过缓

TAB(Tab .) Tabella ① 侧板; 斜板② 片
剂; 锭剂; 糖锭

TAC Preparation Of Tetracycline,
Epinephrine (Adrenaline) , Cocaine 四
环素、肾上腺素、可卡因制剂

Taca Tachycardia 心动过速; 心搏过速

Tacac Tachycardiac 心动过速的; 心搏过
速的; 心搏加速药

Tach Tachometry 流速测定法

Tads Tobacco , Alcohol And Drugs 烟草、
酒精与毒品

Tady Tardive Dyskinesia 迟发性运动障
碍

TAE T Ranscatheter Arterial Embolization
经探管的(肝) 动脉塞栓术【注释】〔进行性肝癌
的优选疗法。大多
数情况下, 与化学疗法并用〕

TAF Tumor Angiogenesis Factor 肿瘤血
管形成因子

TAH Transfusion-Associated Hepatitis
输血相关肝炎

Tah(X) Total Abdominal Hysterectomy

经腹部子宫全切除术

TAIEX Technical Assistance Information Exchange Office 技 术援助信息交
换部

TAL Tendon Achilles Lengthening 阿基里斯跟腱延长术

TAL Tumor Associated Lymphocyte 肿瘤相关淋巴细胞

TAL(TAO) T Riacetyloleandomycin 三乙酰竹桃毒素

TAM Toxoid-Antitoxin Mixture 类 毒素- 抗毒素合剂; 类毒素- 抗毒素混合物

TAM T Ransient Abnormal Myelopoiesis 一过性异常骨髓造血病【注释】〔并发于道恩氏综合征, 表现为
肝脾肿大、白细胞增多、新生儿末梢血中出现幼稚细胞的一过性增多的可自然治愈的疾病。纳入一过性骨髓增殖性综合征〕

Tamet Tarsometatarsal 跗 (骨) 跖(骨) 的

Tana Talonavicular 距 (骨) 舟(骨) 的

T Antigen T Ransplantation Antigen 移 植抗原

T Antigen Tumor Antigen 肿 瘤抗原; T抗原

TAO Thromboangitis Obliterans 血 栓性栓塞性脉管炎【注释】〔易发于吸烟的中年男性, 主要
表现为下肢动脉血管炎症引发的血栓栓塞症状。通常称为伯格氏病〕

Tapa Tail Of The Pancreas 胰腺尾

Tapn Tachypnea 呼吸急促

Tapnc Tachypneic 呼吸急促

TAPS T Ris (Hydroxymethyl) Methylamino-
Propane Sulfonic Acid 三羟甲基
甲氨基丙烷磺酸【注释】〔用于制备 Ph7 .7 ～ 9 .1
范围内
的缓冲液〕

TAPSO 3-[N- Tris (Hydroxymethyl)
Methylamino] 2-Hydroxypropane Sulfonic
Acid 3- [N-(羟甲基) 甲基氨基]
2 羟丙烷磺酸【注释】〔用于制备 Ph7 .0 ～ 8 .2 范
围内
的缓冲液〕

TAPVR (TAPVC) (TAPVD) Total
Anomalous Pulmonary Venous Return
(Connection) (Drainage) 全部肺静脉
血回流异常症【注释】〔为肺静脉血完全回流到
右心系
的先天性异常, 有许多表现形式。多因
心衰致死, 死亡率高达 80%〕

T .A .R . Takata-Ara□s Reaction 高田-
荒反应【注释】〔通过凝胶反应检查脊髓液, 以
用于中枢神经系统疾病诊断〕

TAR Thrombocytopenia-Absent Radii
(Syndrome) 血小板减少-桡骨缺失(综
合征)

TAR Tissue-Air Ratio 组织空中线量比
(值) 【注释】〔为一种放射线剂量的计算法。
即组织深部吸收线量/ 等距空中线量〕

TASS Ticlopidine-Aspirin Strokestudy

抗血小板病疗法之一【注释】〔是一种噻氯匹定和阿斯匹林合

用治疗血小板病的疗法, 现用于脑溢血

发生频率的研究〕

Tasts Tarry Stools 柏油样便

TAT Tetanus Antitoxin 抗 破伤风毒素;

抗破伤风免疫血清【注释】〔为破伤风毒素或其类毒素的抗

体, 属免疫球蛋白 G 类。由于免疫球蛋

白 G 不会造成人血清病等副反应而被

广泛应用〕

TAT Thematic Apperception Test 主 题

统觉测试【注释】〔让受试者观看描绘情绪性场面

的画面, 任意发挥编造故事, 以此诊断

性格的方法〕

TAT Thrombin- Antithrombin Ⅲ 凝血酶-抗凝血酶Ⅲ 【注释】〔为一种血液凝固检查指标。正

常值为 3 .0ng/ Ml 以下〕

TAT Thrombin-Antithrombin (Complex)

凝血酶- 抗凝血酶(复合物)

TB Thymol Blue 麝酚蓝

TB Total Bilirubin 总 胆红素

TB Tracheobronchitis 气管支气管炎

TB Tuberculosis 肺 结核; 结核(病) ; 痨病

TAL 532 TB

TBA Thiobarbituric Acid 硫代巴比土酸

TBA Thoroughbred Breeders□Associa -

Tion 纯种动物种畜协会

Tba Tubercle Bacillus 结核杆菌

TBBM Total Body Bone Mineral 全身骨
无机物; 全身骨矿物质

TBC Texas Beef Council 得克萨斯牛肉
委员会

TBC Tuberculosis 肺结核

Tbe (Tbe .) Tuberculosis 肺结核

TBF Tick-Borne Fever 蜱 传播性发热

TBFB Tracheobronchial Foreign Body
气管支气管异物

TBG Thyroxine Binding Globulin 甲 状
腺素结合球蛋白【注释】〔可与甲状腺激素(T3 ,
T4) 结合
的血清蛋白。在妊娠、急性肝炎、慢性
活动性肝炎、急性卟啉病等情况下增
高, 而肾病(重患除外) 在大量使用激素
类药物治疗时降低〕

TBG Thyroid-Binding Globulin 甲 状腺
结合球蛋白

TBI Total Body Irradiation 放 射线全身
照射【注释】〔在骨髓移植等之前进行的放射
线全身照射〕

TBI Traumatic Brain Injury 外伤性脑损
伤

TBI Tebethion 氨 硫脲; 结核安

T-Bil Total Bilirubin 总 胆红素

TBLB Transbronchial Lung Biopsy 经 支
气管肺活检【注释】〔为末梢肺部病变诊断的常
用手

法。注意避免出血和气胸的发生〕

TBNAB T Ransbronchial Needle Aspiration Biopsy 经支气管针抽吸活检【注释】〔由于肺癌的癌细胞已转移到纵

隔淋巴结, 与支气管壁相接触, 而支气管壁和内腔没有肿瘤的露出和浸润, 通过支气管无法进行诊断的情况下, 在摄像支气管镜的探头上安装注射针, 将其穿刺到支气管壁外, 进行穿刺细胞诊断的方法〕

TBP Thyroxime Binding Protein 甲 状腺素结合蛋白【注释】〔包括甲状腺素结合球蛋白

(TBG) 、甲状腺素结合前蛋白(TBPA)和白蛋白三种类型。血中的 T4 大部分与 TBG 结合〕

TBP Tuberculous Peritonitis 结 核性腹膜炎

TBPA Thyroxin-Binding Prealbumin 甲状腺素结合前白蛋白

TBS Tracheobronchoscopy 气 管支气管镜检查

TBSA Total Body Surface Area 总 体表面积

TBT T Racheobronchial Toilet 气 管内清洗【注释】〔为了清除不能通过咳出的、存在于气管内的黏稠分泌物和异物, 通过气管内插管, 在进行人工呼吸的同时, 反复注入生理盐水清洗气管, 将分泌物或异物清除〕

TBV Total Blood Volume 总血量【注释】〔指全身
的血液容量。正常值为
70～80ml/Kg〕
TBW Total Body Water 体液总量
TC Cytotoxic T Cell 细胞毒性 T 细胞
TC Thrombocyte 血小板
TC Total Cholesterol 总胆固醇
TC Transverse Colon 横结肠〔解〕
Tc Trocar 套针
TC Tubocurarine 筒箭毒碱【注释】〔一种肌松弛
剂〕
TC Tet Racycline 四环素(类)
TCA Terminal Cancer 终末期癌
TCA Thyrocalcitonin 甲状腺降钙素; 降
钙素
Tca Total Calcium 总钙
TCA Total Cholic Acid 总胆酸
TCA T Ricarboxylic Acid 三羧酸
TBA 533 TCA
TCA Trichloroacetic Acid 三氯乙酸; 三
氯醋酸
TCA T Ricyclical Antidepressant 三环抗
抑郁药
Tcb To Cont Rol Bleeding 控制出血
Tcc T Ransitional Cell Carcinoma 移行细
胞癌
TCD Transcranial Doppler Sonography
经头盖的多普勒超声波扫描法【注释】〔是一种
超声波诊断法。最近在
脑神经医学领域中用于发现和观察脑

血管痉挛出现及其过程〕

TC&DB Turn Cough & Deep Breath 转身咳嗽深呼吸

TCDD Tetrachlorodibenzodioxin 四氧二苯二氧杂环己二烯

TCDD Time Controlled Drug Delivery 药剂的控时投与(装置) 【注释】〔有口腔黏膜吸收用和经皮吸收用两种〕

T-Cell Thymus Derived Cell 胸腺衍化细胞; 胸腺来源细胞

T-CELLS Thymus Cells 胸腺细胞

TCES Trans-Cutane Cerebral Elect Ric Stimulation 头皮电刺激法

TCGF T Cell Growth Factor T 细胞生长因子

T .CH Total Cholesterol 总胆固醇

TCH Thiophene-2-Carboxylic Acid Hydrazine (Test) 噻吩-2- 碳酸酰肼(试验)

TCH Total Circulating Hemoglobin 总循环血红蛋白量

TCI Target Cont Rolled Infusion 目标控制注射【注释】〔利用药代动力学知识, 计算出欲治脏器达到效果时所需的药物剂量, 按此剂量进行注射给药的方法。有时也指利用计算机内脏自动注射器注射麻醉药的方法〕

TCO2 Total Carbon Dioxide Content 二氧化碳总含量

Tcp Thrombocytopenia 血小板减少症

TCP Trans-Cutaneous Pacing 经皮起搏

TCP Transmission Control Protocol 传输控制协议

TCP Tropical Canine Pancytopenia 热带犬全血细胞减少症

Tcpc Thrombocytopenic 血小板减少性的

Tcpo2 Trans-Cutaneous Oxygen Pressure 经皮氧分压【注释】〔指利用 PO2 连续测定装置通过
皮肤测定的值。压力(P) 代表透过组织的氧气量, 饱和度(S) 代表血液对氧气的输送能力〕

TCR T Cell Receptor T- 细胞受体【注释】 〔T 细胞通过 TCR 识别抗原, 并
发挥其作用〕

T&Crm Type And Cross-Match (Crossmatch) 血型和交叉配血

TCS Traumatic Cervical Syndrome 颈部扭伤

Tcsz Tonic-Clonic Seizure 强直-阵挛发作

TCT Thrombin Clotting Time 凝血酶凝血时间

TCT Tricarboxylic Acid Cycle 三羧酸循环【注释】 〔也称为柠檬酸三羧酸循环、克雷布氏三羧酸循环。它是机体内有机物完全氧化时的代谢途径, 其产生的能量通过 ATP 储存〕

TD5 / 5 Tolerance Dose Five Per Five (5

年组织) 耐受剂量【注释】〔在 5 年内发生的 5 %
以下的重
度损伤的放射线量〕

TD Tetanus And Diphtheria (Toxoid) 破
伤风和白喉〔类病素〕

TD Thoracic Duct 胸导管〔解〕

TD Tolerance Dose 耐受(剂) 量; 容许剂
量【注释】〔正常组织不受放射线损伤的最
低限度的线量〕

TCA 534 TD

TD Transverse Diameter 横 径〔解〕

TDF Time Dose Fractionation Factor 时
间线量分割因子【注释】〔比较、评价某组织的
放疗效果
时的各种要因和相互关系〕

TDF Tissue Damage Factor 组 织损伤因
子

TDHIA Texas Dairy Herd Improvement
Association 得克萨斯乳兽群促进协会

TDI Therapeutic Donor Insemination 治
疗性供精者人工授精

TDI Total-Dose Insulin 胰 岛素总剂量

TDM Therapeutic Drug Monitoring 治
疗药物浓度测定【注释】〔测定治疗药物的血中
浓度,用
于边观察边确定其适用量〕

TDN Total Digestible Nut Rients 总 消化
养分

TDO Tricho-Dento-Osseou (Syndrome)
毛发-牙齿- 骨(综合征)

TDP Thermal Death Point 热 致死点

Tdp Torsades De Points 心 电图特异波
型之一【注释】〔以基线为中心, 心电图上的
QRS 波呈现扭曲分布的特殊的室性心
动过速〕

TDR Time Dose Relationship 时 间线量
关系【注释】〔指放射量和照射时间的关系〕

TDT Terminal Deoxynucleotide Transferase
末 端脱氧核苷酸转移酶

TDT Thermal Death Time 加热致死时间【注释】
〔在一定条件下所有菌体死亡所
需要的加热时间〕

T & E T Rial And Error 反 复试验(试行
和发现错误试验)

TE Tangential Excision 切向切除

TE Tonsillectomy 扁桃体切除术

Teart Temporal Artery 颞动脉

Tearts Temporal Ar Teritis 巨 细胞性动脉
炎

Teba Temporary Basis 临时基板

Teca Tenckhoff Catheter 坦 基霍夫导管
〔腹膜透析用〕

Tecl Testicle 睾 丸 Orchis 〔拉〕

Tecls Testicles 睾丸

Tecu Tenaculum 持钩

Tecur Temperature Curve 温度曲线

TED Threshold Erythema Dose 红 斑阈
剂量

Tedo Test Dose 试验剂量

TEDP Tetraethyl Dithiopyrophosphate

(Sulfotep)/ Dithionopyrophosphate De
Tétraéthyle 四乙基二硫代焦磷酸酯

TEDS Thromboembolic Disease Suppor T
血栓栓塞性疾病支持疗法

TEE Transesophageal Echocardiography
经食管超声心动图术

Teel Tennis Elbow 网 球肘

Tee (X) Transesophageal Echocardiogram
经食管超声心动图

TEF Tracheo- Esophageal Fistula 气 管-
食管瘘; 气管食管瘘; 食管气管瘘

Tefa Tetralogy Of Fallot 法 洛四联症

Tefas Temporalis Fascia 颞肌筋膜

TEG Thromboelastogram 凝血弹性描记
图【注释】〔客观展示一般凝血检查法检测
不了的凝血块的物理指标。可了解血
块的收缩速度、弹性及血块收缩的衰减
状态等〕

TEG Thromboelastography 凝 血弹性描
记法【注释】〔客观地表示不能用普通的凝血
法测定的血凝的理化指标的方法, 通过
其可测出血块收缩速度、血块的弹性、
血块收缩的减衰状态等〕

Tehe Tension Headache 紧张性头痛

Teil Terminal Ileum 回肠末端

TEL Tet Raethyl Lead 四 乙基铅【注释】 〔为无色
透明的煤油状液体。通
过肺和皮肤吸收, 损伤中枢神经系统。
TD 535 TEL
它为汽油的防爆剂〕

TELISA Thermometric Enzyme Linked

Immunosorbent Assay 测 温酶联免疫吸
附试验【注释】〔ELISA 技术的另一种形式, 用
酶热敏电阻单位表示热的形式, 作为酶
作用的结果〕

Telo Temporal Lobe 颞 叶〔解〕Lobus Temporalis
〔拉〕

TEM Transmission Elect Ron Microscope
透射电子显微镜

TEM Transmission Electron Microscopy
透射电子显微镜术

Teme Telemet Ry 遥测术

TEME Thromboembolic Meningoencephalitis
血 栓栓塞性脑膜炎

TEMED N , N , N , N-Tetrame- Thylethylene-
Diamine N , N , N , N 四甲基乙烯二
胺【注释】〔丙烯酰胺聚合反应的诱导剂〕

TEN Toxic Epidermal Necrolysis 中 毒性
表皮坏死病【注释】〔出现伴有烧伤样水泡的局
限疼
痛性红斑或紫斑。一般认为在成人为
药疹, 而在幼儿为黄色葡萄菌的感染
症。也称为病毒综合征〕

Tena Temporonasal 颞鼻的

Tend . Tenderness 触 痛; 敏感

Tene Technetium 锝

Tenit Tendinitis 腱炎

TENS Transcutaneous Elect Rical Nerve
Stimulation 经皮肤电神经刺激

TEP Termination Of Early Pregnancy
抗早孕活性; 早期妊娠终止

TEP Thrombo-Endophlebectomy 血 栓

静脉内膜切除术

TEP Tracheoesophageal Puncture 气 道
食道穿刺术

Tepa Temporoparietal 颞顶的

TEPA Thio-TEPA 噻替派

TEPA Triethylene Phosphoramide 三乙
烯磷酰胺

TEPP Tetraethyl Pyrophosphate 四 乙
基焦磷酸酯

TESE Testicular Sperm Extraction 睾丸
精子取出法

Tesh Tetanus Shot 破伤风注射

Tesp Temperature Spike 体 温波峰

Tesps Temperature Spikes 体 温波峰

TET Tetanus Toxin 破 伤风毒素

TET T Readmill Exercise Test 踏 板运动
试验【注释】〔为一种体力测定装置。受试者
在传送带上逆向等速、维持固定位置地
进行跑动〕

Teta Telangiectasia 毛细(血) 管扩张

TE(Te) Tetanus 破伤风

Tetir Testicular 睾 丸的

Teto Testosterone 睾酮

Tetox Tetanus Toxoid 破 伤风类毒素(生
物制品)

Teve Tenia Versicolor 杂色绦虫

TEVRO Tennessee Equine Veterinary
Research Organization 田 纳西州马兽
医研究机构

Tewa Temporal Wasting 短暂性消瘦

Tf Tension By Finger Palpation 手 指触
诊张力

TF Tissue Factor 组织因子【注释】〔大量存在于
血管内皮下的成纤

维细胞中的细胞膜糖蛋白, 与凝血第Ⅶ
因子共同引发外因性凝血反应〕

TF Total Flow 总 流量; 总消耗量

TF T Ransfer Factor 转移因子【注释】〔收集结核
菌素反应阳性人的白

细胞(含淋巴细胞) , 将冻融、透析后的
透析袋外液注射给阴性者, 可使其转化

为结核菌素反应阳性。TF 即指能够改
变这种反应性的物质〕

Tf Transferrin 转铁蛋白【注释】〔它是在免疫电
泳中的 B 区域形

成沉降线的血清蛋白, 是血中转运铁的

TEL 536 Tf
蛋白质, 即铁的搬运体〕

TFA Total Fatty Acids 总 脂肪酸

TFA T Rifluoroacetic Acid 三 氟乙酸【注释】〔吸
入麻醉药氟烷在体内分解后

所形成的还原性代谢产物, 认为是氟烷
肝炎的一个病因〕

TFCC Triangular Fibrocartilage Complex
三 角形纤维软骨复合物

Tff Tibiofibular Fracture 胫 腓骨骨折

Tfl Tensor Fasciae Latae 阔筋膜张肌

TFN Totally Functional Neutrophil 总 的
功能性白细胞; 总的功能性嗜中性细胞

TFP Therapeutic Feeding Program 治 疗

性喂养计划

TFPI Tissue Factor Pathway Inhibitor
组织因子通道抑制物【注释】〔抑制 TF 与凝血第
Ⅶ 因子结合,
从而抑制随后引发的外因性凝血反应,
其本质是一种蛋白酶抑制剂〕

TFR T Ransferrin Receptor 转 铁蛋白受
体

TFS Testicular Feminization Syndrome
睾丸女性化综合征【注释】〔染色体和激素为男
性, 但雄性
激素受体缺如, 导致男性化受阻, 外生
殖器和乳房女性化〕

TFT Thyroid Function Test 甲 状腺功能
测试

Tfts Thyroid Function Tests 甲 状腺功能
测试

TG Thioguanine 硫鸟嘌呤

TG Tomography X 线断层照相法; X 线
体层照相法

TG T Riacylglycerol 三酰(基) 甘油

TG T Riglyceride 三酸甘油酯; 甘油三脂【注释】
〔一种中性脂肪〕

TGA Transient Global Amnesia 暂 时性
完全性遗忘症

TGA Transposition Of The Great Arteries
大动脉转位症【注释】〔占先天性心脏病的 5% 和
发绀
性疾病的 10 % ～ 20 %。常见的有主动
脉从右心室、而肺动脉从左心室发出,

主动脉在前, 肺动脉在后的位置异常〕

TGE Transmissible Gastroenteritis 可传
播性胃肠炎

TGF Therapeutic Gain Factor (照射) 治
疗效能比值【注释】〔药剂对肿瘤的放疗增益度
(ERT) 与药剂对周围健康组织的放射损
伤增加度(ERN) 之间的比值〕

TGF T Ransforming Growth Factor 转 化
生长因子【注释】〔有结构和功能完全不同的
A 和
B 两种, TGF-A 在肿瘤中大量存在, 一
般情况下, 能大量产生这种蛋白质的肿
瘤, 多为恶性肿瘤。另一方面, 已清楚
TGF-B 具有促进成纤维细胞、成骨细胞
增殖和抑制上皮(血管内皮细胞)、血细
胞增殖的功能。总的来说, TGF-B 大量
存在于血小板和骨髓中, 对于创伤愈合
和组织修复具有促进作用。因此, 临床
上将 TGF-B 试用于创伤、骨折、免疫性
疾病等的治疗〕

TGF Tubuloglomerular Feedback 肾 小
管肾小球反馈【注释】〔所谓 TGF 现象, 是指当向
汉勒
氏袢的流量增加时, 同一肾单位的 GF R
减少。它是肾进行自动调节的固有机
能〕

TGF Tumor Growth Factor 肿 瘤生长因
子

TGPH Total Gross Painless Hematuria
全大体无痛性血尿

TGT Thromboplastin Generation Test
凝血激酶发生实验【注释】〔确定与内因性凝血
激酶生成相

关的血液凝固第 1 相的因子异常的检查
法〕

TGV Thoracic Gas Volume 胸气容量

TGV Transposition Of The Great Vessels
大血管移位

Th Tetrahydrocor Tisone 四氢可的松

TFA 537 Th

TH Therapy 疗法

TH Thyroid 甲 状腺; 甲状的

TH Thyroid Hormone 甲状腺(激) 素

THA 1 , 2 , 3 , 4- Tet Rahydr-5-Aminoacridine
1 , 2 , 3 , 4- 四氢-5- 氨基吖啶【注释】〔抗胆碱脂
酶药。不过也用做呼

吸系刺激药或阿尔茨海默型脑代谢赋
活剂〕

Thab The Abdomen 腹 部

Thabj Therapeutic Abor Tion 治 病流产;
治疗性流产

Thabjs Therapeutic Abor Tions 治 疗性流
产

Thabl Thoracoabdominal 胸 腹的

Thal Thallium 铊

Thalm Thalamus 丘 脑

THAM T Ris-Hydroxymethyla-Minomethane
缓血酸胺; 三羟甲基氨基甲

烷【注释】〔为治疗酸中毒药。在临床上用
其 0 .3M 液。它容易透过细胞膜和血脑
屏障, 使体液碱性化。由于很少在肾小

管重吸收, 所以, 具有一定的利尿作
用〕

Thao The Aor Ta 主动脉

Thaor Thoracic Aor Ta 胸主动脉

Thar Total Hip Arthroplasty 全髋部复位

Thbe Thrombectomy 血栓切除术

Thbeh Threatening Behavior 危险行为

Thbo Thrombosis 血栓形成

Thbod Thrombosed 形成血栓的

Thboe Thrombose 形成血栓

Thbog Thrombosing 血栓形成

Thbow The Bowel 肠 ; 内脏

Thbr The Breast 乳腺

Thbu Thrombus 血栓

Thca The Cavity 腔

Thcat The Catheter 导管

Thcav Thoracic Cavity 胸腔

Thce The Cervix 颈

Thco Thoracotomy 胸 廓切开术

Thcos Thoracoscope 胸腔镜

Thcosy Thoracoscopy 胸腔镜检查

Thcy Thrombocytosis 血小板增多(症)

Thdi Thought Disorder 思维内容障碍

Thdo Thoracodorsal 胸 背的

Thdse Thyroid Disease 甲状腺疾病

Thenl Thyroid Enlargement 甲状腺肿大

Theso The Esophagus 食管

Thet The Etiology 病 因学

THF Tetrahydrocor Tisone 四 氢可的松
(肾上腺皮质激素类药)

THF Tet Rahydrofolic Acid 四氢叶酸

THF Tetrahydrofolic Acid (Methylt Ransferase
) 四 氢叶酸(甲基转移酶)

Thfa The Fascia 筋膜

Thfol Thiamine And Folate 硫 胺素与叶
酸

Thfx The Fracture 骨折

Thg Thigh 大 腿(动) ; 股

Thgb The Gallbladder 胆

Thgl Thyroglobulin 甲状腺球蛋白

Thgla Thyroid Gland 甲 状腺(甲状腺制
剂)

Thglo Thyroglossal 甲状舌(管) 的

Thgra The Graf T 移 植

Thhol Threshold 阈 值(动)

Thinf The Infant 婴 儿; 幼儿

Thins Thought Insertion 思维插入

Thir Thoroughly Irrigated 彻底冲洗

Thje The Jejunum 空 肠

Thjn The Joint 关 节

Thkd Thickened 增 稠的

Thki The Kidney 肾脏

Thkn The Knee 膝 关节

Thli The Liver 血室; 肝脏

Thlum Thoracolumbar 胸 腰的; 脊柱胸
腰段的

Thly Thrombolytic ① 血栓溶解的② 血
栓溶解剂

TH 538 Thl
Thlyts Thrombolytics 溶血栓的
Thma The Mass 肿块

Thme Thyromegaly 甲状腺肿大

Thmi Thalamic 丘脑的

Thmot Thalamotomy 丘脑切开术

Thms The Microscope 显微镜

Thnwa Thin Walled 薄壁的

Thom The Omentum 网膜

Thop The Operation 手术

Thopl Thoracoplasty 胸廓成形术

Thorc Thoracic 胸的, 胸廓的

Thpac Throat Pack 咽部填塞物

Thpan The Pancreas 胰腺

Thpe Therapeutic 治疗的; 治疗学的

Thpel The Pelvis 骨盆; 盆部; 肾盂

Thper The Peritoneum 腹膜

Thph Thrombophlebitis 血栓性静脉炎

Thpl The Placenta 胎盘

Thpla Thyroplasty 甲状软骨成形术

Thpn Thigh Pain 大腿痛

Thpo Three-Pillow Orthopnea 三枕端坐呼吸

THR Threonine (Aminoacid) 苏氨酸

Thra Therapeutic Range 有效药浓度范围

Thre The Remainder 残余物; 剩余的人

Thri Third Rib 第三肋

Thro Thyroxine 甲状腺素

Thrt Threat 威胁; 恐吓; 造成威胁的事物

Thrus Thrush ① 鹅口疮; 真菌性口炎② 蹄叉腐烂③口炎性腹泻

THR(X) Total Hip Replacement 髋关节

置换术【注释】〔人工材料置换髋臼和股骨头缺损部分后再建关节的手术〕

THS Treatment Hormonal Substitutive 激素替代疗法

THS Tucson Herpetological Society 图森两栖爬行类学会

THSC Totipotent Hematopoletic Stem Cell 全能造血干细胞

Thse Thalassemia 珠 蛋白生成障碍性贫血; 地中海贫血

Thsp Thoracic Spine 胸 脊柱

Thsus The Sutures 缝合; 骨缝

Thsys The Symptoms 症状

Thter Through The Emergency Room 通过急诊室

Thto Thyrotoxicosis 甲状腺毒症

Thton The Tourniquet 止 血带

Thtu The Tumor 肿 瘤

Thut The Uterus 子宫

Thva The Vagina 阴道

Thve The Vein 静 脉

Thve- Three-Vessel 三 血管

Thwof The History Was Obtained From 病史由……获得

Thwu The Wound 伤口

Th-X Thorium-X 钍 X

Thxs Therapies 疗法

Thxt Therapist 治疗师

Thydec Thyroidectomy 甲状腺切除术

Thydi Thyroiditis 甲状腺炎

Thyrc Thyroidectomy 甲状腺切除术

THZ Thiacetazone 氨硫脲

THZ Thiazolidomycin 噻唑霉素

TI Inversion Time 倒位时间【注释】〔利用核磁共
振摄像法(MRI) 进
行摄影时, 对于所使用的脉冲的重复时
间进行缩短或延长, 以此强调组织的
T1 缓和时间或成像的重复时间〕

TI T Ransient (Cerebral) Ischemic 短暂
性缺血性发作【注释】〔由于脑循环障碍出现的
短暂性
脑昏迷〕

TI Tricuspidal Insufficiency 三尖瓣闭锁
不全【注释】〔指由于功能性或器质性病变,
在心缩期血液出现由右心室向右心房
逆流的状态〕

Thl 539 TI

Tiag Thymus Independent Antigen 非
胸腺依赖性抗原

Tiar Tibial Artery 胫动脉

Tia(Sx) Transient Ischemic Attacks 短
暂性缺血性发作(一过性缺血发作)

Tib Tibia 胫骨 〔解〕

TIBC Total Iron Binding Capacity 总铁
结合力【注释】〔为血清铁和不饱和铁结合能力
(UIBC) 的总和〕

Tibc(X) Total Iron-Binding Capacity 总
铁结合力

Tibl Tibial 胫骨的; 胫节的

Tica Ticarcillin 替卡西林

Tiex Tissue Expander 组织扩张器

TIF Tumor-Inhibiting Factor 肿瘤抑制
因子

Tife Tibiofemoral 胫 (骨) 股(骨) 的

Tifi Tibiofibular 胫 (骨) 腓(骨) 的

Tifx Tibial Fracture 胫 骨骨折

TIG Tetanus Immune Globulin 破 伤风
免疫球蛋白

Tiio Tincture Of Iodine 碘酊

TIL Tumor Infilt Rating Lymphocytes 肿
瘤浸润淋巴细胞【注释】〔集中于肿瘤部位的淋
巴细胞。
收集这些细胞与 IL-2 共培养, 能提高
对肿瘤的特异性, 刺激被 MHC 抑制的
杀伤细胞增殖。因此共培养后的 TIL,
再返回患者体内可提高治疗效果〕

TIN Tubulointerstitial Nephropathy 小
管间质性肾病

Tipe Tinea Pedis 脚癣

Tiper Tibioperoneal 胫 (骨) 腓(骨) 的

Tipl Tibial Plateau 胫 骨坪

TIPS Transjugular Int Rahepatic Portosystemic
Shunt Placement 经 颈静脉肝内
门脉系统分流术

Tisi Tinel□s Sign 征 ; 提内耳(氏) 征

TISS Therapeutic Intervention Scoring
System 医 疗处置分数制【注释】〔1974 年, 由
Culle N 设计的所谓
医疗处置分数制, 分为 4 个阶段, 通过
其总分评价疾病严重程度的方法〕

TIT T Riiodothyronine 三 碘甲状腺原氨酸

Tita Titanium 钛

Titr Titrate 被 滴定液; 滴定

Titrd Tit Rated 滴定

Titrg Titrating 滴定; 滴定的

Titu Tibial Tuberosity 胫骨粗隆〔解〕

Tium Tinea Unguium 爪 癣; 爪真菌病

Tiup Term Int Rauterine Pregnancy 足月宫内妊娠

TIVC Thoracic Inferior Vena Cava 胸部下腔静脉

Tive Tinea Versicolor 花斑癣

Tivo Tidal Volume 潮 气容量

Tiwr The Instruments Were Removed 器械被移开

TJ Triceps Jerk 肱三头肌反射

TJA Total Joint Arthroplasty 全 关节成形术

Tk Take ① 接受交配(母畜) ② 成活; 接活

TKA Total Knee Arthroplasty 全 膝关节成形术

TKD Tokodynamometer 膝关节置换术【注释】〔用人工材料置换膝关节两个关节面, 并进行膝关节再造的手术〕

TKE Total Knee Extension 全膝牵伸术

TKP Thermokeratoplasty 角 膜加热成形术

Tkrs Total Knee Replacements 全 膝置换

术

Tkr(X) Total Knee Replacement 膝 关节
置换术

TL Thoracic Lumbar 胸腰的

TL Total Laryngectomy 喉全切除术

TL Tubal Ligation 输卵管结扎

TLC Tender Loving Care 轻 柔照料

TIA 540 TLC

TLC Thin-Layer Chromatography 薄 层
层析法

TLC Total Lung Capacity 肺 总量

TLC Total Lymphocyte Count 总淋巴细
胞技术计数

TLCK 7- Amino-1-Chloro-3- Tosylamido-
2-Heptanone 氨基氯代甲苯磺酰氨基庚
酮【注释】〔一种胰蛋白酶的抑制剂, 丝氨
酸蛋白酶的抑制剂〕

TLD Thermoluminescence Dosimeter
热荧光线量计

TLD Tumor Lethal Dose 肿瘤致死剂量

TLD95 Tumor Lethal Dose Ninety-Five
95 %肿瘤致死线量【注释】〔指治愈 95% 肿瘤局
部的放射线
量〕

TLI Total Lymph Node Irradiation 全 身
淋巴结放射线照射【注释】〔对于重度免疫不全
和先天性代
谢异常, 采用骨髓移植疗法前, 有时预
先进行本处置〕

TLI T Ransport-Level Interface 运输层接

口

TLI T Rypsin-Like Immunoreactivity 胰
蛋白酶样免疫活性

TLR Tonic Labyrinthine Reflex 迷 路紧
张反射

TLSO Thoracolumbosacral Or Thosis 胸
腰骶椎部固定器具【注释】〔治疗可动脊椎区域
为目的的固

定装置, 有 Taylor 式和 Steindler 式〕

TLT Tuberculin Line Test 结 核菌素划痕
试验

TLV Total Lung Volume 总 肺容量【注释】〔指气
管至肺所能吸入的气体总

容量。即预备吸气量、一次换气量、预
备呼气量及残气量的总和〕

TM Thalassemia Major 重 型地中海贫血

TM Thrombomodulin 凝 血调节因子【注释】〔存
在于血管内皮细胞上, 能使
凝血酶转化为抗凝血酶的特殊蛋白质〕

TM T Rabecular Meshwork 小 梁网

Tm Tympanic Membrane 鼓 膜〔解〕

Tma T Ransmetatarsal Amputation 经 跖
骨截肢术

Tmax Temperature Maximum 温 度极大
值; 最高温度

Tmax Time To Maximal Concent Ration
(药物) 达到血中最高浓度所需时间【注释】〔药
物代谢动力学研究用语〕

TMB Trimethobenzedrine 三 甲氧苯丙
胺

TME T Ransmissible Mink Encepha-Lopathy
貂传染性脑病

Tmgthiomethyl-B-D-Galactopyranoside
甲硫基-B-D- 吡喃半乳糖苷【注释】〔乳糖的不可
代谢类似物, 被用
来研究大肠杆菌中乳糖转运系统,B 半
乳糖苷酶的安慰诱导物〕

TMJ(X) Temporomandibular Joint 颞
颌关节

TMLR T Ransmyocardial Laser Revascularization
激 光心肌血运重建术【注释】〔做为严重心绞痛
的治疗方法,
从血液供应不足的心肌外侧, 通过激光
照射, 打 20 ～ 30 个孔穴, 以获得来自
心内壁的血液和新血管的再生。是受
蜥蜴等的心肌可直接吸收心脏内血液
的现象启发而设计的一种手术。在用
气囊导管的 PTCA 或搭桥手术不能奏
效的情况下使用〕

TMMSN Texas Marine Mammal
Stranding Network 得克萨斯海洋哺乳
动物搁浅网

TMO T Rimethadione 三 甲□唑烷二酮

TMP 4 , 5′, 8- Trimethylpsorlen 4 , 5′, 8
三甲基补骨酯【注释】〔是一种 DNA 交联剂, 能
检测染
色质构象的探针〕

TMP Trimethaphan 曲 美芬【注释】〔为短时间作
用型神经节阻断

TLC 541 TMP
剂, 也可作为降压剂、低血压麻醉用药

使用〕

TMP-SMX T Rimethoprim Sulfamethoxa -
Zole 甲氧苄鞍嘧啶磺胺□唑

TMR Transmyocardial Revascularization
心肌内血管新生术【注释】〔利用强激光, 在心脏
壁的数处

打孔, 此时心脏外壁可自行止血, 而心
脏内侧孔难以被封堵, 心内血液被注入
到心壁中而提供氧〕

TMS Trace Mineral Salt 微 量天然盐

TMST Treadmill Stress Test 踏 车负荷试
验; 跑台应激试验

Tmts Trans-Mucosal Therapeutic System
经黏膜治疗系统【注释】〔如同皮肤胶布经皮肤
吸收一

样, 药剂可通过黏贴于黏膜(口腔黏膜
等) 吸收而获得药效。 是既不是胶布,
也不是口服和注射给药的新的给药方
式。 从 1994 年开始有文献〕

TN T Rigeminal Neuralgia 三叉神经痛

TNBP Tri-N-Butyl Phosphate 磷 酸三丁
酯

TNBS 2 , 4 , 6-T Rinit Robenzene Sulfonic
Acid 2 , 4 , 6 三硝基苯磺酸【注释】〔在生物膜中
用以检查某些磷脂
的定向剂〕

TNC Thymic Nurse Cell 胸腺保育细胞

Tnd Tendon 跟 腱

Tndos Tendinous 腱的; 腱性的

Tnds Tendons 肌 腱

TNF Tension Normal By Finger (Palpa -

Tion) 手 指触诊张力正常

TNF Tumor Necrosis Factor 肿 瘤坏死因
子【注释】〔最早因发现其具有肿瘤坏死作
用而命名, 以后逐渐发现其具有更丰富
的生物学活性, 通过许多靶细胞受体而
发挥作用〕

TNG (GTN) T Rinitroglycerol (Glyceryl
Trinitrate) 硝酸甘油【注释】〔作为冠状动脉扩张
药用于心绞
痛治疗, 也是贴膏常用的成分, 有时用
于低血压麻醉辅助药〕

TNI Total Nodal Irradiation 全 结节照射

Tnj Talonavicular Joint 距舟关节

TNM Tumor Nodes Metastasis (Classification)
恶 性肿瘤的 TNM(分类) 【注释】〔国际癌症联合
会做出的有关癌
的国际病期分类〕

TNMU Tonic Neuromuscular Unit 紧 张
性神经肌单位【注释】〔由一个紧张性神经元和
其所支
配的肌细胞构成。 它以一个单位构成
紧张性运动活动〕

TNR Tonic Neck Reflex 紧张性颈反射

TNS Transcutaneous Nerve Stimulation
经皮电刺激神经疗法

TNT T Ransnephrectomy Tube 肾 移植切
除管

TNT T Rinit Rotoluene 三硝基甲苯

TNZ Thermoneutral Zone 温热中间带【注释】〔指
机体热量的产生和释放的平

衡, 是靠皮肤血流增减而单纯散发热进行调节的环境温域。一般为 29 ～31 ℃〕

Toa Tubo-Ovarian Abscess 输卵管卵巢脓肿

Toab Tobacco Abuse 烟草滥用

Toac Toothache 牙痛

Toao Tor Tuous Aor Ta 主动脉扭曲

Tob Tobacco 烟草; 烟叶

Toba Tongue Base 舌底部

Tobi Total Bilirubin 总胆红素

Toca Torn Cartilage 软骨撕裂

Toce Tobacco Cessation 停止吸烟

Toch Total Cholesterol 总胆固醇

Tocl Tonic-Clonic 强直-阵挛

Toco Tocometer 分娩力计

TOD Total Oxygen Demand 总需氧量【注释】〔有机物等可氧化物质完全燃烧氧化时所需要的氧总量。用于环境污染调查〕

Todo Toes Are Downgoing 脚趾向下

TOF Tetralogy Of Fallot 法洛四联症

TOF Tet Ralogy Of Fallot (T Rain-Of-Four) 法洛四联症; 紫绀四联症【注释】〔伴有肺动脉狭窄、高位心室中隔缺损、主动脉右侧移位及右心室肥大等四大病变的先天性心畸形。呈现发绀、眼球结膜充血、呼吸困难、红细胞增多等症状〕

T Of A Transposition Of Aor Ta 主动脉的移位

Tofo Tonsillar Fossa 扁 桃体窝〔解〕

Togm Tomogram X 射线断层照片

Togr Tomography X 线断层照相法; X 线体层照相法

TOK Tuberculosis Of Kidney 肾结核

Tolec Tonsillectomy 扁桃体切除术

Toli Tonsillitis 扁桃体炎

Toly Tocolysis 安 宫; 保胎; 子宫收缩抑制

Tonas Toenails 脚趾甲

Toniq Tourniquet 止血带; 压脉器

Toniqs Tourniquets 止血带

Tonr Tonsillar 扁桃体的

Tooc Total Occlusion 全 阻塞

Toos Tor Tuosity 卷曲性(羊毛)

TOP Termination Of Pregnancy 终 止妊娠; 妊娠终止

Topla Toxoplasma 弓 形体

Topls Toxoplasmosis 弓形体病

Topr Total Protein 总 蛋白; 蛋白质总量

Tor The Operating Room 手术室

TORCH Infections Toxoplasma , Others, Rubella Virus , Cytomega Lovirus, Herpes Virus TORCH 感染〔系胎儿感染最常见的几种非细菌性病原体〕

TORCHS Toxoplasmosis, Rubella, Cytomegalovirus, Herpes Simplex , Syphilis (Infection) 弓 浆虫病、风疹、巨细胞病毒、单纯疱疹、梅毒(感染)

Torr (Torr) Torricelli 托 【注释】〔真空单位(压力)〕

Tort Tortuous 迂曲的; 弯曲的

Tosc Toxicology Screen 毒 理学筛选

Tosts Topical Steroids 局 部类固醇

Tosy Thoracic Outlet Syndrome 胸 部出
口综合征【注释】〔由左右第一肋骨所包围的胸
廓
出口处的神经、血管遭到压迫而引起颈
部、肩部、上肢持续性或反复发作的疼
痛、麻木的一组病征〕

Toxo Toxoplasmose 弓 浆虫病

Toxy Toxicology 毒理学

TP Thiamphenicol 硫霉素

Tp Thrombopoietin 血小板生成素

TP Total Protein 总 蛋白; 蛋白质总量

TP Treponema Pallid 苍 白密螺旋体;
梅毒螺旋体

Tp T Rophoblastin / Trophoblastine 胎 盘
促性腺激素

TP Tympanoplasty 鼓 室成形术

TPA Tissue Plasminogen Activator 组 织
纤维蛋白溶解酶原活化剂【注释】〔为血栓病治
疗药, 与标准肝素
疗法和尿激酶疗法一样倍受关注〕

TPA Total Parenteral Alimentation 胃
肠道外全面营养(法)

Tpac Tissue Plasminogen Activator 组织
纤维蛋白溶解酶原活化剂

TPBF Total Pulmonary Blood Flow 总
肺血流量

TPC Thromboplastin Plasma Component

血浆促凝血酶原激酶成分

TPCF T Reponema Pallidum Complement
Fixation Test 梅 毒螺旋体补体结合试
验; T PCF 试验(检梅毒)

TOD 543 TPC

Tpd Third Por Tion Of The Duodenum 十
二指肠第三段

TPHA Treponema Pallidum Haemagglutination
(Test) 梅毒螺旋体红细胞凝集
(反应) 【注释】 〔为一种梅毒血清学检查方法。
利用从梅毒螺旋体(T P) 提取的蛋白抗
原建立的被动血凝检测 TP 抗体方法〕

TPIA Treponema Palladium Immune
Adherence Test 梅 毒螺旋体免疫吸附试
验; TPIA 试验 【注释】 〔以梅毒螺旋体的死菌为
抗原,
将其与梅毒患者的血清和豚鼠补体相
混合时, 通过抗原、抗体和补体复合物,
可使人的 O 型红细胞发生凝集。 不过,
由于还有 TPHA 等简易方法, 所以现已
不使用〕

TPN Total Parenteral Nutrition 完 全
(胃) 肠外营养; 全静脉营养 【注释】 〔由 Dudr Ic
等发明的, 对于所需
的能量均经静脉投与的治疗法。 在家
庭使用的为 HPN〕

Tpo Two-Pillow Or Thopnea 两 枕端坐呼
吸

TPP Thiamine Pyrophosphate 硫 胺素
焦磷酸 【注释】 〔为活性型维生素 B1 , 又称羧辅
酶、 脱羧辅酶或二磷酸硫胺〕

TPQ 2 , 4 , 5- Trihydroxyphenylalanine
Quinone 三羟苯丙氨醌【注释】〔首先从牛血清酶中鉴定的含铜
的胺氧化酶的氧还活性有机辅助因子,
存在于多种植物以及细菌的胺氧化酶
中。从完整蛋白质的天冬酰胺酪天冬
/ 谷氨酸共有序列中的酪氨酸残基经翻
译后修饰衍生而来〕

Tpr Taper 锥 度

TPR Temperature 温度; 体温

T .P .R . Temperature, Pulse And Respiration
体温、脉搏和呼吸【注释】〔可测定的所谓生命特征的身体
状态的三个基本征候〕

TPR Total Peripheral Resistance 总 外周
阻力; 总末梢阻力【注释】〔从左心室驱出的血液承受的阻
力。可用下式求得。TPR (Dynes/ Sec/
Cm3) = 平均动脉压(Mmhg)/ 心输出量
(1/ 分) × 80〕

TPR Total Pulmonary Resistance 总 肺
循环阻力【注释】〔肺在呼吸肌作用下活动时, 必
须克服弹性阻力、黏性阻力和慢性阻
力, 在此指这些阻力的总和。可通过呼
吸过程中的压力气量曲线的解析测定〕

Tprd Tapered 锥 度的; 锥形的; 变断面
的

Tprg Tapering 渐 减量(药物) ; 尖端细的

Tpsc Thallium Perfusion Scan 铊 灌注扫
描

TPT Total Pump Time 总泵时间

TQ Tourniquet 止血带; 压脉器

TQM Total Quality Management TQM
质量管理【注释】〔为预防医疗事故, 提高诊疗水
平的管理设想〕

T .R . Takata Reaction 高田氏反应

TR Therapeutic Ratio 治疗比率【注释】〔用 TD/ T
LD 表示。用于决定采
用放射线疗法治愈病灶的可能性和难
易度〕

Tr Tincture ① 酊; 酊剂② 药酒③ 色泽;
色彩④染料; 颜料⑤气质; 特征

TR Total Resistance 总 电阻; 总阻力

TR Trachea 气 管

TR T Reatment Required For 应…… 要求
治疗

TR Tricuspid Regurgitation 三尖瓣回流

TR Tuberculin Reaction 结核菌素反应

TR Tubular Reabsorption 肾 小管重吸收
(试验)

TR Turnover Rate 更 替速度【注释】〔在成熟的动
物体内, 构成机体
结构的蛋白质和氨基酸之间处于动态
Tpd 544 TR
平衡, 即合成速度和分解速度处于相对
平衡状态。在此指合成-分解速度〕

TRA Tumor Rejection Antigen 肿瘤排斥
抗原

Trab T Ransversus Abdomen 腹 横肌〔解〕

Musculus T R Ansversus Abdominis〔拉〕

Trach Acetylcholine Turnover Rate 乙
酰胆碱周转率

Trachcy Tracheoscopy 气管镜检查

Trachl T Racheal 气管的

Trachy Tracheostomy 气管造口术

Tracj T Raction 牵引

Tracjl Tractional 牵引的

Traeso T Racheoesophageal 气管食管的

Trans T Ransverse ①横的② 横切的③ 横
肌

Transa Transaminase 氨 基转移酶

Transas Transaminases 氨基转移酶

Trauc T Raumatic 创伤的; 外伤的

Traucy T Raumatically 创 伤性的

Traus Traumas 外伤

Trauz T Raumatize 使…… 受外伤

Trauzd Traumatized 外 伤的

Trauzg T Raumatizing 外伤的

TRBF Total Renal Blood Flow 肾血流总
量

Trbr Tracheobronchial 气管支气管的

Trbrs T Racheobronchitis 气管支气管炎

TRC Tanned Red Cell 鞣质红细胞

TRCA Tanned Red Cell Agglutination 鞣
酸处理的红细胞凝集试验【注释】〔抗原吸附于
红细胞, 遇相应抗
体则出现红细胞凝集反应。为使抗原
吸附于红细胞的效率提高, 有时用鞣酸
处理〕

TRCG Thoroughbred Research Consultative

Group 纯 种动物研究咨询协会

Trch Trochanter ① 转子(股骨) ② 转节
〔昆虫〕

Trchc T Rochanteric 转子的

Trchs T Rochanters 转子

TRCI Total Red Cell Iron 总红细胞铁【注释】 〔可
以用 TRCI = (总血量× Hb×

34)/ 100 进行概算。正常值为 2000～

2500mg〕

Trco Transverse Colon 横结肠 〔解〕

Trda Transudate 漏 出液; 漏出物; 渗出
液

Trdg Transfer Diagnosis 转院诊断

Trdu T Ransducer 传感器

TRF Thyrotropin Releasing Factor 促 甲
状腺激素释放因子

Trfa Transversalis Fascia 横筋膜

Trfas Transverse Fashion 横断方式

Trfe T Ransferrin 铁传递蛋白

Trfi Transfix 贯穿; 刺通

Trfid T Ransfixed 贯穿

Trfij T Ransfixion ① 切断术② 贯穿; 刺
通

Trfin T Rigger Finger 板 机指

Trfins T Rigger Fingers 扳机指

Trfu T Ransfuse 输血

Trfud Transfused 输 血

Trfug T Ransfusing 输血

Trfuj Transfusion ① 输血(法) ② 输液
(法) ③转移; 转输

Trfus Transfuses 输血

Trgl Triglyceride 甘油三酯

Trgls Triglycerides 甘油三酯

TRH Thyrotrop (H) In-Releasing Factor
(Hormone) 促甲状腺激素释放激素【注释】〔丘
脑下部合成, 作用于脑垂体
前叶, 促进垂体促甲状腺素的分泌。用
于脑垂体-甲状腺机能检查〕

TRIAC Triiodothyroacetic Acid 三 碘甲
腺乙酸

Trian Triangle ①三角形; 三角关系②牛
胴去除背部的前四分之一(包括肩, 胸及
腿部)

TRIC Trachoma Or Inclusion Conjunctivi-
TRA 545 TRI

Tis (Agent) 沙眼或包涵体性结膜炎

Trich . Trichomonas 毛滴虫属

Tril T Ransilluminate 透视

Trild Transilluminated 透 照的

Trilj T Ransillumination 透照(法)

Trin T Ransverse Incision 横 切口

TRIT T Riiodothyronine 三 碘甲腺原氨
酸

TRITC Tetramethylrhodamine Isothiocyanate
四 甲基罗丹明异硫氰酸盐【注释】〔在荧光抗体
法中所使用的一种
色素, 发出红色荧光〕

Trkes T Race Ketones 微 量酮

Trla Trabeculation 小梁形成

Trlar Triangular 三角的; 三角形的

Trlec T Rabeculectomy 小梁切除术

Trlo Tremulous 震颤的

Trm Tremor 震颤

TRM T Richomycin 面古霉素〔抗滴虫霉
素药〕

Trmo Trichomonad 毛滴虫

Trmos T Richomoniasis 毛滴虫病; 滴虫
病

Trms Tremors 震颤

Trna-MT Transfer Ribonucleic Acid
(Guanine-N2)- Methyl- Transferase 转
运核糖核酸(鸟嘌呤 N2) 甲基转移酶

Trne Trigeminal Neuralgia 三叉神经痛

Trotc The Remainder Of The Case 本病例
其余的人(物)

Trothe The Remainder Of The …… 的残
余物; …… 剩余的人

TRP T Richo-Rhino-Phalangeal (Syndrome
) 毛发鼻指(趾) (综合征) 【注释】 〔特征为头发
粗糙、梨状鼻、人中
长、上唇薄、近端指(趾) 节间关节处斜
指、短缩圆锥骨端等〕

TRP Tryptophan (Aminoacid) 色氨酸

TRP Tubular Reabsorption Of Phosphate
肾小管磷酸盐重吸收【注释】 〔用于甲状旁腺机
能亢进症的诊
断(正常为 80% ~90 %)〕

Trph Trephine 环踞; 用环踞做手术

Trpl Transplant 移植; 移植物; 移植片

Trpla Treatment Plan 治疗计划

Trpld T Ransplanted 移植

Trplj T Ransplantation 移植(术)

Trpos Transposition 转座子; 变换

Trpr T Ransverse Process 横突〔解〕

TRPRC Tulane Regional Primate Research Center Tulane 灵长类动物研究中心

Trprs Transverse Processes 横突

Trpz Trendelenburg Position 特伦德伦堡体位〔垂头仰卧体位〕

Trre Tricuspid Regurgitation 三尖瓣回流

Trres T Reatment Resistant 抗治疗的

Trri T Racheal Ring 气管环〔动〕

Trria Thyroid Radioisotope Assay 甲状腺放射性同位素测定

Trsa Transversalis ①横的②横肌

Trse T Ransect 样条; 横切

Trsed Transected 横断的

Trseg Transecting 横断的

Trsej Transection 横切面; 横断

Trsij Transition 移行; 过渡

Trso Troublesome 讨厌的; 易出故障的; 困难的

Trsph Transsphenoidal 经蝶骨的

Trsu T Raction Suture 牵引缝合

Trsus Traction Sutures 牵引缝合

Trte Treatment Team 治疗小组

Trtes Treadmill Test 平板试验

Trtu Tracheotomy Tube 气管切开插管

TRT(V) Turkey Rhinotracheitis (Virus) 火鸡鼻气管炎(病毒)

Trtvs Turkey Rhinot Racheitis Viruses

土耳其鼻气管炎病毒

Trv T Ransverse ①横的②横切的③ 横肌

Trva T Ricuspid Valve 三尖瓣

Tri 546 Trv

Trvag T Ransvaginal 经 阴道的

Trve Traverse 交叉; 横断; 横穿

Trve- T Riple-Vessel 三管腔

Trved T Raversed 横 断的

Trveg Traversing 横 向进刀; 导线测量;
遍历

Trven Transvenous 经静脉

Trvy Transversely 横着; 横切; 横断

Trzo T Ransformation Zone 变 性带

TS Suppressor T Cell 抑制性 T 细胞

TS Teaching Strategies 教授方略【注释】 〔医学教
育用语〕

TS Teratology Society 畸形学学会

TS Thrombospondin 血 小板反应蛋白【注释】 〔与
血小板间的黏附反应和血小
板凝集反应有关。已确认也存在于其
他脏器组织及结缔组织中〕

TS Tricuspid Stenosis 三尖瓣狭窄

T&S Type And Screen 血 型判定筛选【注释】 〔通
过比较经过交叉适合试验的
血液量(C) 和实际在输血中使用的血液
量(T) , 研究血液的使用率(C/ T 比)
时, 存在有被称为浪费血液使用的现
状。因此, 对于输血实施率限于 30 %
以下, 或平均 2 单位以下的输血手术,
只要确定血型判定不规则抗体阴性, 就

可在有必要输血的情况下, 通过交叉适
合试验, 提供适合血液〕

TSA Tumor-Susceptible Antigen 肿瘤特
异抗原【注释】〔伴随细胞的癌性变化而出现的
肿瘤抗原中, 仅在其癌细胞中特异存在
的抗原〕

TSB Total Serum Bilirubin 总血清胆红
素

TSB Total Spinal Block 全脊髓麻醉【注释】〔在蛛
网膜下腔内注入局部麻醉
药, 导致所有颈部脊髓以下的脊神经及
上位的中枢出现麻醉状态。在高位麻
醉和硬膜外麻醉出错, 麻醉药大量流入
蛛网膜下腔情况下发生。引起呼吸停
止、意识丧失, 但通过人工呼吸, 消除
局部麻醉的效果后, 予后良好〕

TSE Transmissible Spongiform Encephalopathy
传递性海绵状脑病; 传递
性病毒性海绵状脑病

TSEM T Ransmission Scanning Electron
Microscope 透射扫描电子显微镜

Tsf Suppressive T Cell Factor 抑制性 T
细胞因子【注释】〔从抑制性 T 细胞中提取, 它是
由抗原刺激而释放的因子, 具有抑制抗
体产生的作用〕

Tsgf Thrombin-Soaked Gelfoam 浸有凝
血酶的明胶海绵

TSH Thyroid Stimulating Hormone , Thyrot
Ropin 促甲状腺激素【注释】〔一种垂体前叶分
泌的激素〕

TSI Thyroid Stimulating Immunoglobulin
甲状腺刺激免疫球蛋白

TSM Tween Synthetic Medium 吐温合
成培养基

TSP Total Serum Protein 总 血清蛋白质

TSP Tropical Spastic Paraparesis 热带性
痉挛性脊髓麻痹【注释】〔在热带地区很早以前
就知道此
病, 已弄清其发生多半与 HT LV- Ⅰ 有
关, 和 HAM 为同一个疾病。在 1988 年
被 WHO 合在一起命名为 HAM/ TS P〕

TSRBC T Rypsinized Sheep Red Blood Cell
胰蛋白酶处理的绵羊红细胞

TSS Toxic Shock Syndrome 中 毒性休克
综合征

TSST-1 Toxic Shock Syndrome Toxin-1
中毒性休克综合征毒素-1 【注释】〔耐甲氧青霉
素金黄色葡萄球菌
MRSA 性状改变后的产物, 现 TSST-1
产生菌株正在不断增加〕

Tst Testis 睾 丸

TST Thromboplastin Screening Test 凝
血酶原激酶筛选试验【注释】〔测定内因性凝血
激酶生成速度
Trv 547 TST
的检查法〕

TSTA Tumor Specific T Ransplantation
Antigen 肿瘤特异性移植抗原【注释】〔在实验性
肿瘤免疫应答中, 出
现移植排斥现象时, 引起这种免疫排斥
反应的肿瘤抗原〕

Tste Treadmill Stress Test 踏车负荷试验

Tsts Testes 睾丸

TSVR Total Systemic Vascular Resistance 体循环血管总阻力

TT Test Toxoid 测试类毒素

TT Tetanus Toxoid 破伤风类毒素

TT Thrombin Time 凝血酶时间

TT Tolerance Test 耐量试验

TT Total Thyroxine 总甲状腺素

TTA Transt Racheal Aspiration 经气管吸引

TTA Tumor Transplantation Antigen 肿瘤移植抗原【注释】〔来自近交系动物的可移植肿瘤, 能够在近交系宿主中出现免疫应答或肿瘤移植排斥时, 将引起这种反应的抗原称为 TSTA 或 TATA〕

Ttdm Type Ⅱ Diabetes Mellitus Ⅱ 型糖尿病

Tte T Ransthoracic Echocardiogram 经胸超声心动图

Tter To The Emergency Room 到急诊室

TTH Thyrotropic Hormone 促甲状腺激素

TTI Tension-Time Index 张力-时间系数【注释】〔为心肌耗氧量的一个指标, 它是平均收缩压乘以收缩时间所得的数值〕

TTI Tissue Thromboplastin Inhibitor 组织凝血激酶抑制剂

TTN Transitory Tachypnea Of The Newborn

新生儿短暂呼吸急促

Ttotc The Tip Of The Catheter 导管尖端

TTP Thrombotic Thrombocytopenic Purpura
血栓性血小板减少性紫癜【注释】〔1925 年由
Moschowitz 首次报
道。以神经症状、发热、血小板减少、溶
血性贫血及肾功能障碍为主要特征。
予后不良〕

TTS Tarsal Tunnel Syndrome 跗 管综合
征

TTS Temporary Threshold Shift 暂时性
阈移【注释】〔指受到一定时间连续性音响刺
激的听觉器官, 暂时性地听觉阈值升高
的现象〕

TTS Transdermal Therapeutic System
透皮给药系统【注释】〔它是按照药物释放有效
面积,
将药物与具有透皮作用的黏贴剂混合,
制成皮肤敷剂进行治疗的方式。最近
对其利用率在增加〕

TTT Thymo Turbidity Test 麝 香草酚混
合试验【注释】〔为一种检查肝功能的血清胶体
反应〕

TTTS Twin To Twin Transfusion Syndrome
孪 生儿输血综合征

Ttu T- Tube T 形管

TTW Transt Racheal Washes Or Washing
经气管冲洗

TTX Tetrodotoxin 河豚鱼毒素【注释】〔为河豚的
有毒物质, 可引起舌

端、口唇、指尖等的钝麻, 随意肌麻痹,
进而导致延髓中枢的麻痹。在河豚的
卵巢和肝脏中含量很高。可被碱性溶
液破坏〕

TU Toxic Unit 毒素单位

TU Tuberculin Unit 结核菌素单位

Tu Tumor 肿块

Tuad Tubular Adenoma 管状腺瘤

Tuads Tubal Adhesions 输卵管粘连

Tudrs Tubes And Drains 导管与引流

Tufe Tube Feeding 鼻饲(法)

Tufes Tube Feedings 鼻饲

Tuma Tumor Mass 肿块

Tun Tunnel 管

TST 548 Tun

Tunat Turbinate ① 甲介形的② 陀螺状
的③ 鼻甲(的)

Tund Tunneled 通道; 隧道

Tundl Tuohy Needle 图伊针 〔硬膜外腔
持续导管插入用, 前端为直角弯曲的穿刺
针〕

Tuos Tuberosity 粗隆; 结节

Tuov Tubo-Ovarian 输卵管卵巢的

Tuovs Tubes And Ovaries 输卵管与卵巢

Tupg Tubal Pregnancy 输卵管妊娠

TUR Transurethral Resection 经尿道切
除术【注释】〔经尿道的内窥镜操作, 进行膀
胱、前列腺手术的方法。包括 TUR-BT
和 TUR-P 两种方法〕

TURB T Ransurethral Resection Of The

Bladder 经尿道膀胱切除

Turb Turbinate ① 甲介形的 ② 陀螺状的 ③ 鼻甲(的)

Turbc Turbinectomy 鼻 甲切除术

Turbs Turbinates 鼻甲

TURP Transurethral Prostatectomy 经尿道前列腺切除术

TURP T Ransurethral Resection Of The Prostate 经尿道前列腺切除术

Tuu Transureteroureterostomy (横跨中线的) 输尿管- 输尿管吻合术

Tuva Tunica Vaginas 鞘膜

TV Tidal Volume 潮气量【注释】 〔在平静呼吸过程中的 1 次呼吸
的气体量〕

TV Tricuspid Valve 三尖瓣

TV Typhus Vaccine 斑疹伤寒疫苗

TVC Timed Vital Capacity 定 时的肺活量【注释】 〔在测定用力呼气的肺活量时, 增加时间因素的测定值〕

Tvc True Vocal Cord 真声带; 声襞

Tvd Triple-Vessel Disease 三管腔病

TVH Total Vaginal Hysterectomy 全 阴道子宫切除术

TVH Trans-Vaginal Hysterectomy 经 阴道子宫切除术

TVI Tropical Veterinary Institute (University Of Liege, Belgium) 热带兽医学会

TVMA Texas Veterinary Medical Association

得克萨斯兽医医学会

TVMA Thai Veterinary Medical Association
泰国兽医医学会

TVP Thrombose Venous Profundity 深
部静脉血栓形成

TVU Total Volume Urine 全尿; 24 小时
尿量

TWAR Taiwan Acute Respiratory Disease
台湾急性呼吸系统疾病

TWE Tap Water Enema 自来水灌肠

Twfis Two Fingerbreadths 二指宽

TWG Total Weight Gain 总体重的增加

Twi T-Wave Inversion T 波倒置

Twncs There Were No Complications 没
有并发症

Twne There Was No Evidence 没有迹象

Twntb There Was Noted To Be 有 记录表
明

Twpas Two Packs Of Cigarettes 两包烟

TX Thromboxane 血栓素 【注释】 〔在血小板中,
由花生四烯酸经
过 PGG2 所生成的生物学活性物质〕

TXA2 Thromboxane A2 血 栓素 A2 【注释】 〔具
有对平滑肌的收缩作用和血
小板的凝集作用, 因此, 对于机体来说
并非有用的内因性物质。在发生休克
时其含量增加〕

TXB2 Thromboxane B2 血 栓素 B2 【注释】 〔在
血小板破坏时增加, 由尿液
排出〕

Txc Toxic ① (有) 毒的; 毒性的; 中毒的
②毒剂; 毒物

Txcly Toxicology 毒理学

Tun 549 Txc

Txco Toxicosis 中毒

Txcy Toxicity 毒 性; 毒力

Txs Therapies 疗法

Tycr Type And Cross 血 型和血交叉测定

Tycrd Typed And Crossed 血 型和血交叉
测定

Tyfe Typhoid Fever 伤寒

Tyg Typing 分型; 定型; 分类

Tyma Tympanomastoidectomy 鼓 室乳
突切除术

Tymp Tympanometry 鼓 室测压法; 鼓室
压测量法

Tyni Tympanitic 气鼓的; 鼓响的

Tyno Tympanostomy 鼓 室造口术

Tyoa Thank You Once Again 再次感谢

Typla Tympanoplasty 鼓 室成形术

Typly Typically 典型地; 作为特色的

TYR Tyrosine (Aminoacid) 酪氨酸

Tysc Type And Screen 测定和筛选

Tyscd Typed And Screened 测 定和筛选

Tytu Tympanostomy Tube 鼓室造口管＿ T Absolute
Temperature 绝对温度

T Spine Thoracic 胸 脊柱

T + 1 . . Stages Of Increased Intraocular
Tension 表示眼压升高程度的符号

T Temperature 温 度; 体温

T Testosterone 睾 酮

T Tetracycline 四环素

T Thoracic Ver Tebrae 胸 椎 〔解〕

T Thorax 胸 廓

T Thymine 胸腺嘧啶; 胸腺碱

3T Triage- T Retment- Transpor Tation 判
断- 应急处置- 后方运送【注释】 〔在灾害现场所
要三项重要措

施, 3T 就是其三个单词的组合略语〕

T3 T Riiodothyronine 三碘甲状腺原氨酸【注释】
〔表示甲状腺功能的一个指标。

122± 41mg/ Dl〕

T4 Tetraiodothyronine , Thyroxin 甲 状
腺素; 四碘甲腺原氨酸【注释】 〔表示甲状腺功能
的一个指标。

117± 7pg/ Ml〕

TA Temporal Ar Teritis 颞动脉炎

TA Tension Artérielle 动 脉压

Ta Tension By Applanation 扁 平张力

T&A Tonsils And Adenoids 扁桃体与增
殖腺

TA Tricuspid At Resia 三尖瓣闭锁

TAA Tumor Associated Antigen 肿 瘤相
关抗原【注释】 〔来自近交系动物的植入性肿瘤
引起近交系宿主出现免疫应答和肿瘤
移植排斥反应的抗原〕

Taar Tachyarrhythmia 快速型心律失常

TAB Salmonella Typhia And S . Paratyphoid
A And B (Vaccine) 伤 寒杆菌与甲
型和乙型副伤寒杆菌疫苗

Tabr Tachycardia-Bradycardia 心动过速-心动过缓

TAB(Tab .) Tabella ① 侧板; 斜板② 片剂; 锭剂; 糖锭

TAC Preparation Of Tetracycline, Epinephrine (Adrenaline) , Cocaine 四环素、肾上腺素、可卡因制剂

Taca Tachycardia 心动过速; 心搏过速

Tacac Tachycardiac 心动过速的; 心搏过速的; 心搏加速药

Tach Tachometry 流速测定法

Tads Tobacco , Alcohol And Drugs 烟草、酒精与毒品

Tady Tardive Dyskinesia 迟发性运动障碍

TAE T Ranscatheter Arterial Embolization 经探管的(肝) 动脉塞栓术【注释】〔进行性肝癌的优选疗法。大多数情况下, 与化学疗法并用〕

TAF Tumor Angiogenesis Factor 肿瘤血管形成因子

TAH Transfusion-Associated Hepatitis 输血相关肝炎

Tah(X) Total Abdominal Hysterectomy 经腹部子宫全切除术

TAIEX Technical Assistance Information Exchange Office 技术援助信息交换部

TAL Tendon Achilles Lengthening 阿基里斯跟腱延长术

TAL Tumor Associated Lymphocyte 肿

瘤相关淋巴细胞

TAL(TAO) T Riacetyloleandomycin 三
乙酰竹桃毒素

TAM Toxoid-Antitoxin Mixture 类 毒
素- 抗毒素合剂; 类毒素- 抗毒素混合物

TAM T Ransient Abnormal Myelopoiesis
一过性异常骨髓造血病【注释】〔并发于道恩氏
综合征, 表现为
肝脾肿大、白细胞增多、新生儿末梢血
中出现幼稚细胞的一过性增多的可自
然治愈的疾病。纳入一过性骨髓增殖
性综合征〕

Tamet Tarsometatarsal 跗 (骨) 跖(骨) 的

Tana Talonavicular 距 (骨) 舟(骨) 的

T Antigen T Ransplantation Antigen 移 植
抗原

T Antigen Tumor Antigen 肿 瘤抗原; T
抗原

TAO Thromboangitis Obliterans 血 栓性
栓塞性脉管炎【注释】〔易发于吸烟的中年男性,
主要
表现为下肢动脉血管炎症引发的血栓
栓塞症状。通常称为伯格氏病〕

Tapa Tail Of The Pancreas 胰 腺尾

Tapn Tachypnea 呼吸急促

Tapnc Tachypneic 呼吸急促

TAPS T Ris (Hydroxymethyl) Methylamino-
Propane Sulfonic Acid 三羟甲基
甲氨基丙烷磺酸【注释】〔用于制备 Ph7 .7 ～ 9 .1
范围内

的缓冲液〕

TAPSO 3-[N- Tris (Hydroxymethyl)
Methylamino] 2-Hydroxypropane Sulfonic
Acid 3- [N-(羟甲基) 甲基氨基]
2 羟丙烷磺酸【注释】 〔用于制备 Ph7 .0 ～ 8 .2 范围内
的缓冲液〕

TAPVR (TAPVC) (TAPVD) Total
Anomalous Pulmonary Venous Return
(Connection) (Drainage) 全 部肺静脉
血回流异常症【注释】 〔为肺静脉血完全回流到右心系
的先天性异常, 有许多表现形式。多因
心衰致死, 死亡率高达 80%〕

T .A .R . Takata-Ara□s Reaction 高 田-
荒反应【注释】 〔通过凝胶反应检查脊髓液, 以
用于中枢神经系统疾病诊断〕

TAR Thrombocytopenia-Absent Radii
(Syndrome) 血小板减少-桡骨缺失(综
合征)

TAR Tissue-Air Ratio 组 织空中线量比
(值) 【注释】 〔为一种放射线剂量的计算法。
即组织深部吸收线量/ 等距空中线量〕

TASS Ticlopidine-Aspirin Strokestudy
抗血小板病疗法之一【注释】 〔是一种噻氯匹定
和阿斯匹林合
用治疗血小板病的疗法, 现用于脑溢血
发生频率的研究〕

Tasts Tarry Stools 柏油样便

TAT Tetanus Antitoxin 抗 破伤风毒素;

抗破伤风免疫血清【注释】〔为破伤风毒素或其类毒素的抗

体, 属免疫球蛋白 G 类。由于免疫球蛋白 G 不会造成人血清病等副反应而被

广泛应用〕

TAT Thematic Apperception Test 主 题

统觉测试【注释】〔让受试者观看描绘情绪性场面

的画面, 任意发挥编造故事, 以此诊断

性格的方法〕

TAT Thrombin- Antithrombin Ⅲ 凝血酶-抗凝血酶Ⅲ 【注释】〔为一种血液凝固检查指标。正

常值为 3 .0ng/ Ml 以下〕

TAT Thrombin-Antithrombin (Complex)

凝血酶- 抗凝血酶(复合物)

TB Thymol Blue 麝酚蓝

TB Total Bilirubin 总 胆红素

TB Tracheobronchitis 气管支气管炎

TB Tuberculosis 肺 结核; 结核(病) ; 痨病

TAL 532 TB

TBA Thiobarbituric Acid 硫代巴比土酸

TBA Thoroughbred Breeders□Associa -Tion 纯种动物种畜协会

Tba Tubercle Bacillus 结核杆菌

TBBM Total Body Bone Mineral 全身骨无机物; 全身骨矿物质

TBC Texas Beef Council 得克萨斯牛肉委员会

TBC Tuberculosis 肺结核

Tbe (Tbe .) Tuberculosis 肺结核

TBF Tick-Borne Fever 蜱 传播性发热

TBFB Tracheobronchial Foreign Body
气管支气管异物

TBG Thyroxine Binding Globulin 甲 状
腺素结合球蛋白【注释】 〔可与甲状腺激素(T3 ,
T4) 结合
的血清蛋白。在妊娠、急性肝炎、慢性
活动性肝炎、急性卟啉病等情况下增
高, 而肾病(重患除外) 在大量使用激素
类药物治疗时降低〕

TBG Thyroid-Binding Globulin 甲 状腺
结合球蛋白

TBI Total Body Irradiation 放 射线全身
照射【注释】 〔在骨髓移植等之前进行的放射
线全身照射〕

TBI Traumatic Brain Injury 外伤性脑损
伤

TBI Tebethion 氨 硫脲; 结核安

T-Bil Total Bilirubin 总 胆红素

TBLB Transbronchial Lung Biopsy 经 支
气管肺活检【注释】 〔为末梢肺部病变诊断的常
用手
法。注意避免出血和气胸的发生〕

TBNAB T Ransbronchial Needle Aspiration
Biopsy 经支气管针抽吸活检【注释】 〔由于肺癌
的癌细胞已转移到纵
隔淋巴结, 与支气管壁相接触, 而支气
管壁和内腔没有肿瘤的露出和浸润, 通

过支气管无法进行诊断的情况下, 在摄
像支气管镜的探头上安装注射针, 将其
穿刺到支气管壁外, 进行穿刺细胞诊断
的方法〕

TBP Thyroxime Binding Protein 甲 状
腺素结合蛋白【注释】 〔包括甲状腺素结合球蛋
白
(TBG) 、甲状腺素结合前蛋白(TBPA)
和白蛋白三种类型。血中的 T4 大部分
与 TBG 结合〕

TBP Tuberculous Peritonitis 结 核性腹
膜炎

TBPA Thyroxin-Binding Prealbumin 甲
状腺素结合前白蛋白

TBS Tracheobronchoscopy 气 管支气管
镜检查

TBSA Total Body Surface Area 总 体表面
积

TBT T Racheobronchial Toilet 气 管内清
洗【注释】 〔为了清除不能通过咳出的、存
在于气管内的黏稠分泌物和异物, 通过
气管内插管, 在进行人工呼吸的同时,
反复注入生理盐水清洗气管, 将分泌物
或异物清除〕

TBV Total Blood Volume 总血量【注释】 〔指全身
的血液容量。正常值为
70～ 80ml/ Kg〕

TBW Total Body Water 体液总量

TC Cytotoxic T Cell 细胞毒性 T 细胞

TC Thrombocyte 血 小板

TC Total Cholesterol 总胆固醇

TC Transverse Colon 横结肠〔解〕

Tc Trocar 套针

TC Tubocurarine 筒箭毒碱【注释】〔一种肌松弛剂〕

TC Tet Racycline 四环素(类)

TCA Terminal Cancer 终末期癌

TCA Thyrocalcitonin 甲状腺降钙素; 降钙素

Tca Total Calcium 总钙

TCA Total Cholic Acid 总胆酸

TCA T Ricarboxylic Acid 三羧酸

TBA 533 TCA

TCA Trichloroacetic Acid 三氯乙酸; 三氯醋酸

TCA T Ricyclical Antidepressant 三环抗抑郁药

Tcb To Cont Rol Bleeding 控制出血

Tcc T Ransitional Cell Carcinoma 移行细胞癌

TCD Transcranial Doppler Sonography 经头盖的多普勒超声波扫描法【注释】〔是一种超声波诊断法。最近在脑神经医学领域中用于发现和观察脑血管痉挛出现及其过程〕

TC&DB Turn Cough & Deep Breath 转身咳嗽深呼吸

TCDD Tetrachlorodibenzodioxin 四氧二苯二氧杂环己二烯

TCDD Time Controlled Drug Delivery

药剂的控时投与(装置) 【注释】〔有口腔黏膜吸
收用和经皮吸收
用两种〕

T-Cell Thymus Derived Cell 胸腺衍化细
胞; 胸腺来源细胞

T-CELLS Thymus Cells 胸腺细胞

TCES Trans-Cutane Cerebral Elect Ric
Stimulation 头皮电刺激法

TCGF T Cell Growth Factor T 细胞生长
因子

T .CH Total Cholesterol 总胆固醇

TCH Thiophene-2-Carboxylic Acid Hydrazine
(Test) 噻吩-2- 碳酸酰肼(试验)

TCH Total Circulating Hemoglobin 总 循
环血红蛋白量

TCI Target Cont Rolled Infusion 目 标控
制注射【注释】〔利用药代动力学知识,计算出
欲治脏器达到效果时所需的药物剂量,
按此剂量进行注射给药的方法。 有时
也指利用计算机内脏自动注射器注射
麻醉药的方法〕

TCO2 Total Carbon Dioxide Content 二
氧化碳总含量

Tcp Thrombocytopenia 血小板减少症

TCP Trans-Cutaneous Pacing 经 皮起搏

TCP Transmission Control Protocol 传
输控制协议

TCP Tropical Canine Pancytopenia 热带
犬全血细胞减少症

Tcpc Thrombocytopenic 血 小板减少性

的

Tcpo2 Trans-Cutaneous Oxygen Pressure
经皮氧分压【注释】〔指利用 PO2 连续测定装置
通过

皮肤测定的值。压力(P) 代表透过组织
的氧气量, 饱和度(S) 代表血液对氧气
的输送能力〕

TCR T Cell Receptor T- 细胞受体【注释】〔T 细胞
通过 TCR 识别抗原, 并

发挥其作用〕

T&Crm Type And Cross-Match (Crossmatch)
血 型和交叉配血

TCS Traumatic Cervical Syndrome 颈部
扭伤

Tcsz Tonic-Clonic Seizure 强直-阵挛发作

TCT Thrombin Clotting Time 凝 血酶凝
血时间

TCT Tricarboxylic Acid Cycle 三 羧酸循
环【注释】〔也称为柠檬酸三羧酸循环、克
雷布氏三羧酸循环。它是机体内有机
物完全氧化时的代谢途径, 其产生的能
量通过 ATP 储存〕

TD5 / 5 Tolerance Dose Five Per Five (5
年组织) 耐受剂量【注释】〔在 5 年内发生的 5 ％
以下的重
度损伤的放射线量〕

TD Tetanus And Diphtheria (Toxoid) 破
伤风和白喉〔类病素〕

TD Thoracic Duct 胸导管〔解〕

TD Tolerance Dose 耐受(剂) 量; 容许剂

量【注释】〔正常组织不受放射线损伤的最低限度的线量〕

TCA 534 TD

TD Transverse Diameter 横径〔解〕

TDF Time Dose Fractionation Factor 时间线量分割因子【注释】〔比较、评价某组织的放疗效果时的各种要因和相互关系〕

TDF Tissue Damage Factor 组织损伤因子

TDHIA Texas Dairy Herd Improvement Association 得克萨斯乳兽群促进协会

TDI Therapeutic Donor Insemination 治疗性供精者人工授精

TDI Total-Dose Insulin 胰岛素总剂量

TDM Therapeutic Drug Monitoring 治疗药物浓度测定【注释】〔测定治疗药物的血中浓度,用于边观察边确定其适用量〕

TDN Total Digestible Nut Rients 总消化养分

TDO Tricho-Dento-Osseou (Syndrome) 毛发-牙齿-骨(综合征)

TDP Thermal Death Point 热致死点

Tdp Torsades De Points 心电图特异波型之一【注释】〔以基线为中心,心电图上的QRS波呈现扭曲分布的特殊的室性心动过速〕

TDR Time Dose Relationship 时间线量关系【注释】〔指放射量和照射时间的关系〕

TDT Terminal Deoxynucleotide Transferase
末 端脱氧核苷酸转移酶

TDT Thermal Death Time 加热致死时间【注释】
〔在一定条件下所有菌体死亡所
需要的加热时间〕

T & E T Rial And Error 反 复试验(试行
和发现错误试验)

TE Tangential Excision 切向切除

TE Tonsillectomy 扁桃体切除术

Teart Temporal Artery 颞动脉

Tearts Temporal Ar Teritis 巨 细胞性动脉
炎

Teba Temporary Basis 临时基板

Teca Tenckhoff Catheter 坦 基霍夫导管
〔腹膜透析用〕

Tecl Testicle 睾 丸 Orchis 〔拉〕

Tecls Testicles 睾丸

Tecu Tenaculum 持钩

Tecur Temperature Curve 温度曲线

TED Threshold Erythema Dose 红 斑阈
剂量

Tedo Test Dose 试验剂量

TEDP Tetraethyl Dithiopyrophosphate
(Sulfotep)/ Dithionopyrophosphate De
Tétraéthyle 四乙基二硫代焦磷酸酯

TEDS Thromboembolic Disease Suppor T
血栓栓塞性疾病支持疗法

TEE Transesophageal Echocardiography
经食管超声心动图术

Teel Tennis Elbow 网 球肘

Tee (X) Transesophageal Echocardiogram

经食管超声心动图

TEF Tracheo- Esophageal Fistula 气管-食管瘘; 气管食管瘘; 食管气管瘘

Tefa Tetralogy Of Fallot 法洛四联症

Tefas Temporalis Fascia 颞肌筋膜

TEG Thromboelastogram 凝血弹性描记图【注释】〔客观展示一般凝血检查法检测不了的凝血块的物理指标。可了解血块的收缩速度、弹性及血块收缩的衰减状态等〕

TEG Thromboelastography 凝血弹性描记法【注释】〔客观地表示不能用普通的凝血法测定的血凝的理化指标的方法, 通过其可测出血块收缩速度、血块的弹性、血块收缩的减衰状态等〕

Tehe Tension Headache 紧张性头痛

Teil Terminal Ileum 回肠末端

TEL Tet Raethyl Lead 四乙基铅【注释】〔为无色透明的煤油状液体。通过肺和皮肤吸收, 损伤中枢神经系统。

TD 535 TEL
它为汽油的防爆剂〕

TELISA Thermometric Enzyme Linked Immunosorbent Assay 测温酶联免疫吸附试验【注释】〔ELISA 技术的另一种形式, 用酶热敏电阻单位表示热的形式, 作为酶作用的结果〕

Telo Temporal Lobe 颞叶〔解〕Lobus Temporalis〔拉〕

TEM Transmission Elect Ron Microscope

透射电子显微镜

TEM Transmission Electron Microscopy
透射电子显微镜术

Teme Telemet Ry 遥测术

TEME Thromboembolic Meningoencephalitis
血 栓栓塞性脑膜炎

TEMED N , N , N , N-Tetrame- Thylethylene-
Diamine N , N , N , N 四甲基乙烯二
胺【注释】〔丙烯酰胺聚合反应的诱导剂〕

TEN Toxic Epidermal Necrolysis 中 毒性
表皮坏死病【注释】〔出现伴有烧伤样水泡的局
限疼
痛性红斑或紫斑。一般认为在成人为
药疹, 而在幼儿为黄色葡萄菌的感染
症。也称为病毒综合征〕

Tena Temporonasal 颞鼻的

Tend . Tenderness 触 痛; 敏感

Tene Technetium 锝

Tenit Tendinitis 腱炎

TENS Transcutaneous Elect Rical Nerve
Stimulation 经皮肤电神经刺激

TEP Termination Of Early Pregnancy
抗早孕活性; 早期妊娠终止

TEP Thrombo-Endophlebectomy 血 栓
静脉内膜切除术

TEP Tracheoesophageal Puncture 气 道
食道穿刺术

Tepa Temporoparietal 颞顶的

TEPA Thio-TEPA 噻替派

TEPA Triethylene Phosphoramide 三乙
烯磷酰胺

TEPP Tetraethyl Pyrophosphate 四乙
基焦磷酸酯

TESE Testicular Sperm Extraction 睾丸
精子取出法

Tesh Tetanus Shot 破伤风注射

Tesp Temperature Spike 体温波峰

Tesps Temperature Spikes 体温波峰

TET Tetanus Toxin 破伤风毒素

TET T Readmill Exercise Test 踏板运动
试验【注释】〔为一种体力测定装置。受试者
在传送带上逆向等速、维持固定位置地
进行跑动〕

Teta Telangiectasia 毛细(血)管扩张

TE(Te) Tetanus 破伤风

Tetir Testicular 睾丸的

Teto Testosterone 睾酮

Tetox Tetanus Toxoid 破伤风类毒素(生
物制品)

Teve Tenia Versicolor 杂色绦虫

TEVRO Tennessee Equine Veterinary
Research Organization 田纳西州马兽
医研究机构

Tewa Temporal Wasting 短暂性消瘦

Tf Tension By Finger Palpation 手指触
诊张力

TF Tissue Factor 组织因子【注释】〔大量存在于
血管内皮下的成纤
维细胞中的细胞膜糖蛋白, 与凝血第Ⅶ
因子共同引发外因性凝血反应〕

TF Total Flow 总流量; 总消耗量

TF T Ransfer Factor 转移因子【注释】〔收集结核菌素反应阳性人的白

细胞(含淋巴细胞),将冻融、透析后的

透析袋外液注射给阴性者,可使其转化

为结核菌素反应阳性。TF 即指能够改

变这种反应性的物质〕

Tf Transferrin 转铁蛋白【注释】〔它是在免疫电泳中的 B 区域形

成沉降线的血清蛋白,是血中转运铁的

TEL 536 Tf

蛋白质,即铁的搬运体〕

TFA Total Fatty Acids 总 脂肪酸

TFA T Rifluoroacetic Acid 三 氟乙酸【注释】〔吸入麻醉药氟烷在体内分解后

所形成的还原性代谢产物,认为是氟烷

肝炎的一个病因〕

TFCC Triangular Fibrocartilage Complex 三 角形纤维软骨复合物

Tff Tibiofibular Fracture 胫 腓骨骨折

Tfl Tensor Fasciae Latae 阔筋膜张肌

TFN Totally Functional Neutrophil 总 的功能性白细胞; 总的功能性嗜中性细胞

TFP Therapeutic Feeding Program 治 疗性喂养计划

TFPI Tissue Factor Pathway Inhibitor 组织因子通道抑制物【注释】〔抑制 TF 与凝血第 Ⅶ 因子结合,

从而抑制随后引发的外因性凝血反应,

其本质是一种蛋白酶抑制剂〕

TFR T Ransferrin Receptor 转 铁蛋白受

体

TFS Testicular Feminization Syndrome
睾丸女性化综合征【注释】〔染色体和激素为男
性, 但雄性
激素受体缺如, 导致男性化受阻, 外生
殖器和乳房女性化〕

TFT Thyroid Function Test 甲 状腺功能
测试

Tfts Thyroid Function Tests 甲 状腺功能
测试

TG Thioguanine 硫鸟嘌呤

TG Tomography X 线断层照相法; X 线
体层照相法

TG T Riacylglycerol 三酰(基) 甘油

TG T Riglyceride 三酸甘油酯; 甘油三脂【注释】
〔一种中性脂肪〕

TGA Transient Global Amnesia 暂 时性
完全性遗忘症

TGA Transposition Of The Great Arteries
大动脉转位症【注释】〔占先天性心脏病的 5% 和
发绀
性疾病的 10 % ～ 20 %。常见的有主动
脉从右心室、而肺动脉从左心室发出,
主动脉在前, 肺动脉在后的位置异常〕

TGE Transmissible Gastroenteritis 可传
播性胃肠炎

TGF Therapeutic Gain Factor (照射) 治
疗效能比值【注释】〔药剂对肿瘤的放疗增益度
(ERT) 与药剂对周围健康组织的放射损
伤增加度(ERN) 之间的比值〕

TGF T Ransforming Growth Factor 转 化 生长因子【注释】〔有结构和功能完全不同的 A 和 B 两种, TGF-A 在肿瘤中大量存在, 一般情况下, 能大量产生这种蛋白质的肿瘤, 多为恶性肿瘤。另一方面, 已清楚 TGF-B 具有促进成纤维细胞、成骨细胞增殖和抑制上皮(血管内皮细胞) 、血细胞增殖的功能。总的来说, TGF-B 大量存在于血小板和骨髓中, 对于创伤愈合和组织修复具有促进作用。因此, 临床上将 TGF-B 试用于创伤、骨折、免疫性疾病等的治疗〕

TGF Tubuloglomerular Feedback 肾 小管肾小球反馈【注释】〔所谓 TGF 现象, 是指当向汉勒氏袢的流量增加时, 同一肾单位的 GF R 减少。它是肾进行自动调节的固有机能〕

TGF Tumor Growth Factor 肿 瘤生长因子

TGPH Total Gross Painless Hematuria 全大体无痛性血尿

TGT Thromboplastin Generation Test 凝血激酶发生实验【注释】〔确定与内因性凝血激酶生成相关的血液凝固第 1 相的因子异常的检查法〕

TGV Thoracic Gas Volume 胸气容量

TGV Transposition Of The Great Vessels

大血管移位

Th Tetrahydrocor Tisone 四氢可的松

TFA 537 Th

TH Therapy 疗法

TH Thyroid 甲 状腺; 甲状的

TH Thyroid Hormone 甲状腺(激) 素

THA 1 , 2 , 3 , 4- Tet Rahydr-5-Aminoacridine 1 , 2 , 3 , 4- 四氢-5- 氨基吖啶【注释】〔抗胆碱脂酶药。不过也用做呼

吸系刺激药或阿尔茨海默型脑代谢赋

活剂〕

Thab The Abdomen 腹 部

Thabj Therapeutic Abor Tion 治 病流产;

治疗性流产

Thabjs Therapeutic Abor Tions 治 疗性流

产

Thabl Thoracoabdominal 胸 腹的

Thal Thallium 铊

Thalm Thalamus 丘 脑

THAM T Ris-Hydroxymethyla-Minomethane

缓血酸胺; 三羟甲基氨基甲

烷【注释】〔为治疗酸中毒药。在临床上用

其 0 .3M 液。它容易透过细胞膜和血脑

屏障, 使体液碱性化。 由于很少在肾小

管重吸收, 所以, 具有一定的利尿作

用〕

Thao The Aor Ta 主动脉

Thaor Thoracic Aor Ta 胸主动脉

Thar Total Hip Arthroplasty 全髋部复位

Thbe Thrombectomy 血栓切除术

Thbeh Threatening Behavior 危险行为

Thbo Thrombosis 血栓形成

Thbod Thrombosed 形成血栓的

Thboe Thrombose 形成血栓

Thbog Thrombosing 血栓形成

Thbow The Bowel 肠；内脏

Thbr The Breast 乳腺

Thbu Thrombus 血栓

Thca The Cavity 腔

Thcat The Catheter 导管

Thcav Thoracic Cavity 胸腔

Thce The Cervix 颈

Thco Thoracotomy 胸廓切开术

Thcos Thoracoscope 胸腔镜

Thcosy Thoracoscopy 胸腔镜检查

Thcy Thrombocytosis 血小板增多(症)

Thdi Thought Disorder 思维内容障碍

Thdo Thoracodorsal 胸 背的

Thdse Thyroid Disease 甲状腺疾病

Thenl Thyroid Enlargement 甲状腺肿大

Theso The Esophagus 食管

Thet The Etiology 病 因学

THF Tetrahydrocor Tisone 四 氢可的松
(肾上腺皮质激素类药)

THF Tet Rahydrofolic Acid 四氢叶酸

THF Tetrahydrofolic Acid (Methylt Ransferase
) 四 氢叶酸(甲基转移酶)

Thfa The Fascia 筋膜

Thfol Thiamine And Folate 硫 胺素与叶
酸

Thfx The Fracture 骨折

Thg Thigh 大 腿(动) ; 股

Thgb The Gallbladder 胆

Thgl Thyroglobulin 甲状腺球蛋白

Thgla Thyroid Gland 甲 状腺(甲状腺制剂)

Thglo Thyroglossal 甲状舌(管) 的

Thgra The Graf T 移 植

Thhol Threshold 阈 值(动)

Thinf The Infant 婴 儿; 幼儿

Thins Thought Insertion 思维插入

Thir Thoroughly Irrigated 彻底冲洗

Thje The Jejunum 空 肠

Thjn The Joint 关 节

Thkd Thickened 增 稠的

Thki The Kidney 肾脏

Thkn The Knee 膝 关节

Thli The Liver 血室; 肝脏

Thlum Thoracolumbar 胸 腰的; 脊柱胸腰段的

Thly Thrombolytic ① 血栓溶解的② 血栓溶解剂

TH 538 Thl

Thlyts Thrombolytics 溶血栓的

Thma The Mass 肿块

Thme Thyromegaly 甲状腺肿大

Thmi Thalamic 丘脑的

Thmot Thalamotomy 丘脑切开术

Thms The Microscope 显微镜

Thnwa Thin Walled 薄壁的

Thom The Omentum 网膜

Thop The Operation 手术

Thopl Thoracoplasty 胸廓成形术

Thorc Thoracic 胸的, 胸廓的

Thpac Throat Pack 咽部填塞物

Thpan The Pancreas 胰腺

Thpe Therapeutic 治疗的; 治疗学的

Thpel The Pelvis 骨盆; 盆部; 肾盂

Thper The Peritoneum 腹膜

Thph Thrombophlebitis 血栓性静脉炎

Thpl The Placenta 胎盘

Thpla Thyroplasty 甲状软骨成形术

Thpn Thigh Pain 大腿痛

Thpo Three-Pillow Orthopnea 三枕端坐
呼吸

THR Threonine (Aminoacid) 苏氨酸

Thra Therapeutic Range 有效药浓度范围

Thre The Remainder 残余物; 剩余的人

Thri Third Rib 第三肋

Thro Thyroxine 甲状腺素

Thrt Threat 威胁; 恐吓; 造成威胁的事
物

Thrus Thrush ① 鹅口疮; 真菌性口炎②
蹄叉腐烂③口炎性腹泻

THR(X) Total Hip Replacement 髋关节
置换术【注释】〔人工材料置换髋臼和股骨头缺
损部分后再建关节的手术〕

THS Treatment Hormonal Substitutive
激素替代疗法

THS Tucson Herpetological Society 图

森两栖爬行类学会

THSC Totipotent Hematopoletic Stem Cell 全能造血干细胞

Thse Thalassemia 珠蛋白生成障碍性贫血; 地中海贫血

Thsp Thoracic Spine 胸脊柱

Thsus The Sutures 缝合; 骨缝

Thsys The Symptoms 症状

Thter Through The Emergency Room 通过急诊室

Thto Thyrotoxicosis 甲状腺毒症

Thton The Tourniquet 止血带

Thtu The Tumor 肿瘤

Thut The Uterus 子宫

Thva The Vagina 阴道

Thve The Vein 静脉

Thve- Three-Vessel 三血管

Thwof The History Was Obtained From 病史由……获得

Thwu The Wound 伤口

Th-X Thorium-X 钍 X

Thxs Therapies 疗法

Thxt Therapist 治疗师

Thydec Thyroidectomy 甲状腺切除术

Thydi Thyroiditis 甲状腺炎

Thyrc Thyroidectomy 甲状腺切除术

THZ Thiacetazone 氨硫脲

THZ Thiazolidomycin 噻唑霉素

TI Inversion Time 倒位时间【注释】〔利用核磁共振摄像法(MRI) 进

行摄影时, 对于所使用的脉冲的重复时
间进行缩短或延长, 以此强调组织的
T1 缓和时间或成像的重复时间〕

TI T Ransient (Cerebral) Ischemic 短 暂
性缺血性发作【注释】〔由于脑循环障碍出现的
短暂性
脑昏迷〕

TI Tricuspidal Insufficiency 三 尖瓣闭锁
不全【注释】〔指由于功能性或器质性病变,
在心缩期血液出现由右心室向右心房
逆流的状态〕

Thl 539 TI

Tiag Thymus Independent Antigen 非
胸腺依赖性抗原

Tiar Tibial Artery 胫 动脉

Tia(Sx) Transient Ischemic Attacks 短
暂性缺血性发作(一过性缺血发作)

Tib Tibia 胫骨 〔解〕

TIBC Total Iron Binding Capacity 总 铁
结合力【注释】〔为血清铁和不饱和铁结合能力
(UIBC) 的总和〕

Tibc(X) Total Iron-Binding Capacity 总
铁结合力

Tibl Tibial 胫骨的; 胫节的

Tica Ticarcillin 替 卡西林

Tiex Tissue Expander 组织扩张器

TIF Tumor-Inhibiting Factor 肿 瘤抑制
因子

Tife Tibiofemoral 胫 (骨) 股(骨) 的

Tifi Tibiofibular 胫 (骨) 腓(骨) 的

Tifx Tibial Fracture 胫骨骨折

TIG Tetanus Immune Globulin 破伤风
免疫球蛋白

Tiio Tincture Of Iodine 碘酊

TIL Tumor Infilt Rating Lymphocytes 肿
瘤浸润淋巴细胞【注释】〔集中于肿瘤部位的淋
巴细胞。
收集这些细胞与 IL-2 共培养, 能提高
对肿瘤的特异性, 刺激被 MHC 抑制的
杀伤细胞增殖。因此共培养后的 TIL,
再返回患者体内可提高治疗效果〕

TIN Tubulointerstitial Nephropathy 小
管间质性肾病

Tipe Tinea Pedis 脚癣

Tiper Tibioperoneal 胫(骨)腓(骨)的

Tipl Tibial Plateau 胫骨坪

TIPS Transjugular Int Rahepatic Portosystemic
Shunt Placement 经颈静脉肝内
门脉系统分流术

Tisi Tinel□s Sign 征; 提内耳(氏)征

TISS Therapeutic Intervention Scoring
System 医疗处置分数制【注释】〔1974 年, 由
Culle N 设计的所谓
医疗处置分数制, 分为 4 个阶段, 通过
其总分评价疾病严重程度的方法〕

TIT T Riiodothyronine 三碘甲状腺原氨
酸

Tita Titanium 钛

Titr Titrate 被滴定液; 滴定

Titrd Tit Rated 滴定

Titrg Titrating 滴定; 滴定的

Titu Tibial Tuberosity 胫骨粗隆〔解〕

Tium Tinea Unguium 爪 癣; 爪真菌病

Tiup Term Int Rauterine Pregnancy 足月
宫内妊娠

TIVC Thoracic Inferior Vena Cava 胸部
下腔静脉

Tive Tinea Versicolor 花斑癣

Tivo Tidal Volume 潮 气容量

Tiwr The Instruments Were Removed 器
械被移开

TJ Triceps Jerk 肱三头肌反射

TJA Total Joint Arthroplasty 全 关节成
形术

Tk Take ① 接受交配(母畜) ② 成活; 接
活

TKA Total Knee Arthroplasty 全 膝关节
成形术

TKD Tokodynamometer 膝关节置换术【注释】
〔用人工材料置换膝关节两个关
节面, 并进行膝关节再造的手术〕

TKE Total Knee Extension 全膝牵伸术

TKP Thermokeratoplasty 角 膜加热成
形术

Tkrs Total Knee Replacements 全 膝置换
术

Tkr(X) Total Knee Replacement 膝 关节
置换术

TL Thoracic Lumbar 胸腰的

TL Total Laryngectomy 喉全切除术

TL Tubal Ligation 输卵管结扎

TLC Tender Loving Care 轻 柔照料

TIA 540 TLC

TLC Thin-Layer Chromatography 薄 层
层析法

TLC Total Lung Capacity 肺 总量

TLC Total Lymphocyte Count 总淋巴细
胞技术计数

TLCK 7- Amino-1-Chloro-3- Tosylamido-
2-Heptanone 氨基氯代甲苯磺酰氨基庚
酮【注释】〔一种胰蛋白酶的抑制剂, 丝氨
酸蛋白酶的抑制剂〕

TLD Thermoluminescence Dosimeter
热荧光线量计

TLD Tumor Lethal Dose 肿瘤致死剂量

TLD95 Tumor Lethal Dose Ninety-Five
95 %肿瘤致死线量【注释】〔指治愈 95% 肿瘤局
部的放射线
量〕

TLI Total Lymph Node Irradiation 全 身
淋巴结放射线照射【注释】〔对于重度免疫不全
和先天性代
谢异常, 采用骨髓移植疗法前, 有时预
先进行本处置〕

TLI T Ransport-Level Interface 运输层接
口

TLI T Rypsin-Like Immunoreactivity 胰
蛋白酶样免疫活性

TLR Tonic Labyrinthine Reflex 迷 路紧
张反射

TLSO Thoracolumbosacral Or Thosis 胸
腰骶椎部固定器具【注释】〔治疗可动脊椎区域
为目的的固
定装置, 有 Taylor 式和 Steindler 式〕

TLT Tuberculin Line Test 结 核菌素划痕
试验

TLV Total Lung Volume 总 肺容量【注释】〔指气
管至肺所能吸入的气体总
容量。即预备吸气量、一次换气量、预
备呼气量及残气量的总和〕

TM Thalassemia Major 重 型地中海贫血

TM Thrombomodulin 凝 血调节因子【注释】〔存
在于血管内皮细胞上, 能使
凝血酶转化为抗凝血酶的特殊蛋白质〕

TM T Rabecular Meshwork 小 梁网

Tm Tympanic Membrane 鼓 膜〔解〕

Tma T Ransmetatarsal Amputation 经 跖
骨截肢术

Tmax Temperature Maximum 温 度极大
值; 最高温度

Tmax Time To Maximal Concent Ration
(药物) 达到血中最高浓度所需时间【注释】〔药
物代谢动力学研究用语〕

TMB Trimethobenzedrine 三 甲氧苯丙
胺

TME T Ransmissible Mink Encepha-Lopathy
貂传染性脑病

Tmgthiomethyl-B-D-Galactopyranoside
甲硫基-B-D- 吡喃半乳糖苷【注释】〔乳糖的不可
代谢类似物, 被用

来研究大肠杆菌中乳糖转运系统,B 半
乳糖苷酶的安慰诱导物〕

TMJ(X) Temporomandibular Joint 颞
颌关节

TMLR T Ransmyocardial Laser Revascularization
激 光心肌血运重建术【注释】〔做为严重心绞痛
的治疗方法,
从血液供应不足的心肌外侧,通过激光
照射,打 20 ～ 30 个孔穴,以获得来自
心内壁的血液和新血管的再生。是受
蜥蜴等的心肌可直接吸收心脏内血液
的现象启发而设计的一种手术。在用
气囊导管的 PTCA 或搭桥手术不能奏
效的情况下使用〕

TMMSN Texas Marine Mammal
Stranding Network 得克萨斯海洋哺乳
动物搁浅网

TMO T Rimethadione 三 甲□唑烷二酮

TMP 4 , 5′, 8- Trimethylpsorlen 4 , 5′, 8
三甲基补骨酯【注释】〔是一种 DNA 交联剂,能
检测染
色质构象的探针〕

TMP Trimethaphan 曲 美芬【注释】 〔为短时间作
用型神经节阻断

TLC 541 TMP
剂,也可作为降压剂、低血压麻醉用药
使用〕

TMP-SMX T Rimethoprim Sulfamethoxa -
Zole 甲氧苄鞍嘧啶磺胺□ 唑

TMR Transmyocardial Revascularization

心肌内血管新生术【注释】〔利用强激光, 在心脏壁的数处

打孔, 此时心脏外壁可自行止血, 而心

脏内侧孔难以被封堵, 心内血液被注入

到心壁中而提供氧〕

TMS Trace Mineral Salt 微 量天然盐

TMST Treadmill Stress Test 踏 车负荷试

验; 跑台应激试验

Tmts Trans-Mucosal Therapeutic System

经黏膜治疗系统【注释】〔如同皮肤胶布经皮肤吸收一

样, 药剂可通过黏贴于黏膜(口腔黏膜

等) 吸收而获得药效。是既不是胶布,

也不是口服和注射给药的新的给药方

式。从 1994 年开始有文献〕

TN T Rigeminal Neuralgia 三叉神经痛

TNBP Tri-N-Butyl Phosphate 磷 酸三丁

酯

TNBS 2 , 4 , 6-T Rinit Robenzene Sulfonic

Acid 2 , 4 , 6 三硝基苯磺酸【注释】〔在生物膜中用以检查某些磷脂

的定向剂〕

TNC Thymic Nurse Cell 胸腺保育细胞

Tnd Tendon 跟 腱

Tndos Tendinous 腱的; 腱性的

Tnds Tendons 肌 腱

TNF Tension Normal By Finger (Palpa -

Tion) 手 指触诊张力正常

TNF Tumor Necrosis Factor 肿 瘤坏死因

子【注释】〔最早因发现其具有肿瘤坏死作

用而命名, 以后逐渐发现其具有更丰富
的生物学活性, 通过许多靶细胞受体而
发挥作用〕

TNG (GTN) T Rinitroglycerol (Glyceryl
Trinitrate) 硝酸甘油【注释】 〔作为冠状动脉扩张
药用于心绞
痛治疗, 也是贴膏常用的成分, 有时用
于低血压麻醉辅助药〕

TNI Total Nodal Irradiation 全 结节照射

Tnj Talonavicular Joint 距舟关节

TNM Tumor Nodes Metastasis (Classification)
恶 性肿瘤的 TNM(分类) 【注释】 〔国际癌症联合
会做出的有关癌
的国际病期分类〕

TNMU Tonic Neuromuscular Unit 紧 张
性神经肌单位【注释】 〔由一个紧张性神经元和
其所支
配的肌细胞构成。 它以一个单位构成
紧张性运动活动〕

TNR Tonic Neck Reflex 紧张性颈反射

TNS Transcutaneous Nerve Stimulation
经皮电刺激神经疗法

TNT T Ransnephrectomy Tube 肾 移植切
除管

TNT T Rinit Rotoluene 三硝基甲苯

TNZ Thermoneutral Zone 温热中间带【注释】 〔指
机体热量的产生和释放的平
衡, 是靠皮肤血流增减而单纯散发热进
行调节的环境温域。 一般为 29 ～31 ℃〕

Toa Tubo-Ovarian Abscess 输卵管卵巢脓

肿

Toab Tobacco Abuse 烟草滥用

Toac Toothache 牙痛

Toao Tor Tuous Aor Ta 主动脉扭曲

Tob Tobacco 烟草; 烟叶

Toba Tongue Base 舌底部

Tobi Total Bilirubin 总胆红素

Toca Torn Cartilage 软骨撕裂

Toce Tobacco Cessation 停止吸烟

Toch Total Cholesterol 总胆固醇

Tocl Tonic-Clonic 强直-阵挛

Toco Tocometer 分娩力计

Tocol Tor Ticollis 斜颈; 捩颈

Tocoy Total Colonoscopy 全结肠镜检查

TOD Total Denervation 完全失神经支

TMP 542 TOD

配

TOD Total Oxygen Demand 总需氧量【注释】〔有
机物等可氧化物质完全燃烧
氧化时所需要的氧总量。用于环境污
染调查〕

Todo Toes Are Downgoing 脚趾向下

TOF Tetralogy Of Fallot 法洛四联症

TOF Tet Ralogy Of Fallot (T Rain-Of-Four)
法洛四联症; 紫绀四联症【注释】〔伴有肺动脉狭
窄、高位心室中
隔缺损、主动脉右侧移位及右心室肥大
等四大病变的先天性心畸形。呈现发
绀、眼球结膜充血、呼吸困难、红细胞增
多等症状〕

T Of A Transposition Of Aor Ta 主 动脉的
移位

Tofo Tonsillar Fossa 扁 桃体窝 〔解〕

Togm Tomogram X 射线断层照片

Togr Tomography X 线断层照相法; X
线体层照相法

TOK Tuberculosis Of Kidney 肾结核

Tolec Tonsillectomy 扁桃体切除术

Toli Tonsillitis 扁桃体炎

Toly Tocolysis 安 宫; 保胎; 子宫收缩抑
制

Tonas Toenails 脚趾甲

Toniq Tourniquet 止血带; 压脉器

Toniqs Tourniquets 止血带

Tonr Tonsillar 扁桃体的

Tooc Total Occlusion 全 阻塞

Toos Tor Tuosity 卷曲性(羊毛)

TOP Termination Of Pregnancy 终 止妊
娠; 妊娠终止

Topla Toxoplasma 弓 形体

Topls Toxoplasmosis 弓形体病

Topr Total Protein 总 蛋白; 蛋白质总量

Tor The Operating Room 手术室

TORCH Infections Toxoplasma , Others,
Rubella Virus , Cytomega Lovirus, Herpes
Virus TORCH 感染 〔系胎儿感染最常见
的几种非细菌性病原体〕

TORCHS Toxoplasmosis, Rubella, Cytomegalovirus,
Herpes Simplex , Syphilis
(Infection) 弓 浆虫病、风疹、巨细胞病
毒、单纯疱疹、梅毒(感染)

Torr (Torr) Torricelli 托 【注释】 〔真空单位(压
力)〕

Tort Tortuous 迂曲的; 弯曲的

Tosc Toxicology Screen 毒 理学筛选

Tosts Topical Steroids 局 部类固醇

Tosy Thoracic Outlet Syndrome 胸 部出
口综合征【注释】 〔由左右第一肋骨所包围的胸
廓
出口处的神经、血管遭到压迫而引起颈
部、肩部、上肢持续性或反复发作的疼
痛、麻木的一组病征〕

Toxo Toxoplasmose 弓 浆虫病

Toxy Toxicology 毒理学

TP Thiamphenicol 硫霉素

Tp Thrombopoietin 血小板生成素

TP Total Protein 总 蛋白; 蛋白质总量

TP Treponema Pallid 苍 白密螺旋体;
梅毒螺旋体

Tp T Rophoblastin / Trophoblastine 胎 盘
促性腺激素

TP Tympanoplasty 鼓 室成形术

TPA Tissue Plasminogen Activator 组 织
纤维蛋白溶解酶原活化剂【注释】 〔为血栓病治
疗药, 与标准肝素
疗法和尿激酶疗法一样倍受关注〕

TPA Total Parenteral Alimentation 胃
肠道外全面营养(法)

Tpac Tissue Plasminogen Activator 组织
纤维蛋白溶解酶原活化剂

TPBF Total Pulmonary Blood Flow 总

肺血流量

TPC Thromboplastin Plasma Component
血浆促凝血酶原激酶成分

TPCF T Reponema Pallidum Complement
Fixation Test 梅毒螺旋体补体结合试
验; T PCF 试验(检梅毒)

TOD 543 TPC

Tpd Third Por Tion Of The Duodenum 十
二指肠第三段

TPHA Treponema Pallidum Haemagglutination
(Test) 梅毒螺旋体红细胞凝集
(反应) 【注释】 〔为一种梅毒血清学检查方法。
利用从梅毒螺旋体(T P) 提取的蛋白抗
原建立的被动血凝检测 TP 抗体方法〕

TPIA Treponema Palladium Immune
Adherence Test 梅 毒螺旋体免疫吸附试
验; TPIA 试验【注释】 〔以梅毒螺旋体的死菌为
抗原,
将其与梅毒患者的血清和豚鼠补体相
混合时, 通过抗原、抗体和补体复合物,
可使人的 O 型红细胞发生凝集。 不过,
由于还有 TPHA 等简易方法, 所以现已
不使用〕

TPN Total Parenteral Nutrition 完 全
(胃) 肠外营养; 全静脉营养【注释】 〔由 Dudr Ic
等发明的, 对于所需
的能量均经静脉投与的治疗法。 在家
庭使用的为 HPN〕

Tpo Two-Pillow Or Thopnea 两 枕端坐呼
吸

TPP Thiamine Pyrophosphate 硫 胺素

焦磷酸【注释】〔为活性型维生素 B1，又称羧辅酶、脱羧辅酶或二磷酸硫胺〕

TPQ 2 , 4 , 5- Trihydroxyphenylalanine Quinone 三羟苯丙氨醌【注释】〔首先从牛血清酶中鉴定的含铜的胺氧化酶的氧还活性有机辅助因子，存在于多种植物以及细菌的胺氧化酶中。从完整蛋白质的天冬酰胺酪天冬/谷氨酸共有序列中的酪氨酸残基经翻译后修饰衍生而来〕

Tpr Taper 锥 度

TPR Temperature 温度; 体温

T .P .R . Temperature, Pulse And Respiration 体温、脉搏和呼吸【注释】〔可测定的所谓生命特征的身体状态的三个基本征候〕

TPR Total Peripheral Resistance 总 外周阻力; 总末梢阻力【注释】〔从左心室驱出的血液承受的阻力。可用下式求得。TPR (Dynes/ Sec/ Cm3) = 平均动脉压(Mmhg)/ 心输出量 (1/ 分) × 80〕

TPR Total Pulmonary Resistance 总 肺循环阻力【注释】〔肺在呼吸肌作用下活动时, 必须克服弹性阻力、黏性阻力和慢性阻力, 在此指这些阻力的总和。可通过呼吸过程中的压力气量曲线的解析测定〕

Tprd Tapered 锥 度的; 锥形的; 变断面的

Tprg Tapering 渐 减量(药物) ; 尖端细的

Tpsc Thallium Perfusion Scan 铊 灌注扫
描

TPT Total Pump Time 总泵时间

TQ Tourniquet 止血带; 压脉器

TQM Total Quality Management TQM
质量管理【注释】〔为预防医疗事故, 提高诊疗水
平的管理设想〕

T .R . Takata Reaction 高田氏反应

TR Therapeutic Ratio 治疗比率【注释】 〔用 TD/ T
LD 表示。用于决定采
用放射线疗法治愈病灶的可能性和难
易度〕

Tr Tincture ① 酊; 酊剂② 药酒③ 色泽;
色彩④染料; 颜料⑤气质; 特征

TR Total Resistance 总 电阻; 总阻力

TR Trachea 气 管

TR T Reatment Required For 应…… 要求
治疗

TR Tricuspid Regurgitation 三尖瓣回流

TR Tuberculin Reaction 结核菌素反应

TR Tubular Reabsorption 肾 小管重吸收
(试验)

TR Turnover Rate 更 替速度【注释】 〔在成熟的动
物体内, 构成机体
结构的蛋白质和氨基酸之间处于动态
Tpd 544 TR
平衡, 即合成速度和分解速度处于相对
平衡状态。在此指合成-分解速度〕

TRA Tumor Rejection Antigen 肿瘤排斥
抗原

Trab T Ransversus Abdomen 腹 横肌 〔解〕

Musculus T R Ansversus Abdominis 〔拉〕

Trach Acetylcholine Turnover Rate 乙酰胆碱周转率

Trachcy Tracheoscopy 气管镜检查

Trachl T Racheal 气管的

Trachy Tracheostomy 气管造口术

Tracj T Raction 牵引

Tracjl Tractional 牵引的

Traeso T Racheoesophageal 气管食管的

Trans T Ransverse ①横的② 横切的③ 横肌

Transa Transaminase 氨 基转移酶

余物; …… 剩余的人

TRP T Richo-Rhino-Phalangeal (Syndrome) 毛发鼻指(趾) (综合征) 【注释】 〔特征为头发粗糙、梨状鼻、人中长、上唇薄、近端指(趾) 节间关节丛斜指、短缩圆锥骨端等〕

TRP Tryptophan (Aminoacid) 色 氨酸

TRP Tubular Reabsorption Of Phosphate 肾小管磷酸盐重吸收【注释】 〔用于甲状旁腺机能亢进症的诊断(正常为 80% ～90 %)〕

Trph Trephine 环踞; 用环踞做手术

Trpl Transplant 移植; 移植物; 移植片

Trpla Treatment Plan 治疗计划

Trpld T Ransplanted 移植

Trplj T Ransplantation 移植(术)

Trpos Transposition 转 座子; 变换

Trpr T Ransverse Process 横突〔解〕

Trprs Transverse Processes 横突

Trpz Trendelenburg Position 特伦德伦堡体位〔垂头仰卧体位〕

Trre Tricuspid Regurgitation 三尖瓣回流

Trres T Reatment Resistant 抗治疗的

Trri T Racheal Ring 气管环〔动〕

Trria Thyroid Radioisotope Assay 甲状腺放射性同位素测定

Trsa Transversalis ①横的②横肌

Trse T Ransect 样条; 横切

Trsed Transected 横断的

Trseg Transecting 横断的

Trsej Transection 横切面; 横断

Trsij Transition 移行; 过渡

Trso Troublesome 讨厌的; 易出故障的; 困难的

Trsph Transsphenoidal 经蝶骨的

Trsu T Raction Suture 牵引缝合

Trsus Traction Sutures 牵引缝合

Trte Treatment Team 治疗小组

Trtes Treadmill Test 平板试验

Trtu Tracheotomy Tube 气管切开插管

TRT(V) Turkey Rhinotracheitis (Virus) 火鸡鼻气管炎(病毒)

Trtvs Turkey Rhinot Racheitis Viruses 土耳其鼻气管炎病毒

Trv T Ransverse ①横的②横切的③ 横肌

Trva T Ricuspid Valve 三尖瓣

Tri 546 Trv

Trvag T Ransvaginal 经 阴道的

Trve Traverse 交叉; 横断; 横穿

Trve- T Riple-Vessel 三管腔

Trved T Raversed 横 断的

Trveg Traversing 横 向进刀; 导线测量;
遍历

Trven Transvenous 经静脉

Trvy Transversely 横着; 横切; 横断

Trzo T Ransformation Zone 变 性带

TS Suppressor T Cell 抑制性 T 细胞

TS Teaching Strategies 教授方略【注释】〔医学教
育用语〕

TS Teratology Society 畸形学学会

TS Thrombospondin 血 小板反应蛋白【注释】 〔与
血小板间的黏附反应和血小
板凝集反应有关。已确认也存在于其
他脏器组织及结缔组织中〕

TS Tricuspid Stenosis 三尖瓣狭窄

T&S Type And Screen 血 型判定筛选【注释】 〔通
过比较经过交叉适合试验的
血液量(C) 和实际在输血中使用的血液
量(T), 研究血液的使用率(C/ T 比)
时, 存在有被称为浪费血液使用的现
状。因此, 对于输血实施率限于 30 %
以下, 或平均 2 单位以下的输血手术,
只要确定血型判定不规则抗体阴性, 就
可在有必要输血的情况下, 通过交叉适
合试验, 提供适合血液〕

TSA Tumor-Susceptible Antigen 肿 瘤特
异抗原【注释】〔伴随细胞的癌性变化而出现的

肿瘤抗原中, 仅在其癌细胞中特异存在
的抗原〕

TSB Total Serum Bilirubin 总 血清胆红
素

TSB Total Spinal Block 全脊髓麻醉【注释】 〔在蛛
网膜下腔内注入局部麻醉
药, 导致所有颈部脊髓以下的脊神经及
上位的中枢出现麻醉状态。在高位麻
醉和硬膜外麻醉出错, 麻醉药大量流入
蛛网膜下腔情况下发生。引起呼吸停
止、意识丧失, 但通过人工呼吸, 消除
局部麻醉的效果后, 予后良好〕

TSE Transmissible Spongiform Encephalopathy
传递性海绵状脑病; 传递
性病毒性海绵状脑病

TSEM T Ransmission Scanning Electron
Microscope 透 射扫描电子显微镜

Tsf Suppressive T Cell Factor 抑 制性 T
细胞因子【注释】 〔从抑制性 T 细胞中提取, 它是
由抗原刺激而释放的因子, 具有抑制抗
体产生的作用〕

Tsgf Thrombin-Soaked Gelfoam 浸 有凝
血酶的明胶海绵

TSH Thyroid Stimulating Hormone , Thyrot
Ropin 促 甲状腺激素【注释】 〔一种垂体前叶分
泌的激素〕

TSI Thyroid Stimulating Immunoglobulin
甲状腺刺激免疫球蛋白

TSM Tween Synthetic Medium 吐温合
成培养基

TSP Total Serum Protein 总 血清蛋白质

TSP Tropical Spastic Paraparesis 热带性
痉挛性脊髓麻痹【注释】〔在热带地区很早以前
就知道此
病, 已弄清其发生多半与 HT LV- Ⅰ 有
关, 和 HAM 为同一个疾病。在 1988 年
被 WHO 合在一起命名为 HAM/ TS P〕
TSRBC T Rypsinized Sheep Red Blood Cell
胰蛋白酶处理的绵羊红细胞

TSS Toxic Shock Syndrome 中 毒性休克
综合征

TSST-1 Toxic Shock Syndrome Toxin-1
中毒性休克综合征毒素-1 【注释】〔耐甲氧青霉
素金黄色葡萄球菌
MRSA 性状改变后的产物, 现 TSST-1
产生菌株正在不断增加〕

Tst Testis 睾 丸

TST Thromboplastin Screening Test 凝
血酶原激酶筛选试验【注释】〔测定内因性凝血
激酶生成速度
Trv 547 TST
的检查法〕

TSTA Tumor Specific T Ransplantation
Antigen 肿瘤特异性移植抗原 【注释】 〔在实验性
肿瘤免疫应答中, 出
现移植排斥现象时, 引起这种免疫排斥
反应的肿瘤抗原〕

Tste Treadmill Stress Test 踏车负荷试验

Tsts Testes 睾 丸

TSVR Total Systemic Vascular Resistance
体循环血管总阻力

TT Test Toxoid 测 试类毒素

TT Tetanus Toxoid 破 伤风类毒素

TT Thrombin Time 凝血酶时间

TT Tolerance Test 耐量试验

TT Total Thyroxine 总甲状腺素

TTA Transt Racheal Aspiration 经气管吸引

TTA Tumor Transplantation Antigen 肿
瘤移植抗原【注释】〔来自近交系动物的可移植
肿
瘤, 能够在近交系宿主中出现免疫应答
或肿瘤移植排斥时, 将引起这种反应的
抗原称为 TSTA 或 TATA〕

Ttdm Type Ⅱ Diabetes Mellitus Ⅱ 型糖
尿病

Tte T Ransthoracic Echocardiogram 经 胸
超声心动图

Tter To The Emergency Room 到 急诊室

TTH Thyrotropic Hormone 促 甲状腺激
素

TTI Tension-Time Index 张力-时间系数【注释】
〔为心肌耗氧量的一个指标, 它
是平均收缩压乘以收缩时间所得的数
值〕

TTI Tissue Thromboplastin Inhibitor 组
织凝血激酶抑制剂

TTN Transitory Tachypnea Of The Newborn
新生儿短暂呼吸急促

Ttotc The Tip Of The Catheter 导 管尖端

TTP Thrombotic Thrombocytopenic Purpura
血栓性血小板减少性紫癜【注释】 〔1925 年由
Moschowitz 首次报

道。以神经症状、发热、血小板减少、溶
血性贫血及肾功能障碍为主要特征。
予后不良〕

TTS Tarsal Tunnel Syndrome 跗 管综合
征

TTS Temporary Threshold Shift 暂时性
阈移【注释】〔指受到一定时间连续性音响刺
激的听觉器官, 暂时性地听觉阈值升高
的现象〕

TTS Transdermal Therapeutic System
透皮给药系统【注释】 〔它是按照药物释放有效
面积,
将药物与具有透皮作用的黏贴剂混合,
制成皮肤敷剂进行治疗的方式。最近
对其利用率在增加〕

TTT Thymo Turbidity Test 麝 香草酚混
合试验【注释】〔为一种检查肝功能的血清胶体
反应〕

TTTS Twin To Twin Transfusion Syndrome
孪 生儿输血综合征

Ttu T- Tube T 形管

TTW Transt Racheal Washes Or Washing
经气管冲洗

TTX Tetrodotoxin 河豚鱼毒素【注释】 〔为河豚的
有毒物质, 可引起舌
端、口唇、指尖等的钝麻, 随意肌麻痹,
进而导致延髓中枢的麻痹。在河豚的
卵巢和肝脏中含量很高。可被碱性溶
液破坏〕

TU Toxic Unit 毒素单位

TU Tuberculin Unit 结核菌素单位

Tu Tumor 肿块

Tuad Tubular Adenoma 管状腺瘤

Tuads Tubal Adhesions 输卵管粘连

Tudrs Tubes And Drains 导管与引流

Tufe Tube Feeding 鼻饲(法)

Tufes Tube Feedings 鼻饲

Tuma Tumor Mass 肿块

Tun Tunnel 管

TST 548 Tun

Tunat Turbinate ① 甲介形的② 陀螺状
的③鼻甲(的)

Tund Tunneled 通道; 隧道

Tundl Tuohy Needle 图伊针〔硬膜外腔
持续导管插入用, 前端为直角弯曲的穿刺
针〕

Tuos Tuberosity 粗隆; 结节

Tuov Tubo-Ovarian 输卵管卵巢的

Tuovs Tubes And Ovaries 输卵管与卵巢

Tupg Tubal Pregnancy 输卵管妊娠

TUR Transurethral Resection 经尿道切
除术【注释】〔经尿道的内窥镜操作, 进行膀
胱、前列腺手术的方法。包括 TUR-BT
和 TUR-P 两种方法〕

TURB T Ransurethral Resection Of The
Bladder 经尿道膀胱切除

Turb Turbinate ① 甲介形的②陀螺状的
③鼻甲(的)

Turbc Turbinectomy 鼻甲切除术

Turbs Turbinates 鼻甲

TURP Transurethral Prostatectomy 经
尿道前列腺切除术

TURP T Ransurethral Resection Of The
Prostate 经尿道前列腺切除术

Tuu Transureteroureterostomy (横跨中
线的) 输尿管- 输尿管吻合术

Tuva Tunica Vaginas 鞘膜

TV Tidal Volume 潮气量【注释】〔在平静呼吸过
程中的 1 次呼吸
的气体量〕

TV Tricuspid Valve 三尖瓣

TV Typhus Vaccine 斑疹伤寒疫苗

TVC Timed Vital Capacity 定 时的肺活
量【注释】〔在测定用力呼气的肺活量时,
增加时间因素的测定值〕

Tvc True Vocal Cord 真声带; 声襞

Tvd Triple-Vessel Disease 三管腔病

TVH Total Vaginal Hysterectomy 全 阴
道子宫切除术

TVH Trans-Vaginal Hysterectomy 经 阴
道子宫切除术

TVI Tropical Veterinary Institute
(University Of Liege, Belgium) 热带
兽医学会

TVMA Texas Veterinary Medical Association
得克萨斯兽医医学会

TVMA Thai Veterinary Medical Association
泰国兽医医学会

TVP Thrombose Venous Profundity 深
部静脉血栓形成

TVU Total Volume Urine 全 尿; 24 小时

尿量

TWAR Taiwan Acute Respiratory Disease
台湾急性呼吸系统疾病

TWE Tap Water Enema 自来水灌肠

Twfis Two Fingerbreadths 二指宽

TWG Total Weight Gain 总体重的增加

Twi T-Wave Inversion T 波倒置

Twncs There Were No Complications 没
有并发症

Twne There Was No Evidence 没有迹象

Twntb There Was Noted To Be 有 记录表
明

Twpas Two Packs Of Cigarettes 两包烟

TX Thromboxane 血栓素【注释】〔在血小板中,
由花生四烯酸经
过 PGG2 所生成的生物学活性物质〕

TXA2 Thromboxane A2 血 栓素 A2 【注释】 〔具
有对平滑肌的收缩作用和血
小板的凝集作用, 因此, 对于机体来说
并非有用的内因性物质。 在发生休克
时其含量增加〕

TXB2 Thromboxane B2 血 栓素 B2 【注释】 〔在
血小板破坏时增加, 由尿液
排出〕

Txc Toxic ① (有) 毒的; 毒性的; 中毒的
②毒剂; 毒物

Txcly Toxicology 毒理学

Txco Toxicosis 中毒

Txcy Toxicity 毒 性; 毒力

Txs Therapies 疗法

Tyfe Typhoid Fever 伤寒

Typly Typically 典型地; 作为特色的

TYR Tyrosine (Aminoacid) 酪氨酸

Japanese

略語　日本語の意味　　　スペル

T　　温度、体温　Temperature
胸椎の、胸髄の　　Thoracic
胸部、胸郭　Thorax
原発腫瘍　　Tumor
側頭の　　　Temporal
T 波　T-Wave
分娩予定日　Termin(独)
横　　Transverse

TA　三尖弁閉鎖（症）　Tricuspid Atresia
前脛骨の　　Tibialis Anterior(ラ)
総動脈幹　Truncus Arteriosus
側頭動脈炎　Temporal Arteritis
腸チフス　　Typhus Abdominalis(ラ)
毒素・抗毒素　　Toxin-Antitoxin

T&A　扁桃摘出（術）とアデノイド切除（術）
Tonsillectomy And Adenoidectomy

TAA　胸部大動脈瘤　　Thoracic Aortic
Aneurysma
腫瘍関連抗原　　Tumor Associated
Antigen

Tab　錠剤　Tablet

Tachy　頻脈　Tachycardia

TAE　経カテーテル肝動脈塞栓（術）
Transcatheter Arterial Embolization

TAH　完全人工心臓　　Total Artiflcial Heart
腹式子宮全摘術　　Total Abdominal
Hysterectomy

TAI　肝動脈注入療法　　Transhepatic Arterial Infusion

TAO　閉塞性血栓性血管炎、バージャー病　　Thromboangiitis Obliterans

TAP　三尖弁輪形成（術）　　Tricuspid Annuloplasty

TAR　人工足関節置換術　Total Ankle Replacement

TB　　結核　Tuberkulose(独)

　　　総ビリルビン　　Total Bilirubin

　　　沐浴　Tub Bathing

TBAB 経気管支針吸引生検　　Transbronchial Aspiration Biopsy

Tbc　結核　Tuberculosis(ラ)

T-Bil　総ビリルビン　　Total Bbilirubin

TBL　気管支洗浄　Tracheobronchial Lavage

TBLB 経気管支肺生検　　Transbronchial Lung Biopsy

TBLC 満期出産、出生児　Term Birth, Living Child

TBT　気管気管支内洗浄　Tracheobronchial Toilet

TBV　全血液量　　Total Blood Volume

TBW　体内総水分（両）　Total Body Water

TC　　総コレステロール　Total Cholesterol

　　　テトラサイクリン　Tetracycline

T&C　血液型判定および交差試験　　Type And Cross Match

TCA　三環系抗うつ薬　　Tricyclic Antidepressant

TCI　一過性脳虚血　　Transient Cerebral Ischemia

TCIE　一過性脳虚血発作　Transient Cerebral Ischemic Episode

Tcpaco2　　経皮的動脈血二酸化炭素分圧
　　　　　Transcutaneous Partial Pressure Of Arterial
Carbon Dioxide
Tcpao2　　経皮的動脈血酸素分圧
　　　　　Transcutaneous Partial Pressure Of Arterial
Oxygen
T-CPAP　　気管内挿管持続陽圧呼吸　Tube
Continuous Psitive Airway Pressure
TCS　テトラサイクリン系抗生物質
　　　　Tetracyclines
TDA　血中薬物濃度測定　Therapeutic Drug Assay
Tds　１日３回服用
TEE　経食道エコー心電図　　　Transeophageal
Echocardiogram
Temp　温度、体温　Temperature
TESPA　　　トリエチレンチオホスホラミド（チ
オテパ）
　　　　　Triethylenethiophosphoramide(Thiotepa)
Tetra　四肢麻痺　　Tetraplegia
TF　　経管栄養　　Tube Feeding
TF，T/F　　ファロー四徴（症）　　　Tetralogy
Of Fallot
TFLX　トスフロキサシン　Tosufloxacin
TG　　中性脂肪、トリグリセリド
　　　　Triglyceride
TGA　一過性全健忘　　　Transient Global
Amnesia
　　　　大血管転位症　　　Transposition Of The
Great Arteries
TGV　大血管転位（症）　Transpotion Of Great
Vessel
TH　　視床（内側）出血　Thalamic Hemorrhage

甲状腺ホルモン　　Thyroid Hormone

Th　　胸椎の、胸髄の　　Thorasic

視床　Thalamus

Th(1～12)　　（第 1 ～12）胸椎　Thorasic
Vertebral

THA　終末肝動脈枝　　Terminal Hepatic
Arteriole

人工股関節全置換術　　Total Hip
Arthroplasty

THR　人工股関節全置換術　　Total Hip
Replacement

TI　　三尖弁閉鎖不全（症）　　Tricuspid
Insufficiency

TIA　一過性脳虚血発作　Transient
Ischemic(Cerebral)Attack

TICO 急性冠動脈閉塞の血栓溶解
　　　　　Thrombolysis In Acute Coronary Occlusion

TIE　一過性虚血発作　　Transient Ischemic
Episode

TIG　破傷風免疫グロブリン　　Tetanus Immune
Globulin

TIMI　心筋梗塞の血栓溶解　　Thrombolysis In
Myocardial Infarction

TIN　間質性腎炎　Tubulointerstitial Nephritis

TJR　関節全置換術　　Total Joint Replacement

TKA　膝関節全置換術　　Total Knee Arthroplasty

TKR　人工膝関節置換術　Total Knee Replacement

TL　　側頭葉　Temporal Lobe

TLC　全肺気量　Total Lung Capasity

TLV　全肺容量　Total Lung Volume

TM　腫瘍マーカー　　Tumor Merker

Tmax　最高血中濃度到達時間　　Time Of
Maximum Concentration

TN　　三叉神経痛、三叉神経　　Trigeminal
Neuralgia, Trigeminal Nerve

TNG　トリニトログリセリン　　Trinitroglycerin

TNM　TNM（腫瘍・リンパ節転移・遠隔転移）

分類　Tumor, Node, Metastasis(Classification)

TNT　トロポニン TTroponin T

TOB　トブラマイシン　　Tobramycin

TOF　ファロー四徴（症）　　Tetralogy Of
Fallot

Tomo, TomoX 線断層撮影（法）
　　　　Tomography

TOP　妊娠の終結、妊娠中絶　　Termination Of
Pregnancy

TOPV 経口ポリオワクチン　　Trivalent Oral
Poliovirus Vaccine

Torr, Torr　トール（圧力の単位）　　Torricelli

TP　　総蛋白　　Total Protein
　　　タキソール、シスプラチンの併用化学療法
　　　Taxol, Cisplatin(CDDP)

Tp　　温度、体温　Temperature

TPA　完全経静脈栄養　　Total Parenteral
Alimetation

TPH, TPHA 完全経静脈栄養　　Total Parenteral
Hyperalimentation

TPHA 梅毒トレポネーマ赤血球凝集試験
　　　Treponema Pallidum Hemagglutination(Test)

TPI　梅毒トレポネーマ運動抑制試験
　　　Treponema Immobilization(Test)

TPIA　梅毒トレポネーマ免疫付着試験
　　　Treponema Immune Adherence(Test)

TPN　完全静脈栄養法　　Total Parenteral
Nutririon

TPP　血小板減少性紫斑病
　　　　Thrombocytopenic Purpura

TPR　全肺血管抵抗　　Total Pulmonary
Resistance

　　　全末梢血管抵抗　　Total Peripheral
Vascular Resistance

　　　体温、脈拍、呼吸　Temperature-Pulse-
Respiration

TPV　終末門脈枝　Terminal Portal Venule

　　　全血漿量　　Total Plasma Volume

TPVR 全肺血管抵抗　　Total Pulmonary
Vascular Resistance

TR　　三尖弁逆流（症）　Tricuspid Regurgitation

　　　ツベルクリン反応　Tuberculin Reaction

　　　トラコーマ　Trachoma

Tr　　気管　Trachea

　　　治療、処置　Treatment

Tr　　牽引　Traction

Transpl　　移植する、移植　　Transplant,
Transplantation

TRM　トリコマイシン　　Trichomycin

TS　　三尖弁狭窄（症）　Tricuspid Stenosis

TSB　全脊（椎）麻（酔）（法）　　Total
Spinal Block

TSI　　三尖弁狭窄兼閉鎖不全症　Tricuspid
Stenoinsufficiency

TSPR 全末梢（血管）抵抗　　Total Systemic
Pripheral Resistance

TSR　三尖弁狭窄兼閉鎖不全症　Tricuspid
Stenosis And Regurgitation

TT　　トロンビン時間　　Thrombin Time

　　　トロンボテスト　　Thrombo Test

TTA　経気管吸引　Transtracheal Aspiration

TTN(B)　　新生児一過性頻呼吸　　Transient Tachypnea Of Newborn

TTP　血栓性血小板減少性紫斑病

　　　Thrombotic Thrombocytopenic Purpura

TTTS 双胎（胎児）児間輸血症候群　Twin-To-Twin Transfusion Syndrome

TTX　テトロドトキシン　Retrodotoxin

TUR　経尿道的切除（術）　　Transurethral Resection

Turbn 経尿道的膀胱頸部切除（術）

　　　Transurethral Resection Of Bladder Neck

Turbt,　TUR-Bt　　経尿道的膀胱腫瘍切除（術）

　　　Transurethral Resecsion Of Bladder Tumor

Turcap 経尿道的前立腺癌切除（術）

　　　Transurethral Resecsion Of Carcinoma Of Prostate

TURP 経尿道的前立腺切除（術）

　　　Transurethral Resecsion Of Prostate

TUV　全（24 時間）尿量　Total Urine Volume

TV　　1 回換気量　　Tidal Volume

　　　三尖弁　　　　Tricuspid Valve

Tv　　胸椎　Thoracic Vertebrae

TVD　三枝病変　　Triple Vessel Disease

TVH　膣式子宮全摘（術）　　Total Vaginal Hysterectomy

TVP　三尖弁形成（術）　Tricuspid Valvuloplasty

TVR　三尖弁置換術　　Tricuspid Valve Replacement

Tx　　治療　Treatment

U
French

UGD Ulcère Gastroduodénal
UP Unité Plaquettaire

English

UAU Uterine Activity Unit

UB Ultimobranchial Body; Unna Boot; Upper
Back; Urinary Bladder

UB 82 Universal Billing Document [1982]

UBA Undenaturated Bacterial Antigen;
Ureidoisobutyric
Acid

UBB Ubiquitin B

UBBC Unsaturated Vitamin B12 Binding Capacity

UBC Ubiquitin C; University Of British Columbia

UBE Ubiquitin-Activating Enzyme

UBF Uterine Blood Flow

UBG, Ubg Urobilinogen

UBI Ultraviolet Blood Irradiation

UBL Undifferentiated B-Cell Lymphoma

UBM Ultrasound Backscatter Microscopy;
Ultrasound Biomicroscopy

UBN Urobilin

UBO Unidentified Bright Object

UBP Ureteral Back Pressure

UBPS Ultrasound Bone Profile Score

UBS Unidentified Bright Signal

UBT Urea Breath Test

UBW Usual Body Weight

UC Ulcerative Colitis; Ultracentrifugal; Umbilical
Cord; Unchanged; Unclassifiable;
Unconscious; Undifferentiated Carcinoma;
Undifferentiated
Cells; Unit Clerk; Unsatisfactory
Condition; Untreated Cells; Urea Clearance;
Urethral Catheterization; Urinary Catheter;
Urinary Catheterization; Urine Concentrate;

Urine Culture; Usual Care; Uterine Contractions

U&C Urethral And Cervical; Usual And Customary

UCA Ultrasound Contrast Agent

UCAID University Corporation For Advanced
Internet Development

UCARE, U-CARE Unexplained Cardiac Arrest
Registry Of Europe

UCB Unconjugated Bilirubin

UCBC Umbilical Cord Blood Culture

UCBT Umbilical Cord Blood Transplantation

UCC Uniform Code Council

UCD Urine Collection Device; User-Centered
Design; Usual Childhood Diseases

UCDS Uniform Clinical Dataset

UCE Urea Cycle Enzymopathy

UCG Ultrasonic Cardiography; Urinary Chorionic
Gonadotropin

UCHD Usual Childhood Diseases

UCI Unusual Childhood Illness; Urethral
Catheter In; Urinary Catheter In

UCL Ulnar Collateral Ligament; Upper Collateral
Ligament; Upper Confidence Limit; Upper
Control Limit; Urea Clearance

UCLP Unilateral Cleft Of Lip And Palate

UCO Ultrasonic Cardiac Output; Urethral
Catheter Out; Urinary Catheter Out

UA Absorption Unsharpness; Ultraaudible;
Ultrasonic Arteriography; Umbilical Artery;
Unauthorized Absence; Unicystic Ameloblastoma;
Unit Of Analysis; Unstable Angina; Upper
Airways; Upper Arm; Uric Acid; Uridylic Acid;
Urinalysis; Urinary Aldosterone; Uronic Acid;
Uterine Activity; Uterine Aspiration

U/A Uric Acid; Urinalysis

Ua Urinalysis

UAC Umbilical Artery Catheter; Unusualappearing
Child; Uric Acid
UA/C Uric Acid/Creatinine Ratio
UAE Unilateral Absence Of Excretion; Urine
Albumin Excretion; Uterine Artery Embolization
UAEM University Association For Emergency
Medicine
UAGA Uniform Anatomical Gift Act
UAI Uterine Activity Interval
UAI-C Unprotected Anal Intercourse With
Casual Partners
UAL Ultrasound-Assisted Lipoplasty; Ultrasound-
Assisted Liposuction
U-AMY Urinary Amylase
UAN Uric Acid Nitrogen
UAO Upper Airway Obstruction
UAP Unlicensed Assistive Personnel; Unstable
Angina Pectoris; Urinary Acid Phosphatase;
Urinary Alkaline Phosphatase
UAPA Unilateral Absence Of Pulmonary
Artery
UAR Upper Airway Resistance; Uric Acid Riboside
UAS Upper Abdomen Surgery; Upstream

Activating Sequence; Upstream Activation Site

German
UA - Unterarm
US - Unterschenkel
USGS - Unterschenkelgipsschiene

Italian
U
Uranio
Utiunità Terapia Intensiva

Russian

U/A
Urinalysis
Анализ Мочи
UGI
Upper Gastrointestinal
Верхние Отделы Желудочно-Кишечного Тракта
URAC
Uric Acid
Мочевая Кислота
URI
Upper Respiratory Tract Infection
Инфекция Верхних Дыхательный Путей
USP
United States Pharmacopeia
Фармакопея Соединных Штатов Америки
UTI
Urinary Tract Infection
Мочевая Инфекция
UV
Ultraviolet
Ультрафиолет

Chinese

U

UA Umbilical Artery 脐动脉

UA Urinalysis 尿液分析

U/ A Urine Analysis 尿液分析

Uac Uric Acid 尿酸

Uaco Using A Combination Of 联合使用

......

UAF User Authorize File 用户授权文件

UAL Urinary Albumin 尿白蛋白

Uamo Using A Mixture Of 使用……的混合物

UAN Uric Acid Nit Rogen 尿酸氮

Uap Unstable Angina Pectoris 不稳定型心绞痛

Uax Urinalysis 尿液分析

UB Urine Bilirubin 尿胆红素

Ubc Using Bipolar Cautery 使用双极烧灼术

UBF Uterine Blood Flow 子宫血流量

UBW Usual Body Weight 平时体重

UC Ulcerative Colitis 溃疡性结肠炎

UC Urinary Catheter 导尿管

UCA Ultracentrifugal Analysis 超离心分析

UCD University College Dublin 都柏林大学院

UCG Ultrasonic (Ult Rasound) Cardiogra -
Phy(-M) 心脏超声波检查法(心超声波

图)【注释】〔利用超声波法记录心脏壁和瓣膜动态的检查法〕

UCG Urethrocystography 尿 道膀胱 X 射线照相术

UCL Upper Control Limit 上 限界; 控制上限

UCL Urea Clearance 尿 素廓清率; 尿素清除率

Ucr Urine Creatinine 尿 肌酐

UCS Universal Character Set 通 用字符集

UD Ulcerative Dermatosis 溃 疡性皮肤病

UD Uterine Delivery 子宫分娩

UDCA Ursodeoxycholic Acid 熊 脱氧胆酸【注释】〔为一种利胆药〕

UDP Uridine Diphosphate 尿苷二磷酸

UDPG Uridine Diphosphate Glucuronic
Acid 尿 (嘧啶核) 苷二磷酸葡糖醛酸

UE Ulcerative Enteritis 溃疡肠炎

UE Ult Rasonic Endoscope 超声波内窥镜【注释】
〔在纤维镜的前端装上超声探
头, 用超声波照射胃等体腔, 观察周围
脏器〕

Ue Upper Ext Remity 上肢

Uec Using Electrocautery 使用电烙术

UEP United Egg Producers 蛋类联合生
产商

UES Upper Esophageal Sphincter 上部
食道括约部【注释】〔位于食道上端环状咽头肌
的下
方约 3cm 处, 为横纹肌, 静止时处于关
闭状态〕

Ues Upper Extremities 上肢

UEVH Union Of European Veterinary
Hygienists 欧洲兽医卫生工作者联合会

UEVP Union Of European Veterinary
Practitioners 欧洲兽医从业者联合会

UFAW Universities Federation For Animal
Welfare 动物保护大学联盟

Ufc Under Fluoroscopic Cont Rol 荧光镜
下控制

Ufg Under Fluoroscopic Guidance 荧光
镜下指导

UFM Uroflowmetry 尿流测量

UG Urethrogram 尿道造影照片

UG Urethrography 尿 道造影术

UG Urogenital 泌 尿生殖的

U .G .D .P . University Group Diabetes
Program 大 学组糖尿病大纲

U-Gen Urobilinogen 尿 胆素原

UG(I)B Upper Gast Rointestinal Bleeding
上消化道出血

Ugi(S) Upper Gast Rointestinal Series 上
消化道系列(摄影)

UGI(T) Upper Gastrointestinal (T Ract)
上胃肠道

UGT Urogenital Tract 尿 生殖道

UH Umbilical Hernia 脐 疝

UHF Ult Ra-High Frequency 特高频

Uhr Umbilical Hernia Repair 脐 疝修补术

UI Unitéinternationale 国际联合会

UIBC Unsaturated Iron-Binding Capacity
不饱和铁结合力【注释】 〔总铁结合力(TIBC) 和
血清铁之
间的差〕

U .I .E . International Union For Health
Education 国 际卫生教育联合会

UIP Undegraded Intake Protein 未降解
摄入蛋白

U .I .P .P .A . International Union Of
Pure And Applied Physics 国 际理论物
理学与应用物理学联合会

U .I .S .B . International Union Of Biological
Science 国 际生物科学联合会

U .I .S .N . International Union Of Nut
Ritional Science 国际营养科学联合会

UK Urokinase 尿激酶【注释】〔为一种血栓溶解药〕

UKA Unicompartmental Knee Ar Throplasty
单 侧人工膝关节置换术【注释】〔由于以往的全
膝关节置换 TKR
不能让日本人以传统的卷膝正坐坐姿
就坐, 因此, 开发了仅置换膝内侧面的
人工关节〕

UKASTA United Kingdom Agricultural
Supply Trade Association 英 国农业供
应贸易联合会

UKERF University Of Kentucky Equine
Research Foundation 肯 塔基州马研究
基金会大学

UKFOMPO UK Federation Of Milk
Producing Organizations 英 国牛奶业
制造协会

UKROFS United Kingdom Register Of
Organic Food Standards 英 国有机食
品标准注册

UKWCT UK Wolf Conservation Trust
英国野生狼保护协会

UL Upper Limit 上 限

UL Upper Lobe 上部凸角

Ulan Under Local Anesthesia 局部麻醉下

Ular Ulnar Artery 尺 动脉〔解〕

Ulas Ulnar Aspect 尺骨外观

Ulcg Ulcerating 溃烂

Ulcj Ulceration ① 溃烂; 溃疡形成② 腐
败

Ulcjs Ulcerations 溃疡

Ulco Ulcerative Colitis 溃 疡性结肠炎

Ulcv Ulcerative ① 溃疡的; 溃疡性的②
腐败的

Ulde Ulnar Deviation 尺 骨偏斜

Uldse Ulcer Disease 溃 疡病

Ules Upper And Lower Ext Remities 上下
肢

Ulfi Ultrafiltration 超 滤法

Uln Ulnar 尺 骨的; 尺侧的

ULN Upper Limit Of Normal 正 常植上
UFA 552 ULN
限

Ulne Ulnar Nerve 尺神经〔解〕

ULPE Upper Lobe Pulmonary Edema 肺
上叶水肿

Ulrad Ulcerated 成 为溃疡的; 形成溃疡
的

ULS Ultrasonic Laparoscope 超 声波腹腔
镜【注释】〔通过在腹腔镜的前端安装 5 ～
10 兆赫兹的超声波振动器, 由此获得
腹腔脏器断层图像的仪器〕

ULSI Ultra-Large Scale Integration 超 大
规模

ULV Ult Ra- Low Volume 超 低容量

Um Umbilicus 脐

Umco Umbilical Cord 脐 带

Umhe Umbilical Hernia 脐疝

Umin Umbilical Incision 脐带切开

Uml Umbilical ① 脐的; 脐带的② 近脐
的; 近脐带的③中心的; 中央的

UMLS Unified Medical Language System
综合型医学用语系统【注释】〔电子化了的各种
情报档案, 例
如对于医学文献、临床记录、症状数据、
常识等的各种情报源, 能够随意地进行
下载的医学用语系统〕

UMN Upper Motor Neuron (S) 上 运动
神经元【注释】〔在运动神经元当中, 支配头颈
部、下肢等的体上部肌肉的神经元〕

UMP Uridine Monophosphate 尿 甙一
磷酸盐

Umta Umbilical Tape 脐型

UN Ulnar Nerve 尺神经〔解〕

UN Urea Nitrogen 尿素氮

Unan Unstable Angina 不 稳定型心绞痛

Unane Under Anesthesia 麻 醉下

Unas Unassociated 未 缔合的; 无缔合性
的

Unbos Unna Boots 乌 那糊靴〔静脉曲张
性溃疡敷料〕

Unci Uncircumcised 未 受割礼的; 非犹
太人的; 异邦人的

Undi Undifferentiated 分 化不良型的;
未分化的; 无差别的

UNEP United Nations Environment
Program 联合国环境计划

Unfe Undesired Fertility 不 愿生育

UNFPA United Nations Fund For Population
Activities 联 合国人口基金会

Unga Unsteady Gait 步 态不稳

Unlyg Underlying 垫 底焊; 下伏的; 在
下面的

Unma Underlying Malignancy 潜 在恶性
病变

Unmig Undermining 底 部冲刷; 潜挖

Unorg Unorganized 无 结构的; 无器官
的; 无条理的

UNOS United Network Of Organ Sharing
Score 器官共享联合记分网【注释】〔它是美国为
了决定肝脏移植手
术受体的优先顺序所进行的严重度分
类记分方法。根据全身状态, 分Ⅰ～Ⅴ
级, 严重度依次增加, 由此来确定优先
者。Ⅰ 度为可通勤或上学者, Ⅴ 为在
ICU 护理下需要人工呼吸者〕

Unpre Unpredictable 不可预见的; 不能
预料的; 无法预言的

Unte Undescended Testicle 隐 睾

Untes Undescended Testicles 隐睾

UO Urinary Output 尿排出量

U/ O Urine Output 尿 量

Uol Utero-Ovarian Ligament 子 宫卵巢韧
带; 子宫卵巢索

Uols Utero-Ovarian Ligaments 子 宫卵巢
韧带

Uoq Upper-Outer Quadrant 外上象限

UP Ureteropelvic 输 尿管肾盂的

U/ P Urine/ Plasma Ratio 尿 液/ 血浆比

U/ P Urine-To-Plasma Ratio 尿血浆比

UP Uroporphyrin 尿卟啉

Uln 553 UP

Upa Urokinase Plasminogen Activator 尿激酶型纤维蛋白溶解酶原活化剂【注释】〔对于纤维蛋白溶解酶原具有作用并使其转化为具有活性的血浆蛋白溶解酶的一种激活剂。临床上常用作血栓溶解剂。这个物质由于能够溶解细胞外基质, 与癌细胞的浸润和转移密切相关而倍受关注〕

Upe Urine Protein Electrophoresis 尿 蛋白电泳

Upeny Upper Endoscopy 上 内窥镜检查

Upenys Upper Endoscopies 上 内窥镜检查

UPI Uteroplacental Insufficiency 子 宫胎盘机能不全【注释】〔指胎盘的气体交换和营养供应能力下降为原因的胎儿呼吸营养障碍〕

UP Junction Ureteropelvic Junction 输尿管肾盂连接

Uplo Upper Lobe 上 部凸角

UPP Urethral Pressure Profile 尿 道内压曲线【注释】〔将带有侧孔的导尿管插入膀胱内, 按照一定的速度边向其内注入水 (或 CO_2), 边将导尿管向尿道外口牵引, 在这个过程中连续记录的尿道各部位内压的曲线〕

UPPP Uvulopalatopharyngo Plasty 软腭咽形成术【注释】〔对造成打呼噜、睡眠呼吸暂停

综合征的咽部多余黏膜组织进行切除的手术方法〕

UPS Uninterrupted Power Supply 不间断电源

Upsto Upset Stomach 胃部不适

UR Upper Respiratory 上呼吸道的

UR Utilization Review 医疗费内容审查【注释】〔做为医疗费用支付方的企业或保险公司所作的各种医疗内容的审查〕

Urbi Urobilinogen 尿胆素原

Urbl Urinary Bladder 膀胱〔解〕

Urca Urethral Catheter 输尿管导管

Urcal Urticarial 荨麻疹的

Urcar Ur Ticaria 荨麻疹

Urcas Urethral Catheters 输尿管导管

Urce Ureterocele 输尿管疝

Urcl Urology Clinic 泌尿科门诊部

Urco Urine Collection 尿液收集

Urcu(S) Urine Culture(S) 尿培养

Urcut Urethrocutaneous 尿道皮肤的

U .R .D . Unspecific Respiratory Diseases 非特异性呼吸道疾病

Urdi Urinary Diversion 尿流改道

Ure Ureter 输尿管

Uregm Ureterogram 输尿管造影片

Ur(E)L Urethral 输尿管的

Urels Urine Elect Rolytes 尿电泳

Urfr Urinary Frequency 尿频

Urgr Urethrogram 尿道造影照片

Urhe Urinary Hesitancy 排尿犹豫

Uril Ureteroileal 输尿管回肠的

Urin Urinary Incontinence 尿失禁

URI(S) Upper Respiratory Infection 上
呼吸道感染【注释】〔所谓的感冒综合征。扁桃
体
炎、咽炎、喉炎等鼻咽喉的感染症〕

Urli Urolithiasis 尿 石形成; 尿石病

Urly Ureterolysis 输 尿管破裂; 输尿管麻
痹; 输尿管松解术

Urme Urethral Meatus 尿道

Urnaj Urination 排尿

Urny Urinary ①泌尿的; 泌尿器的②尿
的; 含尿的③尿池

Uro Urology 泌尿外科学

Uroc Urologic 泌 尿学的

UROD Uroporphyrinogen Decarboxylase
尿卟啉原脱羧酶

Urok Urokinase 尿激酶; 蛋白分解酶

Urol Urology 泌尿学

Uror Urethral Orifice 输尿管口

Urors Urethral Orifices 输 尿管口

Upa 554 Uro

Uros Urosepsis 尿 脓毒症(病)

Urosc Uroseptic 尿 脓毒病的; 尿脓毒症
的

Urosm Urine Osmolality 尿 渗透压

Urosy Urostomy 尿 道再生术; 泌尿道造
口术

Urot Urologist 泌 尿科医师; 泌尿学家

Urots Urologists 泌尿科学家; 泌尿科医

师

Urou Urine Output 尿量

URR Urea Reduction Rate 尿素减少率

Urre Urinary Retention 尿潴留

Urscy Urethroscopy 尿道镜检查术

Urst Urethral St Ricture 尿 道狭窄

Urste Urethral Stent 尿 道支架

Urstr Urinary Stream 尿线

Ursv Urology Service 泌尿科

Ursys Urinary Symptoms 泌尿症状

URT Upper Respiratory Tract 上 呼吸道

Urth Urethra 尿道

Urthe Urothelium 膀胱上皮

Urthl Urethral 尿道的

Urthp Urethropexy 尿道固定术

Urthpl Urethroplasty 尿 道成形术

Urthv Urethrovesical 尿 道膀胱的

Urtr Urinary T Ract 泌尿道

Urur Urinary Urgency 尿 急

Urves Ureterovesical 输尿管膀胱的

Ury Urology 泌尿外科学

US Ult Rasound 超 声(波)

U/ S Ultrasound , Ult Rasonogram, Ultra -
Sonography 超声波, 超声波图, 超声波
检查法

USAHA United States Animal Health
Association 联合国动物健康联合会

USDA United States Depar Tment Of Agriculture
美国农业部

Usf Usual Sterile Fashion 正常消毒方式

USFWS United States Fish And Wildlife

Service 美国鱼类与野生动物管理局

USG Ultrasonography 超声波扫描术;
超声波检查(法)

Usgu Ultrasound Guidance 超声引导

Usi(N) Urinary St Ress Incontinence 腹
部压迫性尿失禁; 应激性失禁

Usl(I) Uterosacral Ligament 子宫韧带

Usls Uterosacral Ligaments 子宫韧带

Usm Usual Sterile Manner 正常消毒方
式

USMEF United States Meat Expor T
Federation 美国肉类出口联盟

USMLE United States Medical Licensing
Examination 美国医学资格审查
(委员会)【注释】〔为美国医学教育相关的一个
委
员会, 现已将原来 NBME 和 FSMB 纳
入到同一的 USMLE 组织(1992 年以
后)〕

USOGH Usual State Of Good Health 正
常健康状态

U .S .P . United States Pharmacopeia
美国药典

USPCA Ulster Society For The Prevention
Of Cruelty To Animals 阿尔斯特反
虐待动物协会

USPNF United States Pharmacopeia
National Formulary 美国国家药典药
品集

USRDA United States Recommended
Daily Allowance (S) 美国推荐每日津贴

UST Ultrasound Tomography 超声层析成像法

USW Ult Rashort Wave 超 短波

USW Ult Rasonic Wave 超声波

UT Urinary Tract 泌尿道

Ut Uterus 子宫

Utar Uterine Artery 子 宫动脉〔解〕

Utars Uterine Arteries 子宫动脉

Utbl Uterine Bleeding 子 宫出血

Uro 555 Utb

Utca Uterine Cavity 子宫腔

Utco Under The Care Of 在 …… 照管下; 在……管理下

Utcos Uterine Contractions 子 宫收缩

Utfi Uterine Fibroid 子宫纤维瘤

Utfis Uterine Fibroids 子 宫纤维瘤

Utfu Uterine Fundus 子 宫底

Utin Uterine Incision 子宫切开

UTI(X) Urinary T Ract Infection 尿路感染症【注释】〔指一般由非特异性细菌所引发的尿路的感染性炎症。由结核菌、真菌、毛滴虫等及原虫感染而引发的特异性尿路感染症, 和一般细菌性感染相区别〕

UTJ Utero-Tubal Junction 子 宫输卵管接合部

Utle Uterine Leiomyosarcoma 子 宫平滑肌瘤

Utma Uterine Manipulation 子宫推拿

Utn Uterine ①同母异父的②子宫的

Utos Uterus, Tubes And Ovaries 子宫、输
卵管和卵巢

UTP Uridine Triphosphate 尿（嘧啶核)
苷三磷酸

UTP Uridylt Ransferase Phosphate 磷酸
尿苷酰转移酶

Utpo Uterine Polyp 子宫息肉

Utpos Uterine Polyps 子宫息肉

Utpr Uterine Prolapse 子宫脱垂

Utsa Uterosacral 子宫荐骨的

Utsc Urine Toxicology Screen 尿液毒理
学筛选

Utse Uterine Segment 子宫分段

Uttu Uterine Tumor 子宫肿瘤

Utves Uterine Vessels 子宫血管

Utwa Uterine Wall 子宫壁

UU Urine Urobilinogen 尿中尿胆原

UUN Urine Urea Nit Rogen 尿中尿素氮

UV Ulcus Vent Riculi 胃溃疡

UV Umbilical Vein 脐静脉

UV Urine Volume 尿容量

UVI Ultraviolet Irradiation 紫外线照射

UVJ Ureterovesical Junction 输尿管膀
胱连接

Uvj Uterovesical Junction 膀胱子宫结合
部

Uvp Uterovesical Peritoneum 膀胱子宫
腹膜

UVR Ult Raviolet Radiation 紫外(线)辐
射

UV(R) Ultraviolet (Radiation) 紫外线【注释】
〔为 10 ～ 400nm 的电磁波, 以
310nm 为界, 波长比它短时, 称为近紫
外线, 290～ 310nm 之间者, 称为 Dorno
线。250 ～320nm 之间呈现灭菌作用〕

Japanese

U   単位   Unit
       尿素   Urea
UA   臍動脈   Umbilical Artery
       尿酸   Uric Acid
UA(P) 不安定狭心症   Unstable
Abgina(Pectoris)
U/A   検尿   Urinalysis
UAC   臍動脈カテーテル   Umbilical Artery
Catheter
UB   尿潜血   Uric Blood
       膀胱   Urinary Bladder
UBF   子宮血流   Uterine Blood Flow
UC   潰瘍性大腸炎   Ulcerative Colitis
       子宮収縮   Uterine Contraction
       未分化癌   Undifferentiated Carcinoma
UCG   心エコー法   Ultrasound Cardiography
       尿道膀胱造影（法）
       Urethrocystography
Ucpmax   最高尿道閉鎖圧   Maxmum
Urethral Closure Pressure

UCPP 尿道閉鎖圧曲線　　Urethral Closure
Pressure Profile
UCR　無条件反射　Unconditioned Reflex
UCS　無条件刺激　Unconditioned Stimulus
UD　十二指腸潰瘍　　Ulcus Duodeni（ラ）

UDT　停留睾丸　　Undescended Testicle
U/E　上肢　Upper Extremity
UFA　遊離脂肪酸　Unesterified Fatty Acid
UFTMユーエフティー、マイトマイシンＣの併
用化学療法　UFT，Mitomycin C
UG　尿道造影（法）　　Urethrography
UGI（S）　上部消化管（撮影）　　Upper
Gastrointestinal (Series)
UHDF超短時間血液透析濾過（法）　　Ultrashort
Hemodiafiltration
UHL　片側性肺門リンパ節腫大　Unilateral Hilar
Lymphnode Enlargement
UI　潰瘍係数　Ulcer Index
UIP　通常型間室性肺炎　Usual Interstitial
Pneumonia
UK　ウロキナーゼ　　Urokinase
Ul　潰瘍　Ulcer
ULBW　　極端な低出生体重児　　Ultra Low
Birth Weight
UN　尺骨神経　Ulnar Nerve
UO　尿量　Urinary Output
UP　尿蛋白　Urinal Protein
UPI　子宮胎盤機能不全　Uteroplacental
Insufficiency
UPJ　腎盂尿管移行部　Uretero Pelvic Junction

UPPP 口蓋垂軟口蓋咽頭形成（術）
Uvulopalatopharyngoplasty

URI 上気道感染（症） Upper Respiratory
Infection

Uro 泌尿器科 Urology

US 下腿 Unterschenkel（独）
超音波 Ultrasound
尿糖 Urinal Sugar

USB 不安定膀胱 Unstable Bladder

USL 超音波砕石術 Uitrasonic Lithotripsy

USN 超音波ネブライザー Ultrasonic
Nebulizer

UT 尿路 Urinary Tract

UTCA、Utca 子宮癌 Cancer Ob Uterus

UTI 尿路感染（症） Urinary Tract Infection

UV 胃潰瘍 Ulcus Ventriculi（ラ）
臍静脈 Umbilical Vein
紫外線 Ultraviolet Light, Ultraviolet
Ray
尿量 Urine Volume

V
French

VAT
Vaccin Anti-Tétanique
VBEH
Voies Biliaires Extra-Hépatiques
VBIH

Voies Biliaires Intra-Hépatiques
VCI
Veine Cave Inférieure
VCS
Veine Cave Supérieure
VIH
Virus De L'immundéficience Humaine
VPN
Valeur Prédictive Négative
VPP
Valeur Prédictive Positive
VS
Vitesse De Sédimentation
VSH
Veines Sus-Hépatiques
VZV
Varicella-Zoster Virus (Virus Varicelle-Zona)

English

V0 No Evidence Of Venous [Tumor] Invasion

V0.5 Midpoint Voltage

V1 Primary Visual Area; Venous [Tumor] Invasion Assessed

V1 Mean Flow Velocity

V1 To V6 Ventral 1 To Ventral 6 [Chest Leads In ECG]

V Rate Of Reaction Catalyzed By An Enzyme; Specific Volume; Valve; Vein; Velocity; Venous; Ventricular; Versus; Very; Virus; Vision; Volt; Volume

VA Alveolar Ventilation; Vacuum Aspiration; Valproic Acid; Vasodilator Agent; Ventricular Aneurysm; Ventricular Arrhythmia; Ventriculoatrial; Ventroanterior; Veterans Administration; Veterans Affairs; Vincristine, Adriamycin; Viral Antigen; Visual Acuity; Visual Aid; Visual Axis; Volt-Ampere; Volume Average

VA Alveolar Ventilation

V/A Volt/Ampere

V-A Venoarterial

Va Activated Factor V

Va Alveolar Ventilation

Va Volt-Ampere

VAAE Vaccine-Associated Adverse Events

VAB Vincristine, Actinomycin D, And Bleomycin; Violent Antisocial Behavior

VAB-6 Vincristine, Actinomycin, Bleomycin, Cisplatin, Cytoxan

VABP Venoarterial Bypass Pumping; Ventilator-

Associated Bacterial Pneumonia
VABS Vineland Adaptive Behavior Scales
VAC Vacuum-Assisted Closure; Ventriculoatrial
Conduction; Vincristine, Doxorubicin,
And Cyclophosphamide; Virus Capsid Antigen
Vac Vacuum
VACA Valvuloplasty And Angioplasty Of
Congenital Anomalies [Registry]
Vacc Visual Acuity With Correction
Vacc Vaccination
VACO Veterans Affairs Central Office
VACS Veterans Administration Cooperative
Study
VACSDM Veterans Affairs Cooperative
Study On Glycemic Control And Complications
In Non-Insulin Dependent Diabetes
Mellitus
VACT Veterans Administration Cooperative
Trial
VACTERL Vertebral Abnormalities, Anal
Atresia, Cardiac Abnormalities, Tracheoesophageal
Fistula And/Or Esophageal Atresia, Renal
Agenesis And Dysplasia, And Limb Defects
[Association]
VACV Vaccinia Virus
VAD Venous Access Device; Ventricular
Assist Device; Vinblastine And Dexamethasone;
Virus-Adjusting Diluent; Vitamin A Deficiency
Vad Vascular Dementia
VADD Vitamin A Deficiency Disorder
VAE Venous Air Emboli; Vertical Attachment
Energy
VA-ECMO Venoarterial Extracorporeal Membrane
Oxygenation
VAEG Visual And Auditory Environment

Generator
VAERS Vaccine Adverse Events Reporting
System
VAEV Vearoy Virus
VAF Viral-Free Antigen
VAFC Vacuum-Assisted Fascial Closure
VAG Vibroarthrography
Vag Vagina, Vaginal, Vaginitis
VAG HYST Vaginal Hysterectomy
VAH Vertebral Ankylosing Hyperostosis;
Veterans Affairs Hospital; Virilizing Adrenal
Hyperplasia
VA-HIT Veterans Affairs High-Density Lipoprotein
Intervention Trial
VAHS Virus-Associated Hemophagocytic
Syndrome
VAIN Vaginal Intraepithelial Neoplasm
Vak Atrial Volume Constant
VAL Valproate
Val Valine
Val Valine; Valve
VALE Visual Acuity, Left Eye
Val-Heft Valsartan-Heart Failure Trial
VALIANT Valsartan In Acute Myocardial
Infarction [Study]
VALID Velocity Assessment For Lesions Of
Intermediate Severity [Trial]
VALID II Velocity Assessment For Lesions
Of Indeterminate Severity [Trial]
VASP Vasodilator-Stimulated Phosphoprotein
VASPNAF Veterans Administration Stroke
Prevention In Nonrheumatic Atrial Fibrillation
[Study]
VAS RAD Vascular Radiology
VAST Visual Analysis Systems Technology

VAST/STT Visual Analysis Systems Technology/
Space-Time Toolkit
VAT Variable Antigen Type; Vasoocclusive
Angiotherapy; Ventricular Accommodation
Test; Ventricular Activation Time; Vesicular
Amine Transformer; Video-Assisted Thoracoscopy;
Visceral Adipose Tissue; Visual
Action Therapy; Visual Action Time; Visual
Apperception Test; Vocational Apperception
Test
VATER Vertebral Defects, Imperforate Anus,
Tracheoesophageal Fistula, And Radial And
Renal Dysplasia [Association]
V-Atpase Vascular Adenosine Triphosphatase
VATS Veterans Administration Medical Center
Transference Syndrome; Video-Assisted
Thoracic Surgery
Vats Surface Variable Antigen
VATT Vascular Anatomy Teaching Tool
VAV Variable Air Volume
VAWC Vacuum-Assisted Wound Closure
VB Vaginal Bulb; Valence Bond; Venous
Blood; Ventrobasal; Veronal Buffer; Vertebrobasilar;
Viable Birth; Vinblastine; Virus Buffer;
Voided Bladder
Vb Vinblastine
VBAC Vaginal Birth After Cesarean Section
VBAIN Vertebrobasilar Artery Insufficiency
Nystagmus
VBAS Viewsite Brain Access System
VBC Vincristine, Bleomycin, And Cisplatin;
Visualization In Biomedical Computing; Volumetric-
Based Capnometry
VBD Vanishing Bile Duct; Veronal-Buffered
Diluent

VBE Visualized Bronchus Endoscope
VBF Variable Bandwidth Filter
VBG Vagotomy And Billroth Gastroenterostomy;
Venous Blood Gases; Venous Bypass
Graft; Vertical-Banded Gastroplasty
VBI Ventral Blood Island; Vertebrobasilar
Insufficiency;
Vertebrobasilar Ischemia
VBL Vinblastine
VBM Voxel-Based Morphometry
Vbmf Vinblastine, Methotrexate, 5-Fluorouracil
VBNC Viable But Nonculturable [Microorganism]
Vbns Very-High-Bandwidth Network Service;
Very-High-Performance Backbone Network
Service
Valrs Valyl Ribonucleic Acid Synthetase
VALUE Valsartan Antihypertensive Long-
Term Use Evaluation
VAM Ventricular Arrhythmia Monitor; Virtual
Archive Manager
VAMC Veterans Affairs Medical Center
VAMCS Veterans Affairs Medical Center
Score
VAMP Venous Arterial Blood Management
Protection [System]; Vincristine, Amethopterine,
6-Mercaptopurine, And Prednisone
VAN Value-Added Network; Vein, Artery,
Nerve
VANQWISH Veterans Affairs Non-Q-Wave
Infarction Strategies In-Hospital [Study]
VAP Vaginal Acid Phosphatase; Variant Angina
Pectoris; Venous Access Port; Ventilatorassociated
Pneumonia; Virulence-Attenuated
Pool
Vap Vapor

VAPP Vaccine-Associated Paralytic Poliomyelitis
VAPS Visual Analog Pain Score
VAPSE Variation Affecting Protein Structure Or Expression
VAPSHCS Veterans Affairs Puget Sound Health Care System
Va/Q Alveolar Ventilation/Perfusion Ratio
VA/QC Ventilation/Perfusion Ratio
VAR Vector Autoregressive [Model Algorithm]; Venoarteriolar Reflex; Visual-Auditory Range
Var Variable; Variant, Variation, Variety; Varicella
Var Variable; Variant, Variation, Variety; Varicose
VARE Visual Acuity, Right Eye
VARETA Variable-Resolution Electromagnetic Tomography
VA RNA Virus-Associated Ribonucleic Acid
VARPRO Variable Projection
VARS Valyl-Transfer Ribonucleic Acid Synthetase
VARV Variola Virus
VAS Vagal Afferents; Vascular; Vascular Access Service; Ventricular Assist System; Ventriculoatrial Shunt; Verapamil Angioplasty Study; Vesicle Attachment Site; Vestibular Aqueduct Syndrome; Veterans Adjustment Scale; Vibroacoustic Stimulation; Videoassisted Surgery; Viral Arthritis Syndrome; Visual Analog Scale
VASC Vascular; Verbal Auditory Screening For Children; Visual-Auditory Screening
Vasc Visual Acuity Without Correction
Vasc Vascular
VASD Vascular Access Service Database

VASER Vibration Amplification Of Sound
Energy At Resonance [Study]
VACA Valvuloplasty And Angioplasty Of
Congenital Anomalies [Registry]
Vacc Visual Acuity With Correction
Vacc Vaccination
VACO Veterans Affairs Central Office
VACS Veterans Administration Cooperative
Study
VACSDM Veterans Affairs Cooperative
Study On Glycemic Control And Complications
In Non-Insulin Dependent Diabetes
Mellitus
VACT Veterans Administration Cooperative
Trial
VACTERL Vertebral Abnormalities, Anal
Atresia, Cardiac Abnormalities, Tracheoesophageal
Fistula And/Or Esophageal Atresia, Renal
Agenesis And Dysplasia, And Limb Defects
[Association]
VACV Vaccinia Virus
VAD Venous Access Device; Ventricular
Assist Device; Vinblastine And Dexamethasone;
Virus-Adjusting Diluent; Vitamin A Deficiency
Vad Vascular Dementia
VADD Vitamin A Deficiency Disorder
VAE Venous Air Emboli; Vertical Attachment
Energy
VA-ECMO Venoarterial Extracorporeal Membrane
Oxygenation
VAEG Visual And Auditory Environment
Generator
VAERS Vaccine Adverse Events Reporting
System
VAEV Vearoy Virus

VAF Viral-Free Antigen
VAFC Vacuum-Assisted Fascial Closure
VAG Vibroarthrography
Vag Vagina, Vaginal, Vaginitis
VAG HYST Vaginal Hysterectomy
VAH Vertebral Ankylosing Hyperostosis;
Veterans Affairs Hospital; Virilizing Adrenal
Hyperplasia
VA-HIT Veterans Affairs High-Density Lipoprotein
Intervention Trial
VAHS Virus-Associated Hemophagocytic
Syndrome
VAIN Vaginal Intraepithelial Neoplasm
Vak Atrial Volume Constant
VAL Valproate
Val Valine
Val Valine; Valve
VALE Visual Acuity, Left Eye
Val-Heft Valsartan-Heart Failure Trial
VALIANT Valsartan In Acute Myocardial
Infarction [Study]
VALID Velocity Assessment For Lesions Of
Intermediate Severity [Trial]
VALID II Velocity Assessment For Lesions
Of Indeterminate Severity [Trial]
V0 No Evidence Of Venous [Tumor] Invasion
V0.5 Midpoint Voltage
V1 Primary Visual Area; Venous [Tumor] Invasion
Assessed
V1 Mean Flow Velocity
V1 To V6 Ventral 1 To Ventral 6 [Chest Leads
In ECG]
V Rate Of Reaction Catalyzed By An Enzyme;
Specific Volume; Valve; Vein; Velocity; Venous;
Ventricular; Versus; Very; Virus; Vision;

Volt; Volume

VA Alveolar Ventilation; Vacuum Aspiration; Valproic Acid; Vasodilator Agent; Ventricular Aneurysm; Ventricular Arrhythmia; Ventriculoatrial; Ventroanterior; Veterans Administration; Veterans Affairs; Vincristine, Adriamycin; Viral Antigen; Visual Acuity; Visual Aid; Visual Axis; Volt-Ampere; Volume Average

VA Alveolar Ventilation

V/A Volt/Ampere

V-A Venoarterial

Va Activated Factor V

Va Alveolar Ventilation

Va Volt-Ampere

VAAE Vaccine-Associated Adverse Events

VAB Vincristine, Actinomycin D, And Bleomycin; Violent Antisocial Behavior

VAB-6 Vincristine, Actinomycin, Bleomycin, Cisplatin, Cytoxan

VABP Venoarterial Bypass Pumping; Ventilator-Associated Bacterial Pneumonia

VABS Vineland Adaptive Behavior Scales

VAC Vacuum-Assisted Closure; Ventriculoatrial Conduction; Vincristine, Doxorubicin, And Cyclophosphamide; Virus Capsid Antigen

Vac Vacuum

German

Ven - Venös

Vent(R) - Ventral

VES - Ventrikuläre Extrasystole

VHF - Vorhofflimmern

Virol - Virologisch, Virologie

VKB - Vordere Kreuzband

VKBP - Vordere Kreuzbandplastik

VKU - Verkehrsunfall

VO - Verordnung

VSD - Ventrikelseptumdefekt

Vv. - Venen

Italian

Va

(Simbolo Chimica) Vanadio (Vanadium In Inglese)

VAP

(Acronimo Inglese) Ventilator-Associated Pneumonia
(Polmonite Associata A Ventilatore Meccanico)

VAS

(Acronimo Inglese) Visual Analogic Scale (Scala
Analogica Visiva)

VC

(Acronimo Italiano) Volume Corrente

VDRL

(Acronimo Inglese) Venereal Diseases Research
Laboratory (Un Test Per La Sifilide)

VGM

(Acronimo Italiano) Volume Globulare Medio

VILI

(Acronimo Inglese) Ventilator-Induced Lung Injury
(Danno Polmonare Indotto Da Ventilatore Meccanico)

VLDL

(Acronimo Inglese) Very Low Density Lipoprotein
(Lipoproteine A Densità Molto Bassa)

VM

(Acronimo Italiano) Volume Minuto

V/O

(Abbreviazione) Vigile Ed Orientato

Russian

V

Volume

Объем

VD

Veneral Disease

Венерическое Заболевание

VC

Vital Capacity

Жизненная Емкость [Легких]

VF

Ventricular Fibrillation

Фибрилляция Желудочков [Сердца]

VIP

Vasoactive Intestinal Polypeptide

Вазоактивный Интестинальный Полипептид (ВИП)

VLDL

Very Low Density Lipoprotein

Липопротеид Очень Низкой Плотности (ЛОНП)

VMA

Vanillylmandelic Acid

Ванилилминдальная Кислота (ВМК)

VPC

Ventricular Premature Contraction

Желудочковая Экстрасистола

VP-16

Epipodophyllotoxin

Эпидофиллотоксин

Vs

Visit

Визит

VS

Vital Signs

Показатели Жизнедеятельности (Обычно
Включают В Себя Частоту Сер- Дечных
Сокращений, Частоту Дыхания, Артериальное
Давление, Температуру Тела, Сатурацию
Кислорода. В Большинстве Случаев Измеряются
Средним Медперсоналом И Заносятся В
Специальные Бланки (Сходные С
Температурными Листами))

VSD

Ventricular Septal Defect

Дефект Межжелудочковой Перегородки [Сердца]

VT/VF

Ventricular Tachycardia/Fibrillation

Желудочковая Тахикардия/Фибрилляция

Chinese

V

V V Factor , Co-Enzyme I V 因子; 辅酶

I

V Gas Volume/ Unit Time (Flow Velocity)
单位时间内的气体量〔气流速度〕【注释】〔通
常用电子呼吸速度计测定〕

V Venous Blood 静脉血

VA Alveolar Ventilation 肺 泡换气量

VA Ventricular Arrhythmia 室 性心律失
常(不齐)

VA Ver Tebral Artery 椎动脉〔解〕

VA Viral Antigen 病毒抗原

VA Visual Acuity 视敏(锐) 度

V A Ventilation ① 通风; 换气②通风量

③通风装置④ 透气性

V A Vent Ricular Aneurysm 心 室动脉瘤

V A Vent Ricular Arrhythmia 室 性心律
失常; 室律不齐

VAAJ Veterinary Association For Arbit
Ration And Jurisprudence 兽 医仲裁与
法学协会

Vabl Variable 变 量

Vable Vaginal Bleeding 阴 道出血

Vabls Variables 变 量

Vablty Variability 变异度; 变异性

VAC Veterinary Advisory Committee
兽医咨询委员会

Vacag Vacationing 休 假

Vaccj Vaccination 接 种

Vace Varicocele 精 索静脉曲张

Vacel Varicella 水 痘

Vacl Vascular Clamp 血管镊; 血管夹

Vacls Vascular Clamps 血管钳

Vaco Varicose 肿胀的; 曲张的

Vacos Varicosities 静 脉曲张

Vacoy Varicosity 精 索静脉曲张 〔解〕

Va Ricosit As 〔拉〕

Vacuf Vaginal Cuff 阴 道口

Vacui Vasculitis 脉 管炎

Vacuzd Vascularized 血 管化的; 形成血
管的

VAD Ventricular Assist Device 辅 助人
工心(脏) 【注释】 〔与 IABP 的压力辅助相比,
VAD 具有流量辅助的直接效果, 是强

有力的辅助循环法, 适用于 IABP 无效
病例]

VAD Vitamin A Deficiency 维 生素 A 缺
乏

Vade Vas Deferens 输 精管

Vadel Vaginal Delivery 阴道分娩

Vadep Vasodepressor ① 血管抑制剂②
血管减压的

Vades Variable Decelerations 变异减速

Vadi Vaginal Discharge 阴道排出物

Vadil Vasodilator ① 血管扩张剂② 血管
扩张神经③ 血管扩张的

Vadse Valvular Disease 心瓣病

VAF Veterinary Anatomy Forum
(Japan) 兽 医解剖论坛

Vag Vagina 阴道

VAG Vertebral Arteriography 椎 动脉造
影术

Vagc Vaginectomy 睾 丸鞘膜切除术; 阴
道切除术

Vag Exam Vaginal Examination 阴 道检
查

Vag Hyst Vaginal Hysterectomy 阴 道子
宫切除术

Vagl Vaginal ①鞘的②阴道的③ 睾丸鞘
膜的

Vagls Vaginalitis 睾丸鞘膜炎

Vago Vaginitis 阴道炎

VAHS Virus-Associated Hemophagocytic

Syndrome 病 毒相关血细胞吞噬综合征【注释】〔与全身病毒感染相关, 以显著血细胞吞噬相的全身性组织细胞增殖为特征〕

Vahy Vaginal Hysterectomy 阴 道子宫切除术

VAIN Vaginal Intraepithelial Neoplasia 阴道上皮肉瘤形成

VAL Valine (Aminoacid) 缬氨酸

Vala Vastus Lateralis 股 外侧肌〔解〕

Musculus Vastus Late Ralis 〔拉〕

Valec Valvulectomy 瓣 膜切除术

Valo Vasculopathy 血 管病

Valot Valvulotomy 瓣 膜切开术

Vamo Vasomotor ① 血管舒缩的② 血管舒缩药

Vamu Vaginal Mucosa 阴 道黏膜

VAOD Visual Acuity , Oculus Dexter 右眼视力; 右眼视敏度

VAP Variant Angina Pectoris 变 异型心绞痛

Vapa Vaginal Packing 阴道压缩术

Vapat Vascular Pat Tern 血 管型

Vapl Valvuloplasty 瓣膜成形术

Vapr Vasopressor ①血管加压的② 血管加压药

Vapro Vascular Prominence 血管隆突

VAPS Visual Analogue Pain Scale 可 视性模拟式疼痛评价【注释】〔将主观的疼痛程度划分成 10

级, 用于评价治疗过程的方法〕

VAPS Volume Assisted Pressure Support
容量辅助血压支持(系统) 【注释】 〔为一种人工
呼吸器的换气式

样, 由 CMV 和 PSV 组合构成, 可同时
开始换气〕

VA / Q(C) Alveolar Ventilation Perfusion
换气血流比【注释】 〔肺部的气体交换, 通过换气
和

肺血流间的相对平衡来保持高效率, 在
此指这个比率。对于全肺来讲, 最适换
气血流比为 4l/ 5l = 0 .8〕

Varble Variceal Bleed 曲张静脉出血

Vare Vancomycin Resistant 抗 万古霉素

VAS Visual Analogue Scale 可视模拟尺
度【注释】 〔用于患者的疼痛记分, 在 10cm
长线的左端, 记上" 完全没有疼痛"或在
右端记上"无超过此以上疼痛", 在此尺
度线上, 求得被自己认为与其相符的疼
痛度, 用从左端开始的 Mm 单位的测定
值确定所得的分数。为客观地表示个
人疼痛程度为目的而被使用〕

Vasc Vascular 血管的; 脉管的

Vascg Vascularizing 血管化

Vascs Vannas Scissors 维纳(氏) 剪

Vasctr Vasculature 脉管系统

Vascty Vascularity 多 血管(状态) ; 血管
供应

Vascz Vascularize 形成血管; 血管化

Vasczj Vascularization 血 管形成; 血管

化

Vasec Vasectomy 输精管切除术

Vasecs Vasectomies 输 精管切除术

V-A Shunt Ventriculo- Atria Shunt 脑 室
心房短路术【注释】〔针对脑压亢进, 将侧脑室的脑
脊液引导到右心房。与其他方法相比,
由于脑脊液回流到静脉系, 不出现水分
和电解质丧失〕

Vasp Vasospasm 血 管痉挛

Vasu Vascular Surgery 血管手术

VAT Vent Ricular Activation Time 心 室
兴奋时间【注释】〔指兴奋横穿心室内膜至心室外
膜之间的心肌层的时间。由 ECG 上的
Vag 558 VAT
Q 波开始点到 R 波峰为止的时间〕

VAT Video Assisted Thoracoscopy 影 像
辅助胸腔镜检查

Vato Valvulotome 心瓣膜刀

VATS Video-Assisted Thoracoscopic
Surgery 摄像机辅助的胸腔镜下的手术
疗法【注释】〔指利用摄像机, 在胸腔镜下通
过 CO_2 激光对肺胸膜表面进行的烧灼
手术, 用于囊泡性肺气肿症等的外科疗
法〕

Vaves Varicose Veins 曲张静脉

Vawa Vaginal Wall 阴 道壁

Vazo Varicella Zoster 水痘带状疱疹

VB Venous Blood 静脉血

VB6 Vitamin B6 维生素 B6 (维生素类药)

VBAC Vaginal Birth After Cesarean Section 剖腹产后阴道分娩

VBF Veterinary Benevolent Fund 兽医慈善基金会

VBI Ver Tebrobasilar Insufficiency 椎基底动脉供血不足

VBM Vincristine , Bleomycin , Methotrexate 长春新碱、博莱毒素、氨甲喋呤(化疗方案)

VBMA Veterinary Botanical Medicine Association 兽医植物性医药协会

VBN Volatile Basic Nitrogen 挥发碱性氮

VBS Veronal Buffered Saline 巴比妥钠缓冲盐水

VB12 Vitamin B1 2 维生素 B12

VC Vital Capacity 肺活量【注释】 〔从深吸气位持续性地尽量呼气
时, 能够呼出的气体量, 称为肺活量,
它是一个缓慢的过程, 而不是一种强制
快速的过程。 也称为二段肺活量〕

Vc Vocal Cord 声带

VCA Viral Capsid Antigen 病毒壳体抗原

VCF Mean Fiber Shor Tening Rate 平均纤维缩短率(心功率)

VCF Veterinary Christian Fellowship 基督教兽医奖学金

VCFS Velo-Cardio-Facial Syndrome 咽

心面综合征

VCG Voiding Cystography 排 尿膀胱造
影术

VCI Veterinary Council Of Ireland 爱
尔兰兽医委员会

VCM Vancomycin 万 古霉素 〔抗生素类
药〕

VCM Volume Compensation Method 容
积补偿法【注释】〔新型血压计采用的一种瞬时
血
压测定原理〕

VCNZ Veterinary Council Of New
Zealand 新 西兰兽医委员会

VCO
2
CO2 Production (Output) 二 氧化
碳产生量(排出量) 【注释】 〔在 1 分钟内由血液
向肺泡中排
出的二氧化碳的量。 不能通过该项指
标直接判断肺机能障碍, 但是, 在进行
呼吸死腔和 RQ 的计算过程中有用〕

VCR Vincristine 长 春新碱; 安可平【注释】 〔为一
种抗肿瘤药〕

VCS Vasoconstrictor Substance 缩 血管
物质; 血管收缩物质

VCS Veterinary Cancer Society 兽 医
癌症协会

VCU Veterinary Computer Users 兽 医
计算机用户

Vcu(Gx) Voiding Cystourethrogram 排

尿期膀胱尿道摄影片

VCV Volume Cont Rolled Ventilation 容积控制通气

VD Vasodilator ①血管扩张剂②血管扩张神经③血管扩张的

VD Venereal Disease 性病

VD Vent Ral-Dorsal 腹背的

VAT 559 VD

VD Virus Diarrhea 病毒性腹泻

VD Volume Of Dead Space 死腔量【注释】〔生理学性死腔是解剖学性死腔
(VD Anat) 和肺泡死腔(VDA) 之和。其中肺泡死腔随肺的换气血流不均匀分布的增加而增加〕

VDA Visual Discriminatory Acuity 视觉辨别敏度

VDDR Vitamin D-Dependent Rickets 维生素 D 依赖性佝偻病

VDDRI Vitamin D-Dependent Rickets, Type Ⅰ 维生素 D 依赖性佝偻病Ⅰ型

VD(E)M Vasodepressor Material 血管扩张物质; 血管减压物质【注释】〔在休克不全期由肝脏、骨骼肌和脾脏向血液内排出, 降低毛细血管移行部对于肾上腺素的反应性, 发挥降低血压的作用。见于动物的出血性休克时〕

VDH Valvular Disease Of The Hear T 心脏瓣膜病【注释】〔以心瓣膜和瓣膜口的损伤为基础的疾病, 由于心脏的泵机能下降, 导

致循环机能障碍。可分为闭锁不全和
狭窄两类〕

VDM Vasodepressor Mechanism 血管
减压剂机理

VDS Veterinary Deer Society 鹿兽医
协会

VDS Veterinary Defense Society 兽医
防御协会

VDSS Volume Of Distribution Steady
State (药物血中)分布容量【注释】〔为一种药物
代谢动力学中的解
析用语〕

VD/ VT Dead Space Ventilation/ Total
Ventilation (Ratio) 残剩通气/ 总通气
(比率)

VE Expired Gas Volume Per Minute 每
分换气量【注释】〔为 1 分钟内呼出的气体量。
即
1 次换气量乘每分钟的呼吸次数, 平均
值为 6l/ 分〕

VE Vacuum Extraction 胎头吸引术; 真
空抽提

VE Vacuum Extractor 真空提取器; 真
空抽提器

VE Vaginal Examination 阴道检查

VE Ventricular Escape 室性逸搏

VE Ventricular Extrasystole 室性期外
收缩

VE Volume Of Expired Gas 呼气量

Veac Venous Access 静脉通路

Vear Vent Ricular Arrhythmia 室性心律
失常(不齐)

VEB Vent Ricular Ectopic Beat 室性异位
搏动

Veba Vertebrobasilar 脊椎基底动脉的

Vebo Vertebral Body 椎体 Corpus Ver T Ebr
Ale 〔拉〕

Vebos Ver Tebral Bodies 椎体

Vebr Ver Tebra 椎骨

Vebrc Ver Tebrectomy 椎骨切除术

Vebrl Vertebral 椎骨的; 脊椎的

Vebrs Vertebraes 椎骨〔解〕

Veca Vena Cava 腔静脉; 下腔静脉口

Vecal Vena Caval 腔静脉的

VECG Vector Electrocardiogram 矢量
心电图

VECP Visual Evoked Cortical Potential
视力激发皮质电位

Vede Ventilator Dependent 呼吸器依赖
的

VEDP Ventricular End-Diastolic Pressure
心室扩张终期压【注释】 〔做为对心室的前负荷
的指标来
使用。特别是左心室的这个指标, 成为
对整个血液循环动态评价的一个指标。
可用 PAWP 进行间接测定〕

VEDV Ventricular End-Diastolic Volume
心室扩张终期容量【注释】 〔它不仅是心脏扩张
能力的一个

VD 560 VED
指标, 又是整个心脏机能的一个指标。

指标增大, 表明心脏的机能在逐渐下
降〕

VEE Venezuelan Equine Encephalitis
委内瑞拉马脑炎

VEE Venezuelan Equine Encephalomyelitis
委内瑞拉马脑脊髓炎

VEERU Veterinary Epidemiology And
Economics Research Unit 兽医流行病
学与经济学研究所

Vefi Ventricular Fibrillation 心室纤颤

Veg Vegetation 赘生物; 植被

VEGF Vascular Endothelial Growth Factor
血管内皮生长因子

Vegi Vestigial ①遗迹的; 残遗的② 发育
不全的; 萎缩的; 退化的

Vegr Vein Graft 静脉移植

Vegrm Vent Riculogram 心室造影片

Vegv Vegetative ① 植物性的② 营养的;
生长的③ 静止的④无性生殖的

Vehe Vent Ral Hernia 腹壁疝; 腹疝

Veinc Vertical Incision 垂直切口

Veinsu Venous Insufficiency 静脉机能
不全

Veis Veins 静脉

Velit Vestibulitis 前庭炎

Veln Venous Line 静脉输血导管

Velo Vessel Loop 血管攀

Velog Ventriculography 心室造影片

Velos Vessel Loops 血管攀

VEM Vasoexcitor Mechanism 缩血管
药物机理

Vema Vertical Matt Ress 垂直褥垫

VEN Viral Erythrocytic Necrosis 病毒性
红细胞坏死

Ventl Ventral 腹侧的; 腹面的

Veot Venotomy 静脉切开

VEP Visual Evoked Potential 视 觉诱发
电位【注释】 〔视觉刺激在大脑中形成的脑诱
发电位, 用它可以诊断其径路的损伤部
位〕

Vepr Ver Tex Presentation 顶先露

Vepu Venipuncture 静 脉穿刺(术)

Veru Verumontanum 精阜

VES Vent Ricular Extrasystole 室 性期外
收缩; 室性早搏

VES Vesicular Exanthema Of Swine 猪
水泡疹病

Ves Vessel 导 管

VES Voluntary Euthanasia Society 自
愿安乐死协会

Vesta Venous Stasis 静脉停滞

Vestl Vestibule 前 庭

Vestr Vestibular 前庭的

VES(V) Vesicular Exanthema Of Swine
(Virus) 猪 水泡疹(病毒)

Veta Ventricular Tachycardia 室 性心动
过速

VETCPD Veterinary Education Trust
For Continuing Professional Development
兽医继续职业发展教育机构

Vethr Venous Thrombosis 静脉血栓形成

Veti Ver Tigo 头昏

Vetis Vertiginous 眩晕的

VETNNET Veterinary Nursing Network
(Europe-Wide) 兽医护理网(欧
洲范围内)

Veur Vesicourethral ① 膀胱尿道的② 膀
胱与尿道相通的

Veut Vesicouterine ① 膀胱子宫的② 膀
胱与子宫相通的

VF (Vifi) Visual Field 视野

Vf Vent Ricular Fibrillation 心室纤维性
颤动; 心室纤颤【注释】 〔心室不接受来自上位中
枢的支
配, 而是许多心室固有肌的无节律兴奋
状态。在心电图上呈现细动波, 不出现
P 波、QRS 棘和 T 波。心脏射血停止〕

VF Ventricular Flutter 心室扑动(同心
VEE 561 VF
室纤颤)

VF Visual Field / Champ Visual 视野

Vfa Ventricular Fibrillation Arrest 心室
纤颤性心脏停搏

VFA Volatile Fat Ty Acids 挥发性脂肪酸

VFC Venous Flow Controller 静脉流量
控制器

VFC Vent Ricular Function Curve 心室功
能曲线【注释】 〔用 X 轴为前负荷, Y 轴为左心
室工作量所获得的曲线〕

VFD Veterinary Feed Directive 兽医
饲养指南

V Fib Ventricular Fibrillation 心室纤颤

VFIB Ventricular Fibrillation 心室纤维
性颤动; 心室纤颤

Vfib/ CA Vent Ricular Fibrillation Or Cardiac
Arrest 心室纤颤或心脏停搏

VFR Virulent Foot Rot 毒性足腐烂

VG Ventricular Gallop 心室性奔马律

VG Ventriculography 脑室造影片

VGRR Vitamin D-Resistant Rickets 维
生素 D 抗性佝偻病

VH Vent Ricular Hypert Rophy 心室肥大

VH Viral Hepatitis 病毒性肝炎

VH Vaginal Hysterectomy 阴道子宫切
除术

VHD Viral Hemorrhagic Disease 病毒性
出血性疾病

VHD Valvular Heart Disease 瓣膜性心
脏病

VHDL Very High Density Lipoprotein
极高密度脂蛋白

VHF Viral Hemorrhagic Fever 病毒性出
血热

VHI Veterinary Heart Institute 兽医
心脏研究所

VHMA Veterinary Hospital Management
Association (USA) 兽医院管理
协会〔美国〕

VHS Veterinary History Society 兽医
病史协会

VI Ventilation Index 换气指数

VI Veterinary Ireland 爱尔兰兽医

VI Video Image 视频图像

VI Visual Inspection 目 视检查; 外观检查; 肉眼鉴定

VI Volume Index 体 积指标; 容积指数; 卷末索引; 卷索引

VIA Virus Inactivating Agent 病 毒灭活剂; 病毒灭活因子

Viab Viable ①活的; 能活的② 能生存的 ③能发芽的

Viac Visual Acuity 视敏(锐) 度

Viad Villous Adenoma 绒 毛状腺瘤

Viax Visual Axis 视轴

Vica Vitreous Cavity 玻璃体腔

VICH Veterinary International Cooperation On Harmonization (EU) 兽 医国际合作与协调(委员会)

VIC(Or VI Centre) Veterinary Investigation Cent Re 兽医研究中心

Vicu Vit Reous Cutter 玻璃体切除器

Vide Vitamin Deficiency 维生素缺乏

Videt Vit Reous Detachment 玻 璃体分离

Vidis Visual Disturbances 视 觉障碍

VIDRL Victorian Infectious Diseases Reference Laboratory (Aust Ralia) 维多利亚感染性疾病相关实验室 〔澳大利亚〕

Viend Video-Endoscope 影像-内窥镜

VIEU Veterinary Informatics And Epidemiology Unit 兽 医信息学与流行病学研究所

Vifis Visual Fields 视野

Vifl Vitreous Fluid 玻璃体液

Vig Vigorous 精 神饱满; 猛; 猛烈的; 旺
盛

Vihas Visual Hallucinations 视幻觉

Vihe Vitreous Hemorrhage 玻 璃体出血

Viin Viral Infection 病 毒感染

VF 562 Vii

Vilo Visual Loss 视 觉丧失

VIN Vagina Int Raepithelial Neoplasia 阴
道上皮内肿瘤

VIN Veterinary Information Network
兽医信息网

Vinus Visiting Nurses 出 诊护士; 巡查护
士

VIP Vasoactive Intestinal (Poly) Peptide
血管活化肠多肽【注释】〔在肠壁内神经丛内, 存
在有多
种肽神经元, 参与肠运动调节过程中的
重要黏膜内反应、蠕动反射或肠内反
射, VIP 对于环行肌有直接的抑制作
用, 而对纵行肌则通过胆碱能运动神经
元起促进作用〕

VIP Ventilation-Infusion-Pump 换 气- 输
液- 泵【注释】〔对于" 重要人物"配置的在休克
苏醒过程中的必备三大治疗手段, 即所
谓 VIP 疗法〕

Viprs Visual Problems 视觉问题

VIQ Verbal Intelligence Quotient 言 语
智商

Vira-A Vidarabine 阿 糖酰苷; 腺嘌呤阿

糖苷〔抗病毒药〕

Visen Vibratory Sensation 振动感

Visis Vital Signs 生命体征

Visn Vital Sense 视觉

Visy Viral Syndrome 病毒综合征

Vit B12 Cobalamin (Cyanocobalamin)
维生素 B12 ; 氰钴胺; 钴胺素

Vit Vitamin 维 生素

Vit B6 Pyridoxine 维 生素 B6 ; 吡哆醇;
吡哆素

Vitb Vitamin B 维生素 B

Vitc Vitamin C 维生素 C

Vitd Vitamin D 维生素 D

Vite Vitamin E 维生素 E

Vitk Vitamin K 维生素 K

Vitr Vit Reous ① 玻璃状的; 透明的② 玻
璃体

Vits Vitamins 维生素类

VK Vitamin K 维生素 K; 凝血维生素

VKC Vernal Keratoconjunctivitis 春 季
角膜结膜炎

Vode Volume Depletion 血容量不足

Vofos Vocal Folds 声襞

Vog Vomiting 呕吐

VP Variegate Porphyria 杂色卟啉症

VP Vasopressin 抗 利尿激素; 后叶加压
素

VP Venous Pressure 静 脉压

VR Valve Replacement 瓣膜替换术

VR Vascular Resistance 血管阻力

VR Venous Return 静脉血回流

VR Ventilation Rate 通 风率; 换气率

VRI Viral Respiratory Infection 病 毒性
呼吸道感染

Vrl Viral 病 毒(性) 的

Vrs Virus 病 毒

VS Vital Sign 生命指征【注释】 〔也称为生命征象。
它是死征候
的相反语, 指脉搏、 呼吸、 体温等的生理
现象正常运行〕

医专家网

Vsn Vision 视觉; 视力

Vss Vital Signs 生 命体征

VTH Vaginal Total Hysterectomy 经 阴
道全子宫切除术

VUR Vesico Urethral Regurgitation 膀
胱输尿管逆流【注释】 〔指膀胱尿液经输尿管, 甚
至肾
盂逆流的现象〕

Vuva Vulvovaginal 外阴阴道的

Vv Vaginal Vault 阴道穹隆

VV Varicose Veins 曲 张静脉

VV Ventricular Volume 心室容积

医写作指导

VWD Vomiting And Wasting Disease 呕
吐与消耗性疾病

VZA Varicella-Zoster Antigen 水 痘-带
状疱疹抗原

VZIG Varicella-Zoster Immune Globulin
水痘- 疱疹免疫球蛋白

VZV Varicella Zoster Virus 水痘带状疱
疹病毒

Japanese

略語　日本語の意味　　　スペル

V　　静脈　Vein

　　　静脈血　　　　Venous(Blood)

　　　ビタミン　　　Vimamin

VA　　視床前腹側核　　　　(Nucleus)Ventralis
Anterior

　　　視力　Visual Acuity

　　　心室瘤　　　　Vntricular Aneurysma

　　　椎骨動脈　　　Vertebral Artery

　　　肺胞換気量　Alveolar Ventilation

V-A　静脈動脈バイパス（法）　　Venoarterial
Bypass

　　　脳室心房シャント　Ventriculo-Atrial(Shunt)

VA(P) 異型狭心症　Variant Angina Pectoris

VA　　分時肺胞換気量　　　Alveolar Ventilation Per
Minute

VAD　心室補助装置　　　Ventricular Assist
Device

VAG　椎骨動脈造影（法）　　　Vertebral
Angiography

VAHS ウィルス関連赤血球貪食症候群
　　　Virusassociated Hemophagocytic Syndrome

VA/Q 肺換気血流比　　　Ventilation-Perfusion
Quotient(Ratio)

VAS　心室補助装置　　　Ventricular Assist
System

VAT　心房同期型心室ペーシング
　　　Ventricular Pacing，Atrial Sensing,
Triggered Mode

VATS 胸腔鏡下手術　　　　Video-Assisted Thoracic
Surgery

VAZ　奇静脈　　　Vena Azygos（ラ）

VBA　椎骨脳底動脈　　　Vertebrobasilar Artery

VBI　椎骨脳底動脈循環不全（症）
Ventebrobasilar Insufficiency

VBR　側脳室-大脳比、脳室比　　　Ventricular-Brain
Ratio

VC　肺活量　　　Vital Capacity

VCD　右結腸静脈　Vena Colica Dextra（ラ）

VCDA副右結腸静脈　　　Vena Colica Dextra
Accessoria（ラ）

VCG　排尿時膀胱尿道造影（法）　　　Voiding
Cystourethrography

VCM　中結腸静脈　Vena Colica Media（ラ）
　　　バンコマイシン　　　Vancomycin

VCO2 二酸化炭素排出量　Carbon Dioxide Output

VCR　ビンクリスチン　　　Vincristine

VCS　上大静脈　Vena Cava Superior（ラ）

VD　死腔量　　　Volume Of Dead Air Space

VDD　心室抑制心房同期型心室ペーシング
　　　Ventriclke-Double-Double(Pacing)

VDN　ビンデシン　　　Vindesine

VDS　Zielke(チールケ）法による脊柱前方固定術
　　　Ventral Derotating Spinal Fusion

VDT/I 心房同期型心室ペーシング　　　Ventricle-
Doublr-Trigger/Inhibit

VD/VT　　　死腔換気率　Dead-Space Gas Volume
To Tidal Volume Ratio

VE　吸引分娩（術）　Vacuum Extraction
　　　分時換気量　Pulmonary Ventilation Per
Minute

VEDP 心室拡張終（末）期圧　　Ventricular
Endodiastolic Pressure

VEDV 心室拡張終（末）期量　　Ventricular
Endodiastolic Volume

VF　　換気不全　　Ventilatory Failure
　　　心室粗動　　Ventricular Flutter
　　　心室細動　　Ventricular Fibrillation

VG　　脳室造影（法）　　Ventriculography

VGED 右胃大網静脈　　　Vena Gastroepiploica
Dextra（ラ）

VI　　換気指数　　Ventilation Index
　　　容積指数　　Volume Index

VIP　　エトポシド、イホスファミド、シスプラチ
ンの併用化学療法　Etoposide(VP-16),
Ifosfamide, Cisplatin(CDDP)

VLB　　ビンカロイコブラスチン（ビンブラスチン）
　　　Vincaleukoblastine(Vinblastine)

VLBW(I)　　極低出生体重（児）　　Very Low
Birth Weight(Infant)

VLDL 超低比重リポ蛋白　Very Low Density
Lipoprotein

VM　　ビオマイシン　　Viomycin

Vmax 最大呼気流量　　Maximal Expiratory
Flow

VMCP ビンクリスチン、メルファラン、シクロホ
スファミド、プレドニゾロンの併用化学療法
　　　Vinctistine, Melphalan,
Cyclophosphamide, Prednisolone

VMP　　ビンクリスチン、メトトレキサート、プレ
ドニゾロンの併用化学療法　　Vincristine,
Methotrexate, Prednisolone

VMS　上腸間膜静脈　　　Vena Mesenterica Superior

Vol　容積　Volume

Vol%　容積パーセント　　Volume Per Cent

VP　静脈圧　　　Venous Pressure

　　脳室圧　　　Ventricular Pressure

　　バソプレシン　　　Vasopressin

　　ビンクリスＴリン、プレドニゾロンの併用化学療法　　Vincristine, Prednisolone

　　ビンデシン、シスプラチンの併用化学療法　Vindesine, Cisplatine

　　門脈

V-P　脳室腹腔シャント　Ventriculo-Peritoneal(Shunt)

VPB　心室期外収縮　　　Ventricular Premature Beat

VPC　心室期外収縮　　　Ventricular Premature Contraction(Beat)

VPDIA　　　前下膵十二指腸静脈

V/Q　換気/血流比　Ventilation-Perfusion Ratio

VR　換気予備率　Ventilation Resarve

VS, V/S, Vs　　バイタルサイン、生命兆候　Vital Sign

VSA　血管攣縮性狭心症　Vasospastic Angina

VSD　心室中隔欠損（症）　　　Ventricular Septal Defect

VSP　心室中隔穿孔　　　Ventricular Septal Perforation

VSR　心室中隔破裂　　　Ventricular Septal Rupture

VT　心室頻拍　Ventricular Tachycardia

VT, Vt　　　1回換気量　Tidal Volume

VVI　デマンド型心室ペーシング　　　Ventricle
Demand Inhibited(Pacemaker Code)

W

French

English

W Dominant Spotting [Mouse]; Energy; Section Modulus; Series Of Small Triangular Incisions In Plastic Surgery [W-Plasty]; Tryptophan; Tungsten [Ger. Wolfram]; Wakefulness; Ward; Water; Watt; Weber [Test]; Week; Wehnelt; Weight; White; Widowed; Width; Wife; Wilcoxon Rank Sum Statistic; Wistar [Rat]; With; Word Fluency; Work; Wound

W3 World Wide Web

W+ Weakly Positive

W Velocity (M/S); Water; Watt; While; With

WA When Awake; White Adult; Wiskott-Aldrich [Syndrome]

W/A Watt/Ampere

W&A Weakness And Atrophy

WAAT Warfarin Plus Aspirin Vs. Aspirin Trial

WAB Western Aphasia Battery

WACS Women's Atherosclerosis Cardiovascular Study

WAF Weakness, Atrophy, And Fasciculation; White Adult Female

WAFUS Warfarin Anticoagulation Followup Study

WAGR Wilms Tumor, Aniridia, Genitourinary Abnormalities, And Mental Retardation

WAI Web Accessibility Initiative

WAIS Wechsler Adult Intelligence Scale; Western Angiographic And Interventional Society; Wide Area Information Server; Workplace Advocacy Information System

WAIS-R Revised Wechsler Adult Intelligence

Scale
WAK Wearable Artificial Kidney
WALK Walking With Angina-Learning Is
The Key [Program]
WALV Wallal Virus
WAM White Adult Male; Work Area Model;
Worksheet For Ambulatory Medicine
WAN Wide Area Network
WANV Wanowrie Virus
WAP Wandering Atrial Pacemaker; Whey
Acid Protein
WAR Wasserman Antigen Reaction; Without
Additional Reagents
WARCRY Wegener And Related Diseases
Compassionate Regimen Yield [Study]
WARF Warfarin; Wisconsin Alumni Research
Foundation
WARIS Warfarin Reinfarction Study
WARIS II Warfarin-Aspirin Reinfarction
Study–Norwegian
WARSS Warfarin-Aspirin Recurrent Stroke
Study
WARV Warrego Virus
WAS Weekly Activities Summary; Wiskott-
Aldrich Syndrome
WASH Warfarin-Aspirin Study Of Heart
Failure
WASID Warfarin-Aspirin Symptomatic Intracranial
Disease [Study]
WASP Weber Advanced Spatial Perception
[Test]; Wiskott-Aldrich Syndrome Protein
Wass Wasserman [Reaction]
WAST Woman Abuse Screening Tool
WAT Word Association Test
WATCH Warfarin Antiplatelet Trial In

Chronic Heart Failure; Worcester-Area Trial
For Counseling In Hyperlipidemia
WATSMART Waterloo Spatial Motion
Analysis And Recording Technique
WAVE Women's Angiographic Vitamin And
Estrogen [Trial]
WAXS Wide-Angle X-Ray Scattering
WB Waist Belt; Washable Base; Washed
Bladder; Water Bottle; Wechsler-Bellevue
[Scale]; Weight-Bearing; Well Baby; Western
Blot; Wet Bulb; Whole Blood; Whole
Body; Willowbrook [Virus]; Wilson-Blair
[Agar]
Wb Weber; Well-Being
WBA Wax Bean Agglutinin; Western Blot
Assay; Whole-Body Activity
Wb/A Webers/Ampere
WBAPTT Whole-Blood Activated Partial
Thromboplastin Time
WBAT Weight Bearing As Tolerated
WBC Well-Baby Care; Well-Baby Clinic;
White Blood Cell; White Blood Cell Count;
Whole Blood Cell Count
WBCT Whole-Blood Clotting Time
WBDC Whole-Body Digital Scanner
WBE Whole-Body Extract
WBF Whole-Blood Folate
WBGT Wet Bulb Global Temperature
WBH Whole-Blood Hematocrit; Whole-Body
Hyperthermia
WBI Web-Based Instruction; Whole Bowel
Irrigation
WBLT Watson-Barker Listening Test
Wb/M2 Weber Per Square Meter
WBMP Wireless Bitmap

WBN Whole-Blood Nitrogen
WBPTT Whole-Blood Partial Thromboplastin Time
WBR Whole-Body Radiation
WBRT Whole-Blood Recalcification Time; Whole-Breast Radiation Therapy
WBS Wechsler-Bellevue Scale; Wholeblood Serum; Whole-Body Scan; Whole-Body Scintiscan; Wiedemann-Beckwith Syndrome;

German

WHO - World Health Organisation, Weltgesundheitsorganisation
WHO Homepage
WK - Wirbelkörper
WS - Wirbelsäule
WS-KS – Wirbelsäulenklopfschmerz

Italian

W

(Simbolo Chimica) Wolframio O Tungsteno
(Tungsten In Inglese)

Russian

W
White
Белый [Раса]
WBC
White Blood (Cell) Count
Количество Лейкоцитов Крови
W/C
Wheel Chair
Сидячая Каталка, Инвалидное Кресло
WF
White Female
Женщина Белой Расы
WHO
World Health Organization
Всемирная Организация Здравоохранения (ВОЗ)
WPW
Wolff Parkinson White
Вольф-Паркинсон-Уайт (Синдром)
Wt
Weight
Вес

Japanese

略語　日本語の意味　　　スペル
W　　重量、体重　Weight
　　　週　　　Week
　　　創傷　Wound
War　ワッセルマン反応　Wassermann Reaction
WBC　白血球、白血球数　White Blood Cell(Count)
WD　湿布、罨法　Wet Dressing
WDHA　　水様下痢低カリウム血症無胃酸症候群、WDHA症候群 Watery Diarrhea-Hypokalemia-Achlorhydria(Syndrome)
WDLL高分化型小球性悪性リンパ腫　　Well-Differentiated Lymphocytic Lymphoma
WF　ワーファリン　　　Warfarin
WG　ウェゲナー肉芽腫症　　Wegener's Granulomatosis
WHD　ウェルドニッヒ・ホフマン病　　Werdnig-Hoffmann Disease
WHVP　　肝静脈楔入圧　　Wedged Hepatic Venous Pressure
Widal　ヴィダール反応　Widal's Reaction
WK　ウェルニッケ・コルサコフ症候群
　　　Wernicke-Korsakoff(Syndrome）
WMS　ウィルソン・ミキティ症候群　　Wilson-Mikity Syndrome
WNL　正常範囲　Within Nomal Limits
WPW　ウォルフ・パーキンソン・ホワイト症候群
　　　Wolff-Parkinson-White(Syndrome)

WRC　洗浄赤血球　Washed Red Cells

WT　作業療法　Work Therapy

　　腎芽腫、ウィルムス腫瘍　Wilms' Tumor

WT，Ｗ t　体重　Weight

Chinese

W White ①蛋白; 卵白② 白眼(突变型)
③白色动物④ 白带⑤ 白色洗涤物⑥ 精
白(面) 粉⑦白色的; 乳白的
W White Cell 白细胞
WBC White Blood Cell 白细胞
Wbcc White Blood Cell Count 白 血球计
数; 白血细胞计数
WBI Whole Body Irradiation 全 身照射;
全身辐照
WBS Wet Brain Syndrome 湿脑综合征
WBS Wiedemann-Beckwith Syndrome
维得曼贝克威瑟氏综合征; 突脐、巨舌、
巨躯综合征【注释】〔本征是一种遗传性疾病, 属
常
染色体显性遗传, 常发生于有血缘婚姻
史的双亲的子代〕
Wc Wheel Chair 轮椅
WC Whooping Cough 百 日咳
Whce White Cell 白 细胞
Whces White Cells 白 细胞
检查法〕
WL White Lady(Heroin) 海洛因; 二乙
酰吗啡
Wlp Weight- Loss Program 减肥计划
WMD White Muscle Disease 白肌病
WMR Work Metabolic Rate 劳 动代谢
WP Wedge Pressure (肺动脉) 楔压

WPW Wolff-Parkinson-White (Syndrome) 澳-佩-怀综合征; 预激综合征【注释】〔在心电图上, 以 PQ 时间短缩,

QRS 波延长为特征。多数伴发阵发性上室性心动过速。可能与心房室间存在副传导路有关〕

WRC Washed Red Cells 洗 过的红细胞

Wrfx Wrist Fracture 腕 骨骨折

Wrpa Wrist Pain 腕部疼痛

动物研究中心

Wrs Wrists 腕部

Wuca Wound Care 伤 口护理

Wucu Wound Culture 伤 口培养物

Wude Wound Dehiscence 创口裂开

Wueds Wound Edges 伤口边缘

Wuin Wound Infection 伤 口感染; 创伤

French

English

X Sample Mean

X2, X2 Chi-Square

X3 Orientation As To Time, Place, And Person

X Except; Extremity; Horizontal Axis Of A Rectangular Coordinate System; Mole Fraction; Multiplication Symbol; Position; Roentgen [Rays]; Sample Mean; "Times"; Unknown Factor; Xanthine

XA Xanthurenic Acid; X-Ray Analysis

X-A Xylene And Alcohol

Xa Activated Factor X; Chiasma

Xaa Unknown Amino Acid

XAD External Atrial Defibrillation [Trial]

Xam Examination

Xan Xanthine

Xanth Xanthomatosis

Xao Xanthosine

XBP Xanthophyll-Binding Protein; X-Box Binding Protein

XBSN X-Linked Bulbospinal Neuropathy

XC, Xc Excretory Cystogram

XCCL Exaggerated Craniocaudal Lateral [View]

XCE X-Chromosome Controlling Element

X-CGD X-Linked Chronic Granulomatous Disease

Xcv Xanthomonas Campestris Vesicatoria

XD X-Ray Diffraction

XDH Xanthine Dehydrogenase

XDP Xanthine Diphosphate; Xeroderma
Pigmentosum
XDR Extensively Drug-Resistant; Transducer
XDR-TB Extensively Drug-Resistant Tuberculosis
Xe Electric Susceptibility; Xenon
XECT, Xect Xenon-Enhanced Computed
Tomography
XEF Excess Ejection Fraction
XES X-Ray Energy Spectrometry
Xfb Cross-Linked Gibrin
XFD X-Ray Flat Detector
XGP Xanthogranulomatous Pyelonephritis
XGPT Xylosylprotein-4-Beta-Galactosyltransferase
Xi Inactive X Chromosome
XIAP X-Linked Inhibitor Of Apoptosis
XIBV Xiburema Virus
XIC X Chromosome Inactivation Center;
X-Inactivation Center
X-IEP Crossed Immunoelectrophoresis
XINV Xingu Virus
XIP Exchanger Inhibitory Peptide; X-Ray-Induced
Polypeptide; X-Ray In Plaster
XISHF Xamoterol In Severe Heart Failure
[Study]
XIST Inactive X-Chromosome Specific Transcript;
X-Inactivation Specific Transcript
XL Excess Lactate; X-Linked; Xylose-Lysine
XLA, X-LA X-Linked Agammaglobulinemia
XLAS X-Linked Aqueductal Stenosis
XLCM X-Linked Dilated Cardiomyopathy
XLD X-Linked Dominant; Xylose-Lysine-
Deoxycholate
XLH X-Linked Hydrocephalus; X-Linked
Hypophosphatemia
XLHED X-Linked Hypohidrotic Ectodermal

Dysplasia
XLI X-Linked Ichthyosis
XLIF Extreme Lateral Interbody Fusion
XLMR X-Linked Mental Retardation
XLMTM, Xlmtm X-Linked Myotubular
Myopathy
XLOS X-Linked Opitz Syndrome
XLP X-Linked Lymphoproliferative [Syndrome]
XLPD X-Linked Lymphoproliferative Disease
XLR X-Linked Recessive
XLRP X-Linked Retinitis Pigmentosa
XLS X-Linked Recessive Lymphoproliferative
Syndrome
XLSP X-Linked Spastic Paraplegia
XM Crossmatch
XM, Xm Maternal Chromosome X
Xma Chiasma
X-Mas Christmas [Factor]
X-Mat Crossmatch
X-Match Crossmatch
XME Xenobiotic-Metabolizing Enzyme
XML Extensible Markup Language
XMMR Xenopus Molecular Marker Resource
XMP Xanthine Monophosphate
XMR X-Linked Mental Retardation
XMRV Xenotropic Murine Leukemia Virus–
Related Virus
XN Night Blindness
XO Presence Of Only One Sex Chromosome;
Xanthine Oxidase
XOAD X-Linked Ocular Albinism With Deafness
XOM Extraocular Movements
XOP X-Ray Out Of Plaster
XOR Exclusive Operating Room
XP Xanthogranulomatous Pyelonephritis;

Xeroderma Pigmentosum
XP, Xp Paternal Chromosome X; Short Arm
Of Chromosome X
XPA Xeroderma Pigmentosum Group A
XPC Xeroderma Pigmentosum Group C
XPN Xanthogranulomatous Pyelonephritis
XPS X-Ray Photoelectron Spectroscopy;
X-Ray Photoemission Spectroscopy
XPTB Extrapulmonary Tuberculosis
Xq Long Arm Of Chromosome X
XR Extended Release; Xeroradiography; Xlinked
Recessive; X-Ray
X-Rays Roentgen Rays
XRD X-Ray Diffraction
XRE Xenobiotic Response Element
XRF X-Ray Fluorescence
XRFDC X-Ray Film Digitization Console
XRII X-Ray Image Intensifier
XRMR X-Linked Recessive Mental Retardation
XRN X-Linked Recessive Nephrolithiasis
XRS X-Ray Sensitivity
XRT X-Ray Therapy
XS Cross-Section; Excessive; Xiphisternum
X/S Cross-Section
Xs Excess
XSA Cross-Section Area
XSCID X-Linked Severe Combined
Immunodeficiency
[Syndrome]
XSCLH X-Linked Subcortical Laminar Heterotopia
X-Sect Cross-Section
XSP Xanthoma Striatum Palmare
XT Exotropia
Xt Extra Toe
Xta Chiasmata

Xtab Cross-Tabulating
XTE Xeroderma, Talipes, And Enamel Defect
[Syndrome]
XTM Xanthoma Tuberosum Multiplex
XTP Xanthosine Triphosphate
X-TUL External Tumescent Ultrasound Liposculpture
XU Excretory Urogram; X Unit
Xu X-Unit
Xu Cumulative Amount Of Urine
Xu5P, Xu5p Xylulose-5-Phosphate
XUC Extended Use Case [Format]
Xump Xylulose Monophosphate
XX Chromosome X Disomy; Double Strength;
Female Chromosome Type
46,XX 46 Chromosomes, 2 X Chromosomes
(Normal Female)
XXL Xylocaine
XXX Chromosome X Trisomy
XXXX Chromosome X Tetrasomy
XXXXX Chromosome X Pentasomy
XX/XY Sex Karyotypes
XY Male Chromosome Type
46,XY 46 Chromosomes, 1 X And 1 Y Chromosome
(Normal Male)
Xyl Xylose

German

Italian
Xe
(Simbolo Chimica) Xeno (Xenon In Inglese)

Russian

Chinese

X

X X Chromosome Inactivation X 染色体失活

Xala Xanthelasma 黄斑瘤

Xalas Xanthelasmas 黄斑瘤

Xamo Xanthomonas 黄单胞菌

XC X Chromosome X 染色体

X-CGD X-Linked Chronic Granulomatous Disease X 连锁慢性肉芽肿性疾病

X-CI X-Chromosome Inactivation X 染色体失活

XDP Xeroderma Pigmentosum 着色性干皮病; DNA 修复酶缺乏病

Xega Xeroform Gauze 三溴酚铋纱布

Xid X-Chromosome Linked Imune Deficiency X 染色体相关免疫缺陷病

Xist Xiphisternum 剑突

X-Knee Knock-Knee 叉形膝; 膝外翻

XL Excess Lactate 过量乳酸盐

XP Exophoria 外隐斜视

XP Xeroderma Pigmentosum 着色性干皮病【注释】〔由于光线过敏而发病的遗传性疾病〕

Xr X-Ray X 射线; X 光

XRM X-Ray Microscope X 光显微镜

Xrs X-Rays X 光; X 线

XRT X-Ray Therapy X 线疗法

XR(Xr) X-Ray X 射线; X 光

XXXX Four X Syndrome 四 X 综合征

Xyl Xylocaine 赛罗卡因【注释】〔一种局部麻醉药〕

XYY Double Y Syndrome 双 Y 综合征

Y

French

English

Y Coordinate Axis In A Plane; Electrical Admittance; Male Sex Chromosome; Mean Of Y Values; Tyrosine; Year; Yellow; Yersinia; Yield; Yttrium

Y Vertical Axis Of A Rectangular Coordinate System

Y- Yocto- [10−24]

YA Yersinia Arthritis

Y/A Years Of Age

YAC Yeast Artificial Chromosome

YACP Young Adult Chronic Patient

YACV Yacaaba Virus

YADH Yeast Alcohol Dehydrogenase

YAG Yttrium-Aluminum-Garnet [Laser]

YAOV Yaounde Virus

YATAV Yata Virus

Yb Ytterbium

YBOCS Yale-Brown Obsessive Compulsive Scale

YBV Yug Bogdanovac Virus

YCB Yeast Carbon Base

YCMI Yale Center For Medical Informatics

YCT YMCA Cardiac Therapy

YCVDS Yugoslavia Cardiovascular Disease Study

Yd Yard

YDV Yeast-Derived Hepatitis B Vaccine

YDYES Yin Deficiency Yang Excess Syndrome

YE Yeast Extract; Yellow Enzyme

YEH2 Reduced Yellow Enzyme

YEI Yersinia Enterocolitica Infection

Yel Yellow

YEL-AND Yellow Fever Vaccine–Associated
Neurotropic Disease
YEL-AVD Yellow Fever Vaccine–Associated
Viscerotrophic Disease
YF Yellow Fever
YFI Yellow Fever Immunization
YFMD Yellow Fever Membrane Disease
YFV Yellow Fever Virus
YHAP Yale Health And Aging Project
YHV Yaquina Head Virus
YKV Yokapoxvirus
YLC Youngest Living Child
YLD Years Lived With Disability
YLF Yttrium Lithium Fluoride
YLL Years Of Life Lost
YLS Years Of Life Saved
YM Yeast And Mannitol; Yeast And Mold;
Young's Modulus
Ymax Maximum Yield
YMB Yeast Malt Broth
YMRS Young Mania Rating Scale
YMS Young Men's Survey
YMTV Yaba Monkey Tumor Virus
YNB Yeast Nitrogen Base
YNS Yellow Nail Syndrome
YO Year Old
Y/O Years Old
YOB Year Of Birth
Yobs Observed Value
YOGV Yogue Virus
YOKV Yokose Virus
Yops Yersinia Outer Membrane Proteins
YOS Yale Observation Scale
YP Yeast Phase; Yield Pressure
YPA Yeast, Peptone, And Adenine Sulfate

YPAS Yale Preoperative Anxiety Score
Ypka Yersinia Protein Kinase A
YPLL Years Of Potential Life Lost
Yr Year
YRBS Youth Risk Behavior Survey
YRD Yangtze River Disease
YRRM Y Ribonucleic Acid Recognition Motif
YS Yellow Spot; Yield Strength; Yolk Sac
Ys Yellow Spot; Yolk Sac
YSHR Younger Spontaneously Hypertensive Rat
YST Yolk Sac Tumor
Y73SV Y73 Sarcoma Virus
YT, Yt Yttrium
Yts Yoga Therapists
Y-TZP Yttria-Stabilized Tetragonal Zirconia Polycrystalline
Y1V Yaba-1 Virus
Y7V Yaba-7 Virus
Ywacc Younger Woman With Aggressive Cervical Cancer
YWKY Younger Wistar-Kyoto Rat

German
Italian

Y

(Simbolo Chimica) Ittrio (Yttrium In Inglese)

Russian
Chinese

Y

Y Y Chromosome, Male Chromosome

Y 染色体

从业者联合会

YEI Yersinia Enterocolitica Infection
耶尔森菌肠炎

Yein Yeast Infection 酵母感染

Yesp Yellow Sputum 黄痰

YF Yellow Fever 黄热病

YFV Yellow Fever Virus 黄热病病毒

Y-LI Y Linkage Y 染色体连锁

YNS Yellow Nail Syndrome 黄甲综合征

YS(Ys) Yellow Spot 黄斑〔视网膜〕

Y , YAG Yt Trium, Aluminum Garnet
(Laser) 钇、铝石榴石(激光)

Z

English

Z Acoustic Impedance; Atomic Number; Complex
Impedance; Contraction [Ger. Zuckung];
Glutamine; Impedance; Ionic Charge Number;
No Effect; Point Formed By A Line Perpendicular
To The Nasion-Menton Line Through The
Anterior Nasal Spine; Proton Number; Section
Modulus; Standardized Deviate; Standard Normal
Score; Standard Score; Zero; Zone; A Zshaped
Incision In Plastic Surgery
Z Uppercase Greek Letter Zeta
Z Lowercase Greek Letter Zeta
Z- Zetta- [1021]
Z?, Z?? Increasing Degrees Of Contraction
Z Algebraic Unknown Or Space Coordinate;
Axis Of A Three-Dimensional Rectangular
Coordinate
System; Catalytic Amount; Standard
Normal Deviate; Zero
Z- Zepto- [10−21]
ZAG, ZA2G Zinc-Alpha-2-Glycoprotein
ZAM Zhao-Atlas-Marks [Distribution]
ZAMSTAR Zambia, South Africa Tuberculosis
And AIDS Reduction [Program]
ZAP Zeta-Associated Protein [Rabbit]; Zymosan-
Activated Plasma
ZAPF Zinc Adequate Pair-Fed
ZAPS Zonal Air Pollution System
ZAS Zymosan-Activated Autologous Serum
ZB Zebra Body
ZBG Zinc-Binding Group
ZCA Zone Of Cortical Abnormality

ZCAP Zinc-Calcium–Phosphorous Oxide
ZCP Zinc Chloride Poisoning
ZD Zero Defects; Zero Discharge; Zinc Deficiency
Z-D Zamorano-Duchovny [Digitizer]
ZDDP Zinc Dialkyldithiophosphate
Z-DNA Zig-Zag (Left-Handed Helical)
Deoxyribonucleic
Acid
ZDO Zero Differential Overlap
ZDS Zinc Depletion Syndrome
ZDV Zidovudine
ZE Zollinger-Ellison [Syndrome]
ZEBOV Zaire Ebola Virus
ZEBRA Zero Balanced Reimbursement Account
ZEC Zinsser-Engman-Cole [Syndrome]
ZEEP Zero End-Expiratory Pressure
ZEGV Zegla Virus
ZEPI Zonal Echo Planar Imaging
Z-ERS Zeta Erythrocyte Sedimentation Rate
ZES Zollinger-Ellison Syndrome; Zutphen
Elderly Study
ZEST Zocor Early Start Trial
ZF Zero Frequency; Zinc Finger [Protein];
Zona Fasciculata
ZFA N-Benzyloxcarbonyl Phe-Ala
Omefluoromethylketone
ZFF Zinc Fume Fever
ZFP Zinc Finger Protein
ZFX X-Linked Zinc Finger Protein
Zfy Zinc Finger [Protein]
ZG Zona Glomerulosa
ZGM Zinc Glycinate Marker
ZIAR Zona-Induced Acrosome Reaction
ZIFT Zygote Intrafallopian Tube Transfer
ZIG, Zig Zoster Immunoglobulin

ZIKV Zika Virus

ZIP Zoster Immune Plasma

ZIRV Zirqa Virus

Zj Zeptojoule

ZK Zuelzer-Kaplan [Syndrome]

ZLS Zimmerman-Laband Syndrome

Zm Zygomaxillare

ZMA Zinc Meta-Arsenite

ZMC Zygomaticomaxillary Complex

ZN Ziehl-Neelsen [Staining]

ZNF Zinc Finger [Protein]

Znoe Zinc Oxide And Eugenol

Znpp/H Zinc Protoporphyrin/Heme Ratio

ZNS Zonisamide

ZO Zichen-Oppenheim [Syndrome]; Zonula
Occludens; Zuelzer-Ogden [Syndrome]

Zo Impedance; Thoracic Fluid

ZOA Zinc Orthoarsenate

ZOE Zinc Oxide–Eugenol

ZOL Zoladex

ZOMC Zygomatico-Orbito-Maxillary Complex

Zool Zoology

ZOT Zonula Occludens Toxin

ZP Zona Pellucida

ZPA Zone Of Polarizing Activity

ZPC Zero Point Of Change

ZPG Zero Population Growth

ZPO Zinc Peroxide

ZPP Zinc Protoporphyrin

ZPS, Zps Zwitterionic Polysaccharides

ZPT Zinc Pyridinethione

ZR Zona Reticularis

Zr Zirconium

ZRK Zona Receptor Kinase

ZS Zellweger Syndrome; Zutphen Study

ZSC Zone Of Slow Conduction
ZSR Zeta Sedimentation Ratio
ZSV Signature-Tagged Mutagenesis; Zonate
Spot Virus
ZT Zwolle Trial
ZTS Zymosan-Treated Serum
Z-TSP Zephiran-Trisodium Phosphate
ZTT Zinc Turbidity Test
ZTV Zaliv Terpeniya Virus
ZVAD N-Benzyloxcarbonyl Val-Ala-Asp
Omefluoromethylketone
ZVD Zidovudine
ZVT Cell-Binding Test [Ger. Zehlenverbindungstest]
ZW Zellweger [Syndrome]
ZWCHRS Zellweger Cerebrohepatorenal
Syndrome
ZWOLLE Primary Coronary Angioplasty
Compared With Intravenous Streptokinase
[Trial]
ZWS Zellweger Syndrome
ZXF Zero Crossing Frequency
Zy Zygion
Zyc Zymosan Complement
Zyg Zygotene
Zz Ginger [Lat. Zingibar]

German

Italian

Zn
(Simbolo Chimica) Zinco (Zinc In Inglese)
Zr
(Simbolo Chimica) Zirconio (Zirconium In Inglese)

Russian

Зидовудин

Золингер-Эллисон (Синдром)

Chinese

Z Acoustic Impedance 声 阻抗
Z Z-Chromosome Z 染色体
ZCP Zinc Chloride Poisoning 氯 化锌中
毒
ZEC Zinsser-Engman-Cole (Syndrome)
津- 恩- 科三氏综合征; 先天性角化不良
Zedi Zenker□s Diverticulum Zenker 憩室
ZEEP Zero- End-Expiratory Pressure 呼
气终末平压【注释】〔在呼气中不加正压的人工
呼吸
法〕
ZE(S) Zollinger-Ellison (Syndrome)
卓- 艾二氏综合征; 胃泌素瘤【注释】〔由于胃泌
素瘤的存在, 产生过
多的胃泌素, 而引发的难以治愈的消化
性溃疡病〕
ZIG(Zig) Zoster Immune Globulin 带
状疱疹免疫球蛋白【注释】〔用带状疱疹恢复期
患者的分离
血浆制成的 Γ- 球蛋白, 用于带状疱疹患
者的免疫治疗〕
线

津- 拉二氏综合征; 齿龈瘤-指畸形-肝脾肿

大(综合征)

硫酸

锌浊度试验

动物学

整形术

过氧化锌

网 状带

泽 韦格综合征【注释】〔具有特殊的面部长相(眼距过

宽、鼻根扁平、前额突出等) , 肌肉张力

降低, 伴有痉挛, 在哺乳早期死亡。为

隐性遗传病〕

硫酸锌(浊度) 试验【注释】〔也称作康克耳氏试

验, 为肝功

能的一个指标。正常值为 4～ 12 康克耳

单位〕

齐 多夫定〔抗病毒药〕

颧 颞突; 颊骨; 颧骨

颧 弓〔解〕Arcus

〔拉〕

颧骨的

颧额的

颧 的; 颧骨的

颧肌

颧上颌的

颧 骨

About The Author

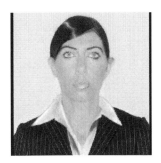

Catherine- Chantal Marango Is A Highly Trained French
Multilingual Professional Who Has Many Years Of
Experience As A Successful Foreign Language Expert And
Pedagogical Pyschologist, Working In Nice, France.

She Celebrates With Her Mediterranean Enthusiasm 10 Years
Being In The Language Business.

Successfully Running Her Linguistic Company Personal
French Teacher (Www.Personalfrenchteacher.Com), She Has
Worked With Thousands Of High-Qualified Global Students
Seeking A Real Language Improvement From General To
Specific Purposes.

Her Real-World Experience, Multilingualism, Extensive
Education, Pragmatic Connection And Pedagogical
Psychology Makes Her The Excellent Choice To Help You
Speak The World With Flying Colors.

Connect With Catherine Chantal Marango On :
Http://Www.Personalfrenchteacher.Com/
Https://Www.Facebook.Com/Catherinechantal.Marango/

Https://Twitter.Com/LEARNFRENCHNICE
Https://Www.Linkedin.Com/In/Personalfrenchteacher/
Https://Www.Instagram.Com/Personalfrenchteacher/
Https://Www.Pinterest.Fr/Catherinec0545/
Https://Catherinechantalmarangoworld.Tumblr.Com/
Https://Www.Reddit.Com/R/Iama/Comments/Fw0keg/Im_Ca
therinechantal_Marango_A_French_Writer_And/
Https://Www.Youtube.Com/Channel/UCY-
Bocxqvywl21hw8vqk_Ja

Catherine Chantal Marango's Books :
Https://Www.Amazon.Com/Catherine-Chantal-
Marango/E/B084LDK21B%3Fref=Dbs_A_Mng_Rwt_Scns_
Share

Https://Books.Google.Fr/

Https://Www.Smashwords.Com/Profile/View/CCM13

Https://Payhip.Com/

Https://Www.Lulu.Com

Back To Top

Printed in Great Britain
by Amazon

16938400R00379